Manual of Dermatologic Therapeutics
With Essentials of Diagnosis

ƆR. B. A. SPILKER

Manual of Dermatologic Therapeutics

With Essentials of Diagnosis

Second Edition

Kenneth A. Arndt, M.D.

Associate Professor of Dermatology,
Harvard Medical School;
Chief, Department of Dermatology,
Beth Israel Hospital,
Boston

Little, Brown and Company · Boston

© 1978

Cover: Scanning electron micrograph of shank skin from a 14-day-old chick embryo cultured for two days in retinoic acid. The epidermal cells are detached from their neighbors, are markedly rounded and bulging, and show pronounced surface microvilli and folds. This illustration of inhibited keratinization, leading eventually to mucous metaplasia, is an indication of the skin's potential to respond to an inductive stimulus with altered morphologic and biochemical differentiation. (Copyright © 1977 by The Williams & Wilkins Company.) From G. L. Peck, P. M. Elias, and B. Wetzel. Effects of retinoic acid on embryonic chick skin. *Journal of Investigative Dermatology* 69:463–476, 1977.

To Anne, David, and Jennifer

Preface

The textual material in this manual was originally prepared in a less detailed form for use by physicians, nurses, and other health-care personnel at the Harvard Community Health Plan. The reception given such practical therapeutic guidelines by clinicians of various specialties, by medical students at the Harvard Medical School, and by house officers at several of the Harvard teaching hospitals encouraged me to write this more comprehensive work.

The first edition of the *Manual of Dermatologic Therapeutics* was greeted enthusiastically. It has been gratifying to realize that such an approach to rational therapeutics has become widely used in the United States, and to know that the information will find good use throughout the world through the Spanish, Portuguese, and Taiwanese editions.

The second edition has been significantly revised and rewritten. It is surprising how much has changed in so short a time, especially in regard to the pathophysiology and approach to the treatment of cutaneous diseases. This edition has been enlarged by the addition of material dealing with several commonly encountered clinical entities and therapeutic problems not previously mentioned, and by the inclusion of information regarding new therapeutic agents as well as structural formulas for most of the medications used in dermatology. I feel that it is important not only to understand how to treat an illness but also to know the composition of the drugs used and their possible modes of action.

The *Manual* should not be used in place of standard dermatologic text-books. Information in greater depth is available in several excellent reference works.* Rather, it should be utilized as an approach to the therapy of the more common cutaneous disorders seen in ambulatory patients. Entities that require specialized therapy, such as malignant tumors of the skin, and conditions seen primarily in the hospitalized patient have been purposely omitted.

The first portion of the *Manual* is organized so that each entity is initially defined and its pathophysiologic features discussed; each disease is then subdivided into subjective data (symptoms), objective data (clinical findings), assessment, and therapy sections, according to the problem-oriented record system in use at many institutions throughout the country. The rest of the text is concerned with procedures, techniques, treatment principles, and discussion of the pharmacodynamics and usage of specific medications employed in treating cutaneous disease.

I would like to express my appreciation to several colleagues across the country for their review of the material for the first edition. Drs. David S. Feingold, Thomas B. Fitzpatrick, and Irwin M. Freedberg of Boston, Dr. Arthur Z. Eisen of St. Louis, Dr. John H. Epstein of San Francisco, and Dr. Silas E. O'Quinn of New Orleans all offered constructive criticism. Dr. Barbara A. Gilchrest carefully reviewed this new edition and made numerous pertinent suggestions. Mrs. Harriet Greenfield is responsible for the excellent new artwork. Jeffrey P. Ross, B.S., R.Ph., offered valuable advice about current pharmaceutical pricing and pharmacy practices. My thanks go to the Schering Corporation, Kenilworth, New Jersey 07033, for permission to reproduce some of the color illustrations. I would also like to acknowledge Dr. Irwin M. Freedberg's continued support. Mrs. Patricia K. Novak skillfully helped prepare the final manuscript. And as always, my wife Anne has been a source of inspiration.

---

* Such references include:

Demis DJ, Crounse RG, Dobson RL, McGuire J (eds): Clinical Dermatology. Hagerstown, Md., Harper & Row, 1972, 4 vols

Fitzpatrick TB, Arndt KA, Clark WC Jr, Eisen AZ, Van Scott EJ, Vaughan JH (eds): Dermatology in General Medicine. New York, McGraw-Hill, 1971, 2048 pp

Moschella SL, Pillsbury DM, Hurley HJ Jr (eds): Dermatology. Philadelphia, Saunders, 1975, 1751 pp

Rook A, Wilkinson DS, Ebling FJG (eds): Textbook of Dermatology. Second Edition. Oxford, Blackwell, 1972, 2118 pp

Contents

Manual of Dermatologic Therapeutics
With Essentials of Diagnosis

NOTICE

The indications and dosages of all drugs in this manual have been recommended in the medical literature and conform to the practices of the general medical community. The medications described do not necessarily have specific approval by the Food and Drug Administration for use in the diseases and dosages for which they are recommended. The package insert for each drug should be consulted for use and dosage as approved by the FDA. Because standards for usage change, it is advisable to keep abreast of revised recommendations, particularly those concerning new drugs.

I
Common Dermatologic Diseases: Diagnosis and Therapy

1
Acne

I. **DEFINITION AND PATHOPHYSIOLOGY** Acne, a very common, self-limited, multifactorial disorder involving the pilosebaceous follicles, is usually first noted in the teenage years. Lesions may begin as early as age 8–10 at "sebarche" and are usually seen 2 years earlier in girls; severe disease affects boys ten times more frequently (up to 15 percent are involved), increases in prevalence steadily throughout adolescence, and then decreases in adulthood.

Severity of involvement can most often be correlated with the amount of sebum secreted; patients with severe acne will usually have large and active sebaceous glands with consequent prominent follicle openings ("pores") and oily skin ("seborrhea"). However, there is much variation and overlap in sebum secretion between unaffected control subjects and acne patients, and no evidence has yet been found that sebum in acne patients differs qualitatively from that of normal persons.

Androgens are the only stimulus to sebaceous gland development and secretion, but acne patients do not have higher plasma levels of androgens. At puberty, hormonal stimuli lead to increased growth and development of pilosebaceous follicles. In those who develop acne there is presumably a heightened responsiveness of these glands to androgenic stimulation. This heightened end-organ response of the sebaceous glands results in increased conversion of testosterone to dihydrotestosterone (DHT) and other 5α reduced metabolites; acne-bearing skin has been shown to produce up to 20 times more DHT than normal skin for corresponding areas. The enlarged gland secretes sebum into a dilated follicle that contains a disproportionately large quantity of normal cutaneous bacteria. Sebum contains free and esterified fatty acids as well as unsaponifiable lipid components. It is the free fatty acid fraction of sebum, produced in the sebaceous follicle by the action of enzymes associated with the anaerobic diphtheroid *Propionibacterium* (*Corynebacterium*) *acnes*, that acts as the primary irritating substance in inflammatory acne. Other as yet unidentified components of sebum induce the pilosebaceous follicle to grow in a hyperkeratotic manner. This results in the intrafollicular desquamation of large numbers of horny cells that, in the acne patient, tend to stick together rather than flow to the surface with sebum. The resultant impacted lipid and keratin mass expands to fill the lumen and form a solid plug in the dilated opening, becoming a closed comedone ("whitehead"). If this comedonal mass protrudes from the follicle, it is recognized as an open comedone ("blackhead"). Its dark color is due to oxidized lipid and to melanin within the mass of horny cells; this plug is *not* dirt. With further distention the follicle walls leak or rupture, releasing sebum, keratin, bacteria, and hair into the dermis and resulting in an inflammatory mass (papule, "pimple," pustule, nodule, cyst, and/or abscess). In adult life the cells lining the follicle presumably become less susceptible to comedogenic materials. The spontaneous disappearance of acne may also be related to a decreased dermal reactivity to irritant substances.

As many as a third of adult women are affected by a low-grade acneform eruption that may start de novo or merge imperceptibly with preexisting adolescent acne. This may be induced by chronic exposure to comedogenic substances present in some cosmetics and moisterizing creams, by androgenic stimuli from progestogens present in some oral contraceptives, by recent cessation of oral contraceptives ("post-pill acne"), or may be from unknown causes.

Acne may lead to pitted or hypertrophic scarring. If left alone, most inflammatory acne tends to disappear slowly in the early twenties in men and somewhat later in women. Adequate therapy will in all cases decrease its severity and may entirely suppress this disease.

II. SUBJECTIVE DATA

A. Patients' presenting complaints may be related to inconspicuous lesions that nevertheless cause considerable social embarrassment. As with all medical and psychological conditions, the patient's perception of the severity of his problem is the most important guide to treatment, and judgmental decisions by the physician about the severity of objective disease must be evaluated in this context.

B. Inflammatory lesions of acne may itch as they erupt and may be very painful on pressure.

C. Pustules and cysts often rupture spontaneously and drain a purulent and/or bloody but odorless discharge.

III. OBJECTIVE DATA (See color insert.)

A. **Noninflammatory lesions** The initial lesion is the closed comedone, visible as a 1–2-mm white dot (whitehead) most easily seen when the skin is stretched. If follicle contents extrude, a 2–5-mm, dark-topped, open comedone results (blackhead).

B. **Inflammatory lesions** Erythematous papules, pustules, cysts, and abscesses may be seen. Patients with cystic acne also tend to show "double" or polyporous comedones, which result from prior inflammation during which epithelial tongues have caused fistulous links between neighboring pilosebaceous units. Acne lesions are seen primarily on the face, but the neck, chest, shoulders, and back may be involved. One or more anatomic areas may be involved in any given patient, and the pattern of involvement, once present, tends to remain constant.

C. The skin, scalp, and hair are frequently very oily.

IV. ASSESSMENT Several points regarding etiology or therapy should be considered with each patient:

A. Are endocrine factors important in this patient?

  1. Are menstrual periods regular? Is there any hirsutism? (Stein-Leventhal syndrome, Cushing's syndrome, and other endocrinopathies are frequently accompanied by acne.)

2. Is there a premenstrual flare-up? The pilosebaceous duct orifice is significantly smaller between days 15–20 of the menstrual cycle, leading to increments in duct obstruction and resistance to flow of sebum. Many of these women tend to do well on anovulatory drugs.

3. Is the patient on oral contraceptives, or has she stopped taking these pills within the past few months? When were the pills started? Which ones? During the first two or three cycles on oral contraceptives acne may flare up. Post-pill acne may continue for as long as a year after birth control pills are stopped. Although anovulatory drugs may provide excellent therapy for acne, the various pills differ enormously in their effect on the sebaceous gland (see p. 13). Oral contraceptives that contain the androgenic and antiestrogenic progestogens norgestrel, norethindrone, and norethindrone acetate may actually provoke an acneform eruption. Ovral® is cited particularly frequently in this regard.

B. What is the effect of seasonal changes? Has the patient recently been in a hot and humid environment? Is sunlight beneficial? Most patients find that summer sunlight will clearly diminish the activity of their acne. However, very humid environments or heavy sweating will lead to keratin hydration, swelling and decrease in the size of the pilosebaceous follicle orifice, and partial or total duct obstruction. It is thus not always good advice to "get out into the sun," unless it's a dry climate. A small number of people overly exposed to sunlight will develop an acneform papular eruption related to abnormal follicular keratinization ("Mallorca," miliary, actinic acne).

C. Is the patient exposed to heavy oils, greases, or tars? These comedogenic agents will initiate lesions, as can some greasy substances used for hair care (pomade acne).

D. Does the patient wear occlusive or tight clothing or have any habits that will initiate or aggravate the disease? Mechanical trauma (pressure, friction, rubbing, squeezing) as from clothing or athletic wear or from behavioral habits will also cause lesions. For example, individuals with the habit of cradling the chin in his or her hand may develop unilateral lesions at that site.

E. Has the patient been on any medications known to cause acne? The most prominent among these are corticosteroids, ACTH, androgens, iodides, and bromides. Other possible stimuli include trimethadione, Dilantin®, INH, lithium, halothane, cobalt irradiation, and hyperalimentation therapy. Corticosteroids, both systemic and topical, are not directly comedogenic; they do appear to sensitize—to "prime"—the follicular epithelium to the comedogenic effects of sebum. Steroid acne starts as uniform red papules, which are then succeeded by closed comedones, and later by open comedones. Chronic steroid acne shows all three types of lesions.

F. How has the patient's acne been treated in the past? Have antibiotics been used? If so, what were the instructions, dosage, duration, and effect of these therapies? Was tetracycline inadvertently taken with meals instead of on an empty stomach? Was the dosage adequate? (see Antibiotics, p. 11).

An unusual complication of chronic tetracycline administration is the development of a **gram-negative folliculitis.** Such patients will notice a sudden change in their acne, with the appearance of pustules or large inflammatory cysts that, on culture, usually grow *Proteus* species. Since acne cysts are sterile on routine bacteriologic culture, a sudden change in morphology warrants gram stain and culture of cyst/abscess contents. Gram-negative folliculitis usually responds to ampicillin, 1 gm daily, after which tetracycline can again be started.

G. Is there any effect of stress or emotional upsets on acne activity? An acutely stressful situation may cause acne to flare up suddenly (but "nerves" are not the cause of the disease!).

H. The number and type of lesions should be roughly quantitated in order to assess further therapeutic responses.

V. THERAPY

A. Mild involvement (few to many comedones)

1. *Antibacterial and comedolytic preparations* These should be applied during the day and/or night to the point of mild dryness and erythema but not discomfort. The alcohol-gel-based benzoyl peroxide preparations are the preparations of choice for the usual case. The 5%

concentration is used initially and the 10% later if tolerated.

Clear alcohol gels: Benzagel®, Desquam-X®, Pan Oxyl®
Clear acetone gel: Persagel®
Clear oil-based lotion: Benoxyl®, Persadox®

a. *Pharmacodynamics* Benzoyl peroxide is effective both as a potent bacteriostat and as a peeling or comedolytic agent. It is hypothesized that benzoyl peroxide, which apparently serves as a depot of free radical oxygen on the skin surface, is decomposed by the cysteine present in skin, after which the oxygen is capable of oxidizing proteins in its vicinity. This would include the bacterial proteins of the sebaceous follicles, thus decreasing the number of *P. acnes* and consequently the amount of free fatty acids (FFA). Topical 5% benzoyl peroxide lowers FFA 50–60% after daily application for 14 days, and decreases aerobic bacteria by 84% and anaerobic bacteria (primarily *P. acnes*) by 98%. Benzoyl peroxide will also reduce the size and number of comedones present. **Topical antibiotics** (*e.g.* clindamycin 1–3%, propylene glycol 10%, in 70% isopropyl alcohol) applied 1–2id also seem to be effective in patients with mild or moderate involvement.

2. *Other peeling and comedolytic preparations* These agents produce irritation and consequent peeling and exfoliation, which is assumed to cause loosening or ejection of comedones. These effects are thought to be secondary to the increased epidermal mitotic activity accompanying irritation. There is no evidence that these medications actually break down keratin.

Not all topical irritants will have the property of decreasing the presence or new formation of comedones. Recent studies show that tretinoin accomplishes this most effectively (almost 100 percent of lesions), followed by 10–15% salicylic acid, and 10% benzoyl peroxide (about 50% reduction).

a. **Abradant cleansers:** Apply 1–2id. These products incorporate finely divided particles with cleansers and wetting agents in order to help remove skin surface debris and promote drying.

Polyethylene particle cleanser: Pernox® scrub or lotion

Aluminum oxide particle cleansers: Brāsivol® (fine, medium, rough)

Sodium tetraboxate decahydrate particle cleanser: Komex®. These particles dissolve on use and thus their abrasiveness is limited.

b. **Clear gels or lotions:** Acne-Aid®, Komed®, Microsyn®, Transact®

Tinted creams: Acne-Aid®, Acnomel®, Fostril®, Sulforcin®

Tinted lotions: Acne-Aid®, Liquimat®, Resulin®

B. **Mild or moderate involvement** (many comedones, some papules and/or pustules)

1. *Benzoyl peroxide gel,* and/or

2. *Tretinoin* (trans-retinoic acid; vitamin A acid) used alone or in combination with benzoyl peroxide gels may offer unique beneficial effects for those who can tolerate its use. This medication has been available for only a few years and its true place in dermatologic therapy is not yet clear. The irritant effects of tretinoin limit its usefulness, but these can be minimized by the correct method of application. Tretinoin, which does not function as a vitamin in its therapeutic applications, increases epidermal cell turnover and decreases the cohesiveness ("stickiness") of horny cells, thus inhibiting the formation of comedones while helping existing comedones to become loosened and expelled. Tretinoin not only changes follicular keratinization, but decreases the normal cell layers of the stratum corneum from 14 to 5. This decrease in thickness of the barrier layer may potentiate the penetration of other topical agents.

a. *Instructions for use*

(1) Erythema and peeling—a mild flush—are the objects of therapy. More severe dryness is to be avoided. It is the achievement of a mild

            facial flush that is important and not the specific adherence to a predetermined course of therapy.

(2)   Fair-complexioned patients with easily irritated skin should start with the 0.05% cream or gel; others may use the 0.1% cream, solution, or pads.

(3)   All other topical acne agents should be stopped prior to initiating retinoic acid therapy. Use mild, gentle soaps no more than twice daily.

(4)   Apply once daily lightly to all areas except around the eyes and lips. Apply approximately 1 hr before bedtime on thoroughly dry skin—wait for at least 15 min after the face has been washed.

(5)   Avoid prolonged, excessive exposure to sun or use an effective sunscreen.

(6)   Expect redness and peeling within a week, lasting 3–4 weeks, and a flare-up in the acne during the first 4–6 weeks. This is explained as the surfacing of lesions onto the skin.

(7)   Clearing requires approximately 3 months. Inflammatory lesions improve more rapidly, but comedones take longer. Effectiveness cannot be judged before 8 weeks and is best assessed at 12 weeks.

(8)   Water-based cosmetics can be used.

(9)   If a patient cannot tolerate the pads or solution, use the 0.05% cream or gel. Also, application can be less frequent—every other night, or skipping every third night, etc.

(10)   Tretinoin application should be continued after the lesions clear.

b.   *Tretinoin products* Retin-A® cream, 0.1% or 0.05%; Retin-A® solution, 0.05%; Retin-A® saturated pads, 0.05%; Retin-A® gel, 0.05%

3. *Combined tretinoin-benzoyl peroxide therapy* With this mode of therapy the tretinoin prevents or removes comedones, while the benzoyl peroxide lowers *P. acnes* and FFA. The tretinoin also enhances absorption of the benzoyl peroxide. Irritant reactions limit the use of this combination therapy but some claim that the two agents used together are less irritating than tretinoin alone.

   a. *Instructions for use*

      (1) Apply tretinoin cream, solution, or pad in the evening as above

      (2) Apply benzoyl peroxide alcohol gel in the morning.

      (3) If irritation is a problem, start with a 5% benzoyl peroxide preparation and tretinoin cream or gel used only every other night.

      (4) After clearing, decrease frequency of therapy and concentration of medication.

C. **Moderate or severe involvement** (inflammatory papules, pustules, cysts, abscesses, and/or scarring) Use topical therapy as discussed above, plus antibiotics or possibly estrogens.

   1. *Antibiotics* Some systemic antimicrobials suppress the growth of normal cutaneous flora (primarily *P. acnes*). As bacteria are decreased and the FFA level slowly diminishes, inflammatory lesions decrease and new lesions stop appearing within 2–6 weeks. Antibiotic therapy cannot be truly evaluated until 6–8 weeks after starting. While sebum composition changes, the secretory rate remains constant. Therapy may need to be continued for months to years.

   One measure of the efficacy of antibiotics is the change in the free fatty acid ratio in sebum. As the ratio goes down, acne should improve. In subjects who are given tetracycline hydrochloride 1 gm/qd, or minocycline 200 mg/qd, or erythromycin 1 gm/qd, or clindamycin 450 mg/qd, the percent decrease after 1 week of oral administration averages 9%, 16%, 22%, and 42%, respectively. This latter is comparable to a decrease of 38% after 1 week of topical administration of 10% benzoyl peroxide alone. After 4 weeks of any of the above four antibiotics, the ratio should decrease by 44%, 38%, 43%, and 58%, respectively, contrasted to a 47% decrease after 2 weeks of topical 10% benzoyl peroxide and tretinoin topical therapy.

a. Tetracycline is the drug of choice. It is the least expensive, has the fewest side-effects, and is best tolerated for long periods of time. Several studies have clearly shown there to be no adverse effects after long-term oral administration. Tetracycline is effective in low doses because high concentrations are achieved within sebaceous follicles, especially when inflammation is present. This antibiotic may also inhibit bacterial lipase directly.

Aside from minor GI tract irritation, *Candida* vaginitis is the only common complication. Although tetracyclines can cause enamel hyperplasia and hence tooth discoloration, by age 12 growth of teeth is essentially complete. Tetracycline should not be used in younger children nor administered during pregnancy. There is drug interaction with the metallic ions Al^{+++}, Mg^{++}, and Ca^{++} present in antacid preparations and dairy products; these products should never be taken at the same time as tetracycline.

Initiate therapy at 250 mg 4id (or 500 mg 2id) taken on an empty stomach ($\frac{1}{2}$ hr before meals or 2 hr after) until there is clear improvement; then decrease the dosage to a maintenance level (250–500 mg qd) or stop it. If inflammatory lesions have not subsided after 4–6 weeks, increase the dose to 1.5 gm qd for 2 weeks, and if necessary to 2 gm qd for the subsequent 2 weeks. Occasionally it is of benefit to use 2–3 gm daily for several weeks in order to induce remission in otherwise unresponsive patients. Once remission is achieved, it is almost always possible to decrease the dosage to a lower level.

b. Erythromycin 1 gm qd is the second drug of choice. The same dose and time responses as noted above also apply to this drug.

c. Minocycline (Minocin®, Vectrin®) 200 mg is very effective in some patients unresponsive to the above antibiotics. There appears to be no cross-resistance with tetracycline. Dizziness, nausea, and vomiting may be a problem if full doses are administered initially. Start at 50 mg qd and slowly increase. Some patients eventually may achieve complete control on 50 mg of minocycline daily.

d. Clindamycin (Cleocin®) 300–450 mg qd is an extremely effective agent for acne. However, the risk of severe colitis limits its systemic use to only very severe cases unresponsive to all other modes of therapy.

e. Trimethoprim/sulfamethoxazole (Bactrim®, Septra®) has also been shown to decrease FFA levels and inhibit inflammatory acne.

2. **Estrogens** (given as anovulatory agents) may be of use in very severe or otherwise unresponsive cases in young women. Most or all of the estrogen effect is the result of adrenal androgen inhibition rather than local suppression at the gland site; small doses of androgen can overcome the sebum-suppressive effects of large doses of estrogen in women as well as in men. There is a direct correlation between the degree of sebaceous gland inhibition and acne improvement. The gland, however, responds variably to estrogen suppression. On the average there will be a decrease of 25% in sebum production on administration of 0.1 mg of ethinyl estradiol. This drug and its 3-methyl ether, mestranol (which has two-thirds the potency of ethinyl estradiol), are the estrogens present in oral contraceptives. With combination therapy it is important to use a pill with adequate estrogenic effect linked with a non-androgenic progestogen.

The preferable pills are Enovid E® (0.1 mg mestranol, 2.5 mg norethynodrel), Enovid 5® (0.075 mestranol, 5.0 mg norethynodrel), Ovulen® (0.1 mg mestranol, 10 mg ethynodiol diacetate), or Demulin® (0.05 mg ethinyl estradiol, 1.0 mg ethynodiol diacetate), in decreasing order of effectiveness. Sequential therapy with Oracon® (0.1 mg ethinyl estradiol, 25.0 mg dimethisterone) was also effective, but this drug is no longer available. Improvement in acne should be noted within 2 months and marked improvement within 4 months of administration. Ovral® should be avoided. Estrogen therapy is rarely needed before age 16, after which time there will be no problems with growth retardation.

D. Adjunctive therapy

1. *Acne surgery*

a. *Comedone expression*   Gentle removal of comedones by pressing over the lesion with a comedone extractor or the opening of an eye dropper not only relieves the patient of unsightly lesions but also may prevent progression to more inflammatory lesions. Occasionally it may be necessary to incise the follicular opening carefully with a #11 scalpel blade or 25-, 27-, or 30-gauge needle. Overrigorous attempts to express comedones may result in an increased inflammatory response.

Recurrence of comedones after removal is common. Open comedones have been shown to recur within 24–40 days, and closed comedones within 30–50 days. Less than 10 percent of comedone extractions are a complete success. Nevertheless this mode of therapy, carefully done, is useful in the appropriate case.

b. *Draining of cysts*   Careful and judicious incision and drainage of cysts and/or abscesses may initiate healing and shorten the duration of lesions.

2. *Intralesional corticosteroids*   The therapy of choice for cystic lesions and acne abscesses is the intralesional injection of small amounts of corticosteroid preparations (triamcinolone acetonide, 2.5 mg/ml). The high local concentration of corticosteroid injected leads to rapid involution of these nonpyogenic, sterile, inflammatory lesions. The stock 10 mg/ml steroid suspension should be diluted 1:3 with lidocaine or saline and only enough injected through a 1-ml syringe with a 27- or 30-gauge needle to distend the cyst slightly (usually 0.025–0.1 ml). Use of undiluted solutions or injections of too great an amount may lead to atrophic depressions in the skin (see p. 294). Most lesions, particularly early ones, will flatten and disappear within 48 hr after injection.

3. **Cryosurgery** Desquamation and involution of lesions will often occur after use of a slush made of precipitated sulfur, powdered dry ice, and acetone; or the use of solid carbon dioxide dipped in acetone; or liquid nitrogen spray for 5–10 sec.

4. **Hot compresses** Hot compresses with Vleminckx's solution (sulfurated lime, available as Vlem-Dome®) used for 10–20 min 1–2id are useful in very active, cystic disease.

5. **Ultraviolet light (UVL)** Exposure to sunlight or UVB sunlamps is very effective in most patients. Administer enough UVL to cause a mild erythema (see p. 247). Patients also using tretinoin may show a heightened sensitivity to UVL.

E. **Patient education about longstanding misconceptions** Neither changes in diet nor use of vitamins or vaccines has been shown to affect sebaceous gland function or acne activity. If a patient finds that certain foods aggravate the eruption, those items alone should be avoided. Strict diets, on the other hand, lead to a great deal of intrafamilial conflict and personal grief, but no improvement in the skin.

REFERENCES

Ad Hoc Committee Report: Systemic antibiotics for the treatment of acne vulgaris. Arch Dermatol 111:1630–1636, 1975

Barranco VP: Effect of androgen-dominant and estrogen-dominant oral contraceptives on acne. Cutis 14:384–386, 1974

Becker FT: Treatment of tetracycline-resistant acne vulgaris. Cutis 14: 610–613, 1974

Frank SB: Acne Vulgaris. Springfield, Ill, Thomas, 1971

Fulton JE Jr, Farzad-Bakshandek A, Bradley S: Studies on the mechanism of topical benzoyl peroxide and vitamin A acid in acne vulgaris. J Cutan Pathol 1:191–200, 1974

Fulton JE Jr, Pablo G: Topical antibacterial therapy for acne. Arch Dermatol 110:83–86, 1974

Kaidbey KH, Kligman AM: The pathogenesis of steroid acne. J Invest Dermatol 62:31–36, 1974

Kaidbey KH, Kligman AM: Effectiveness of peeling agents on experimental open comedones. Cutis 16:53–56, 1975

Mandy SH: The art of tretinoin therapy in acne. Cutis 14:853–857, 1974

Milne JA: Acne vulgaris. In Recent Advances in Dermatology. Edited by A Rook. London, Churchill, 1973, pp 218–244

Pablo GM, Fulton JE Jr: Sebum: analysis by infrared spectroscopy. II. The suppression of fatty acids by systemically administered antibiotics. Arch Dermatol 111:734–735, 1975

Plewig G, Kligman AM: Acne Morphogenesis and Treatment. New York, Springer-Verlag, 1975, 333 pp

Pochi PE: Antibiotics in acne. N Engl J Med 294:43–44, 1976

Pochi PE, Strauss JS: Sebaceous gland suppression with ethinyl estradiol and diethylstilbestrol. Arch Dermatol 108:210–214, 1973

Price VH: Testosterone metabolism in the skin. A review of its function in androgenic alopecia, acne vulgaris, and idiopathic hirsutism including recent studies with antiandrogens. Arch Dermatol 111:1496–1502, 1975

Sebaceous Glands and Acne Vulgaris. Proceedings of the 22nd Annual Symposium on the Biology of Skin. J Invest Dermatol 62:119–339, 1974

The Therapeutic Use of Vitamin A Acid. G Stüttgen, Conference Chairman. Acta Derm Venereol (Stockh) 55(Suppl 74):185 pp, 1975

2
Alopecia Areata

I. **DEFINITION AND PATHOPHYSIOLOGY** Alopecia areata is a unique, often self-limited disorder characterized by plaques of asymptomatic, noninflammatory, nonscarring, complete hair loss most commonly involving the scalp. Children and young adults are most frequently affected and there is a positive family history in 10–20 percent of cases. The cause is unknown but it seems likely that it is due to autoantibodies aimed at hair follicles: the histopathology is similar to that of presumed autoimmune diseases such as Hashimoto's thyroiditis; the disease responds to anti-inflammatory medications; and there appears to be an increased incidence of other autoimmune diseases and circulating antibodies to other tissues in patients with alopecia areata. Emotional stress is often mentioned as another precipitating factor.

The course of alopecia areata is erratic and impossible to predict. In general, the younger the patient at onset and the more widespread the disease, the poorer the prognosis. Cases developing before puberty have a particularly dismal regrowth rate. One patient in 10 has hair loss only in sites other than the scalp—eyelashes, eyebrows, beard, general body hair—and a similar number progress to loss of all scalp hair (alopecia totalis). Regrowth of hair during the first attack takes place within 6 months in 30 percent of cases, within 1 year in 50 percent, and within 5 years in 75 percent; complete recovery occurs in approximately 30 percent; in up to 33 percent the hair never regrows. New lesions reappear within months to years in up to 50 percent of cases. A prolonged and difficult course with poor outlook is associated with total loss of hair from scalp and body (alopecia universalis); with rapid progression of disease; with eyebrow, eyelash, or beard involvement, and with severe associated nail changes.

II. **SUBJECTIVE DATA**   The hair loss is usually without discomfort; rarely, there may be paresthesias in affected areas.

III. **OBJECTIVE DATA**

A. Lesions are well defined, single or multiple, round or oval areas of total hair loss in which the skin seems very smooth and soft. Any hair-bearing area can be affected.

B. In active lesions the "exclamation-point hair" may be seen around the margins. These loose hairs protrude about 3–10 mm above the scalp surface and have a dark, rough, brush-like tip, a narrower, less pigmented shaft, and an atrophic root. These hairs reflect the disturbed keratinization seen after injury to the growing hair follicle and with transition to a resting follicle; they are pathognomonic of expanding alopecia areata.

C. Regrowing hairs appear first as fine, downy, vellus strands which are gradually replaced by normal terminal hair. These new hairs are often lusterless, may break easily, and may be white.

D. Nail changes, present in 10–20 percent of cases, consist of discrete pits in the nail surface usually arranged in horizontal or vertical rows, longitudinal ridging and thickening, or severe dystrophy.

IV. **ASSESSMENT**

A. Careful examination will show no evidence of scarring or inflammation. In tinea capitis, hair loss is not total in the involved areas, hairs present are dull and lusterless, and erythema and scaling are present. Traumatic or self-induced hair loss (trichotillomania) is characterized by only partial hair thinning and hairs that are twisted, broken, and of varying lengths. A mass or traces of preceding inflammation accompany subadjacent furuncles or inflamed cysts. Other differential diagnostic considerations include secondary syphilis and lupus erythematosus. If the diagnosis is in question, a biopsy will be useful: typical findings of alopecia areata would be lymphocytic infiltrate around an affected hair bulb and lower one-third of the follicle, and atrophic hairs.

B. Patients with alopecia areata are generally healthy and do not require investigative laboratory studies.

V. THERAPY

A. Reassurance about the likelihood of spontaneous regrowth and a simple explanation covering the nature and course of the disease, as well as the poor results of most treatments, are usually all that is necessary. When hair loss is extensive or when there is total or universal alopecia, an honest discussion of the chronic nature of alopecia areata is necessary. A wig is useful in extensive cases.

B. Topical medications or stimulants usually induce changes that are no more than a placebo effect. Rarely, use of occlusive topical corticosteroids leads to some regrowth.

C. Intralesional corticosteroid injections can be considered for small areas that are cosmetically disfiguring and persistent, particularly on the scalp or occasionally on the eyebrows. Some regrowth should be evident 4–6 weeks after injections. Up to 33 percent of patients will not regrow hair; failures occur primarily in new and rapidly expanding plaques, or in areas of long-standing hair loss.

   1. Inject plaques at 1–2-cm intervals with a tuberculin syringe and a 27- or 30-gauge needle, or with a needleless jet injector.

   2. Dilute triamcinolone acetonide suspension to 5 mg/ml; 0.05 to 0.1 ml should be placed in each site.

   3. Reinject at 4–6-week intervals. If no growth is present at 3 months, it is not worth continuing the procedure.

   4. Areas of corticosteroid-related regrowth may begin to thin after 3–6 months and can be reinjected again if necessary.

Spontaneous regrowth frequently has occurred during this interval.

D. Treatment with systemic corticosteroids will often stimulate hair regrowth but infrequently alters the basic course and is rarely if ever warranted.

E. Topical immunotherapy utilizing allergic contact sensitization and challenge with dinitrochlorobenzene (DNCB) was recently found useful for inducing hair growth. Enhancement of the T-lymphocyte pool may be the mode of action. The place of DNCB in routine therapy of alopecia areata awaits further study.

REFERENCES

Abell E, Munro DD: Intralesional treatment of alopecia areata with triamcinolone acetonide by jet injector. Br J Dermatol 88:55–59, 1973

Cochran REI, Thomson J, MacSween RNM: An auto-antibody profile in alopecia totalis and diffuse alopecia. Br J Dermatol 95:61–65, 1976

Daman LA, Rosenberg EW, Drake L: Treatment of alopecia areata with DNCB. Arch Dermatol In press, 1978

Ebling FJ, Rook A: Hair. In Textbook of Dermatology (2nd Ed). Edited by A Rook, DS Wilkinson, FJG Ebling. Oxford, Blackwell, 1972, pp 1598–1604

Eckert J, Church RE, Ebling FJ: The pathogenesis of alopecia areata. Br J Dermatol 80:203–210, 1968

Kern F, Hoffman WH, Hambrick GW Jr, Blizzard RM: Alopecia areata: immunologic studies and treatment with prednisone. Arch Dermatol 107:407–412, 1973

Mehlman RD, Griesemer RD: Alopecia areata in the very young. Am J Psychiatry 125:605–614, 1968

Muller SA: Alopecia: syndromes of genetic significance. J Invest Dermatol 60:475–492, 1973

Muller SA, Windelmann RK: Alopecia areata: an evaluation of 736 patients. Arch Dermatol 88:290–297, 1963

Winter RJ, Kern F, Blizzard RM: Prednisone therapy for alopecia areata. Arch Dermatol 112:1549–1552, 1976

3
Aphthous Stomatitis
(Canker Sores)

I. **DEFINITION AND PATHOPHYSIOLOGY** Canker sores are recurrent, painful, mucosal erosions that appear on the inner cheeks, lips, gums, tongue, palate, and pharynx. The prevalence of aphthous ulceration in the general population is about 19 percent, and although they may be found at any age they occur most commonly between 10 and 40 years. Multiple local and systemic triggering factors such as trauma, food and drug allergy, and physical and emotional stress have been implicated in the pathogenesis, but the data are conflicting and the etiology of this syndrome has not been firmly established. Herpes simplex virus has never been isolated from aphthae. Premenstrual flare-ups in women are not uncommon. Most lesions heal without scarring within 2 weeks. Spontaneous complete remission of the disease is uncommon.

One regular finding is the isolation of a pleomorphic alpha-hemolytic streptococcus, *S. sanguis*, from aphthous lesions. These organisms or their cell wall materials can produce lesions in animals that are histologically similar to those found in sections of human lesions, and they may produce a hypersensitivity reaction of a delayed type in animals and humans with recurrent aphthae. Streptococcal cell wall material may be pathogenic in aphthous stomatitis with the cell wall lacking L-form present during remissions. There is considerable support for the theory that cell-mediated immunity to oral mucosal antigens, or to some cross-reacting microbial antigens, may be involved in the pathogenesis of aphthous ulceration. Lymphocytes from patients with recurrent aphthous stomatitis or Behçet's syndrome (oral and genital ulceration associated with iritis) are cytotoxic for gingival epithelial target cells. Also, hemagglutinating antibodies to homogenates of oral mucosa are present in 70–80 percent of patients, and good correlation has been found between clinical features of aphthous stomatitis and lymphocyte transformation.

II. **SUBJECTIVE DATA** Tingling or burning may antedate the appearance of the lesions by 24 hr. During the first 2–3 days the lesions are extremely painful and may interfere with eating and speaking.

III. **OBJECTIVE DATA** Aphthae appear as single or multiple, small —1–10-mm diameter—shallow erosions with clearly defined borders covered by a gray membrane and surrounded by an intense erythematous halo. Rarely, extremely large or exceedingly numerous lesions appear.

IV. **ASSESSMENT** Morphologically similar lesions can be seen with (a) acute herpes simplex gingivostomatitis (see p. 105), (b) candidiasis (see p. 87), (c) Vincent's angina, (d) traumatic ulcers, (e) ulcers in patients with agranulocytosis or cyclic neutropenia, (f) B_{12} or folate-deficient macrocytic anemia. Differential diagnosis from erythema multiforme, erosive lichen planus, pemphigus, pemphigoid, and herpangina should not be difficult. The erosions of Behçet's syndrome may be identical, and it is possible that this syndrome is a severe form of the same entity as aphthous stomatitis.

V.   **THERAPY** Therapy of aphthous stomatitis is aimed at: (a) controlling the pain, (b) shortening the duration of lesions already present, and (c) aborting new lesions. Those objectives may often be attained.

A. **Controlling pain**

1. *Topical anesthetics* Apply dyclonine HCl solution (Dyclone®) to ulcers as often as needed. Onset of anesthesia is rapid, and duration of numbing is up to 1 hr. Lidocaine

(Xylocaine®, ointment 5% or viscous) or diphenhydramine HCl (Benadryl® elixir) may be used in the same
way. Avoid extensive spread of topical medications. If local
anesthetics are used over too wide an area, a disturbing
"cotton-mouth" feeling and total loss of taste results; these
symptoms frequently are worse than those of the original
problem.

2. ***Silver nitrate stick*** application destroys nerve endings
   and may provide relief from pain for the duration of the
   eruption, but the ulcers may enlarge slightly and heal more
   slowly.

B. Aborting lesions and shortening course

1. ***Suppression of oral streptococci by topical antibiotics***
   is a logical approach to therapy and is often successful.

   a. The application of tetracycline compresses is the method
   of choice. Saturate gauze pledgets with 250 mg of tetracycline dissolved in 30 ml of water and apply for 10
   min 4–6id. Alternatively, one can use an oral suspension of tetracycline or the contents of tetracycline capsules; 5 ml (250 mg) of the antibiotic should be held
   in the mouth for 5–10 min 4–6id and then swallowed.
   Nothing should be taken by mouth for the following
   30 min. Continue therapy for 5–7 days. If gastrointestinal side effects develop, they may be eliminated by having the patient expectorate the antibiotic after the oral
   rinse. In many patients this treatment effectively short-
   ens the duration of lesions, decreases pain, and aborts
   early lesions, although, unfortunately, some lesions do
   not respond to this regimen. Patients with recurrent
   lesions should be instructed to initiate therapy as early
   as possible.

   b. Some patients acquire resistance to tetracycline. In
   those instances use a 1% cephalexin monohydrate compress made by dissolving a 250-mg capsule of cephalexin (Keflex®) in 30 ml of water and applying as
   in (a).

2. ***Topical steroids*** also can be useful, especially if applied
   during the prodromal stages. Triamcinolone acetonide 0.1%
   in a base that adheres to mucous membrane (Kenalog® in

Orabase®) or other corticosteroid agents (e.g., Lidex® ointment) should be applied at least 4id. Others advocate use of 2.5-mg tablets of hydrocortisone sodium succinate, or 0.1-mg tablets of betamethasone 17-valerate, allowed to slowly dissolve near the lesion, 3–4id.

3. *Administration of systemic corticosteroids* can abort attacks if taken for 1–3 days during the prodromal period, and it will usually induce healing of lesions in patients with severe erosive lesions.

REFERENCES

Brody HA, Silverman S Jr: Studies on recurrent oral aphthae. I. Clinical and laboratory comparisons. Oral Surg 27:27–34, 1969

Dolby AE: Management of recurrent oral ulcerations. Practitioner 210: 403–408, 1973

Editorial: Recurrent oral ulceration. Br Med J 3:757–758, 1974

Graykowski EA, Barile MF, Lee WB, Stanley HR Jr: Recurrent aphthous stomatitis. Clinical, therapeutic, histopathologic, and hypersensitivity aspects. JAMA 196:637–644, 1966

Lennette EH, Magoffin RL: Virologic and immunologic aspects of major oral ulcerations. J Am Dent Assoc 87:1055–1073, 1973

Rogers RS, Sams WM, Shorter RG: Lymphocytotoxicity in recurrent aphthous stomatitis. Lymphotoxicity for oral epithelial cells in recurrent aphthous stomatitis and Behçet's syndrome. Arch Dermatol 109:361–363, 1974

Ship II, Galili DA: Systemic significance of mouth ulcers. Postgrad Med 49:67–77, 1971

Shore RN, Shelley WB: Treatment of aphthous stomatitis by suppression of intralesional streptococci. Arch Dermatol 109:400–402, 1974

Weathers DR, Griffin JW: Intraoral ulcerations of recurrent herpes simplex and recurrent aphthae: two distinct clinical entities. J Am Dent Assoc 81:81–88, 1970

4
Bacterial Skin Infections

I. DEFINITION AND PATHOPHYSIOLOGY

A. Pyodermas

1. A pyoderma is a purulent infection of the skin. Most are caused by streptococci or staphylococci. Pyodermas occur in up to 10 percent of children in the southeastern United States, in 80 percent of children in endemic areas, and are also very common in adults. Impetigo and folliculitis are the primary bacterial skin infections. Folliculitis may lead to the production of furuncles or carbuncles. Preceding cutaneous lesions, obesity, treatment with steroids and chemotherapeutic agents, dysglobulinemia, white cell dysfunction in leukemia or chronic granulomatous disease, and probably diabetes—all predispose to the development of these infections.

   a. **Nonbullous streptococcal impetigo** is found most often on the face and other exposed areas. It is very contagious among infants and young children but much less so in older persons. Predisposing factors include poor health and hygiene, malnutrition, and a warm climate, as well as antecedent scabies, chickenpox, contact and atopic dermatitis, and other eruptions. The primary lesion is a fragile subcorneal pustule that most frequently contains group A beta-hemolytic streptococci and, less commonly and later in the course of the disease, secondarily colonizing coagulase-positive staphylococci usually not of the group 2 phage type. In patients who ultimately develop impetigo, streptococci may be cultured first from normal skin, then from lesions, and much later from the respiratory tract; staphylococci are initially in the respiratory tract, then on normal skin, and finally in skin lesions. Untreated streptococcal impetigo spontaneously clears both clinically and bacteriologically in about 10 days.

The overall incidence of postpyodermal acute glomerulonephritis is about 2 percent. In tropical climates, nephritogenic strains of streptococci commonly cause impetigo, and in some southern areas of the United States 85 percent of all cases of acute nephritis in preschool children are preceded by cutaneous streptococcal infection.

b. **Bullous staphylococcal impetigo** is seen primarily in children and is caused by phage group 2 staphylococci. These organisms elaborate an exfoliative toxin that induces an intraepidermal subgranular cleavage plane, resulting in blister formation. This organism can also be responsible for an exfoliative dermatitis in infants (**Ritter's disease**) and for toxic epidermal necrolysis (**staphylococcal scalded-skin syndrome**) in infants and children.

c. **Folliculitis** is a staphylococcal infection starting around hair follicles. Superficial folliculitis usually does not represent a serious problem, but deep and/or recurrent lesions of the scalp, nose, and eyelid cilia (styes) are far more distressing.

d. **Furuncles,** or boils, usually develop from a preceding superficial staphylococcal folliculitis. They are most frequently found in areas of hair-bearing skin subject to friction and maceration, especially the face, scalp, buttocks, and axillae. **Recurrent furunculosis** inexplicably develops in an unfortunate few who seem unable to rid themselves permanently of the staphylococcus. There is no evidence that these patients harbor any specific staphylococcal strains or have any definable deficiency in their host defense mechanisms.

    e. **Carbuncles** are staphylococcal abscesses that are larger and deeper than boils and develop in thick inelastic skin. They usually drain at multiple points and are found commonly in the back of the neck, the back, and the thighs.

B. **Erythrasma,** a mild, chronic, localized, superficial bacterial infection involving intertriginous areas of skin, is caused by *Corynebacterium minutissimum*. These organisms are often part of the normal flora, and some change in host-parasite relationship, such as increased heat or humidity, results in the development of the clinical disorder.

II. SUBJECTIVE DATA

A. Impetigo is usually pruritic.

B. All forms of deep folliculitis hurt; styes, boils, and carbuncles may become exquisitely painful.

C. Erythrasma lesions are usually asymptomatic.

III. OBJECTIVE DATA (See color insert.)

A. **Nonbullous streptococcal impetigo** begins as a small erythematous macule that rapidly develops into a fragile vesicle with an erythematous areola. The vesicopustule breaks and leaves a red, oozing erosion capped with a thick golden yellow crust that appears "stuck on." Satellite pustules and lesions are usual. The presenting lesions of bullous staphylococcal impetigo are flaccid bullae which are first filled with clear, then cloudy, fluid and then quickly replaced by a thin, varnish-like crust.

B. **Folliculitis** lesions consist of superficial or deep pustules, or follicular nodules. The face is a common site for deep folliculitis.

C. **Styes** are erythematous swellings around lid cilia.

D. **Furuncles** start as firm, red, tender nodules that become fluctuant, point, and rupture, discharging a core of necrotic tissue.

E. **Carbuncles** appear similar to furuncles, but drain at multiple points.

F. **Erythrasma** may be seen as dry, smooth to slightly creased or scaly, sharply marginated plaques in the inguinal, axillary, or inframammary folds; as mild scaling or fissuring between the 3–4 or 4–5 toe webs; or in generalized scaly patches. Lesions are easily mistaken for those of superficial fungal infection.

IV. ASSESSMENT

A. Factors predisposing to infection should be identified, evaluated, and treated or eliminated.

B. Most cases of impetigo or folliculitis need not be routinely cultured; recalcitrant or unusual cases deserve a gram stain and culture of the exudate.

C. Ninety percent of patients with acute glomerulonephritis secondary to pyoderma will have an elevated serum titer of anti-DNAse B; only 50 percent of similar patients will have elevated levels of anti-streptolysin O.

D. Erythrasma is diagnosed by the characteristic coral red fluorescence of lesions when viewed under the Wood's light. Fluorescence is caused by a water-soluble porphyrin, and hence may be lacking if the patient has bathed recently. The organisms appear as gram-positive rodlike filamentous and coccoid forms and are best viewed under $45\times$ magnification or oil immersion after gram or Giemsa stain of affected scales. Culture is rarely required and needs special media.

V. THERAPY

A. **Impetigo** caused by both streptococci and staphylococci should be treated with systemic antibiotics; such treatment is valid despite the fact that the disease is often self-limited, and that there is no convincing evidence that treating pyodermas will prevent subsequent glomerulonephritis. Systemic treatment is justified for several reasons: first, impetigo sometimes does not resolve for a very long time and may become widespread before it does; second, systemic antibiotics can shorten the healing time and decrease the number of recurrences; third, benzathine penicillin will decrease streptococcal carrier rates for at least 4 weeks and is thus useful both therapeutically as well as prophylactically; fourth, data now accumulated document the ineffectiveness of topical antibiotics in reliably eliminating either staphylococci or streptococci from lesions of streptococcal impetigo. Studies from the southern United States have shown a cure rate of 39 percent for streptococcal impetigo after 2 weeks of therapy with topical hexachlorophene and bacitracin, compared to 99 percent after IM benzathine penicillin or a 10-day course of oral erythromycin, or 98 percent after 10 days of oral phenoxymethyl penicillin.

1. Treat with one injection of IM benzathine penicillin (600,-000 units in children 6 years or younger, 1.2 million units if 7 or older) or 10 days of erythromycin (250 mg 4id) or phenoxymethyl penicillin (250 mg 4id). Bullous staphylococcal impetigo should be treated with a semisynthetic penicillin (dicloxacillin, 250 mg 4id) or erythromycin.

2. The lesions should be soaked 3–4id in warm tap water, saline, or a soap solution to remove the crusts. In addition, it might be useful to have both patient and family bathe at least once daily with a bacteriocidal iodine (e.g., Betadine® skin cleanser) or bacteriostatic soap containing hexachlorophene or other antiseptic agents.

3. Apply an iodine ointment (Betadine®) or simple bland emollient to the base of cleansed lesions after crust has been removed.

B. **Superficial folliculitis** may respond to aggressive topical hygiene and local antibiotics. Folliculitis on the male beard area is unusually recalcitrant and recurrent and should be treated with systemic antibiotics. Simple **furunculosis** needs to be treated only with moist heat. Local ophthalmic antibiotics should be instilled into the eye for styes. Larger boils should be carefully and conservatively incised and drained after they point; after the incision only topical antibiotics are needed. Furuncles or carbuncles associated with a surrounding cellulitis or those associated with fever or located on the upper lip, nose, cheeks, or forehead also are treated with a semisynthetic penicillin, erythromycin, or clindamycin.

C. **Recurrent furunculosis** represents a difficult therapeutic problem, one which should be approached as follows:

1. Assess the organism's antibiotic sensitivity and start on the appropriate drug (most often a semisynthetic penicillin). Continue treatment for 1–3 months and then later as necessary. Long-term systemic therapy will keep new lesions from erupting and sometimes induces the problem to disappear completely.

2. Methods for maintaining rigorous topical hygiene are noted below. However, the use of such programs alone often does not inhibit recurrent furunculosis, and it is now not clear whether topical treatment substantially adds anything of benefit to the care of such patients.

   a. Patient and family should bathe and shampoo 1–2 times daily. Nails should be clipped short and scrubbed as in a surgical prep. Avoid occupational situations that result in occlusion or maceration of skin appendages (dirt, oils, impermeable clothing).

   b. Instill an antibiotic cream or ointment into the anterior nares daily (e.g., Betadine® ointment, Neosporin® ointment).

   c. Precautions during or before shaving must be maintained whenever there are facial lesions. The beard should be soaked with hot water for 5 min prior to shaving. Blades should be discarded daily. As an aftershave, 70% alcohol should be used. The razor should be left in alcohol between shaves or boiled for 5–10 min prior to shaving; similarly, electric razor heads are soaked in alcohol for 1–2 hr between shaves. Use a brushless shaving cream or soap alone.

   d. Separate towels, washcloths, sheets, and clothing should be used; they should be laundered in boiling water and changed daily.

   e. Dressings must be changed frequently and disposed of immediately. Paper tissues instead of handkerchiefs should be used.

   f. Consider bacterial interference treatment when all else fails. In this method a nonpathogenic staphylococcus is inoculated onto multiple sites on the patient's skin after the pathogenic strain has been eliminated by intensive antibiotic administration. After the new organism colonizes the skin, furuncles may cease.

D. **Erythrasma** may be treated topically with keratolytic compounds such as Keralyt® gel or 3% or 6% sulfur and salicylic acid ointment; or it may be treated systemically with erythromycin 250 mg 4id for 2 weeks.

REFERENCES

Dajani AS, Ferrieri P, Wannamaker L: Endemic superficial pyoderma in children. Arch Dermatol 108:517–522, 1973

Dillon HC: Streptococcal infections of the skin and their complications: impetigo and nephritis. In Streptococci and Streptococcal Diseases: Recognition, Understanding and Management. Edited by LW Wannamaker, JM Masten. New York, Academic, 1972, pp 571–587

Dillon HC Jr, Reeves MSA: Streptococcal immune responses in nephritis after skin infection. Am J Med 56:333–346, 1974

Elias PM, Fritsch P, Epstein EH: Staphylococcal scalded skin syndrome. Clinical features, pathogenesis, and recent microbiological and biochemical developments. Arch Dermatol 113:207–219, 1977

Maibach HI, Hildick-Smith G: Skin Bacteria and Their Role in Infection. New York, McGraw–Hill, 1964, 331 pp

Noble WC (Ed): Microbial skin disease. Br J Dermatol 86(Suppl 8):102 pp, 1972

Rasmussen JE: Topical antibiotics. J Dermatol Surg 2:69–71, 1976

Sarkany I, Taplin D, Blank H: Incidence and bacteriology of erythrasma. Arch Dermatol 85:578–582, 1962

Storrs FJ: Treatment of nonbullous impetigo. Cutis 16:886–891, 1975

Strauss WG, Maibach HI, Shinefield HR: Bacterial interference treatment of recurrent furunculosis. II. Demonstration of the relationship of strain to pathogenicity. JAMA 208:861–863, 1969

Wannamaker LW: Impetigo contagiosa. Prog Dermatol 7:11–14, 1973

5
Bites and Stings
(Spiders, Snakes, Insects)

I. DEFINITION AND PATHOPHYSIOLOGY Reaction to bites and stings is initiated by either a toxin or allergen injected by the offending arthropod (spider, tick, scorpion, mite) or snake. The direct toxic mechanisms include contact with venoms, irritating hairs, salivary secretions, or vesicant fluids; indirect contact may result from inhalation or ingestion of debris, particles, body parts, or excretions. Spiders and snakes inject venoms that may be hemolytic or may disturb the clotting system or act as neurotoxins. Intravascular coagulation may account for the clinical picture seen after the recluse spider bite. The vast majority of serious reactions to biting insects, including bees, hornets, wasps, yellow jackets, fleas, mosquitoes, ants, and bedbugs, are caused by an acquired hypersensitivity; over 80 percent of deaths result from anaphylactic reactions and occur within an hour of the sting. Many patients who develop generalized reactions to insect stings have no history of previous systemic or local reaction to a sting. Approximately 50 percent of deaths attributed to venomous animals result from Hymenoptera (bee or wasp) stings; rattlesnake bites account for 20 percent of fatalities, and poisonous spiders, 14 percent. Venom from Hymenoptera contains serotonin, kinins, acetylcholine, lecithinase, hyaluronidase, and phospholipase; exposure to this venom has been shown to release histamine from leukocytes of Hymenoptera-allergic patients.

II. SUBJECTIVE DATA

A. **Spiders** The spiders that cause serious reactions in man in the United States most commonly are the black widow (*Latrodectus mactans*) and the brown recluse spider (*Loxosceles reclusa*). After a short sharp pain at the site of a black widow spider bite, systemic symptoms, including chills, vomiting, pain in abdomen and legs, sweating, and cramps, begin in 15–60 min and usually subside within several hours. Severe local pain associated with local swelling occurs between 4–8 hr after a recluse spider bite. Viscerocutaneous loxoscelism, with severe chills, vomiting, arthralgias, and hematologic abnormalities, is rare.

B. **Snakes** The pit vipers (rattlesnake, moccasin, and copperhead) are the most dangerous snakes in the United States. Local reactions to bites are pain and swelling, which may be accompanied by a tingling sensation around the lips, vertigo, muscular twitching, or bleeding (hematuria, hematemesis).

C. **Insects** The *normal reaction* to the sting of a bee, wasp, hornet, or yellow jacket is itching and pain, both of which subside within a few hours. Severe *local reactions* result in itching, pain, and in an unusual amount of swelling around the site of the sting. *Toxic reactions,* which occur after 10 or more simultaneous stings, are characterized by gastrointestinal symptoms, vertigo, headache, and fever. *Immediate systemic allergic reactions* show the usual manifestations of anaphylaxis: urticaria, laryngeal edema, bronchospasm, abdominal cramps, and shock. *Delayed allergic reactions* occur within hours to 2 weeks following the sting and present with symptoms similar to serum sickness.

The harvester ant and fire ant cause most ant-sting reactions in man. Both are associated with "fire" because of the intense burning and pain associated with their stings. Some patients may develop immediate systemic allergic reactions to fire ant stings.

The immediate allergic reaction to the injected salivary fluids of mosquitoes is itching; the delayed reaction, occurring several hours later, is accompanied by a more severe, intense, burning itch. Flies do not actually bite but pierce through the skin, thus allowing salivary gland fluids to enter and cause toxic and allergic reactions. The little (1 x 5 mm) black fly is renowned for inducing an extremely painful and long-lasting reaction. Flea bites itch.

III. OBJECTIVE DATA

A. **Spiders**   The local reaction to a black widow spider bite is unremarkable. Severely ill patients will have the symptoms described, which may be accompanied by a morbilliform erythema. The bite of the recluse spider is relatively painless; the bite reaction goes through stages, beginning with edema, progressing to bulla formation (0–2 hr), then to surrounding ischemia (2–6 hr), blue-black cyanosis (5–12 hr), and then to extensive necrosis and gangrene (12 hr on).

B. **Snakes**   The bite will usually consist of two fang marks surrounded by intense edema, ecchymosis, and sometimes bullae.

C. **Insects**

1. *Bees, wasps, hornets, yellow jackets*

a. *Normal:* red area with a control punctum gradually surrounded by a white zone and red flare. Later a wheal forms and disappears within hours.

b. *Local reaction:* intense edema around the sting area.

c. *Toxic reactions:* cutaneous signs are usually edema without urticaria.

d. *Immediate systemic allergic reactions* are those of anaphylaxis.

e. *Delayed systemic allergic reactions:* urticaria, accompanied by lymphadenopathy and polyarthritis.

2. *Ants*   Fire ant stings develop as a wheal surmounted by two hemorrhagic puncta and evolve into vesicles and, 8–10 hr later, umbilicated pustules. Crusts and scar tissue gradually form over the next week.

3. *Mosquitoes*   The immediate reaction is production of a wheal; a swollen papular lesion may appear as delayed reaction several hours later.

4. **Flies** The blackfly sting causes either nodular vesicular lesions or firm, rough pruritic nodules. Both reactions may last weeks to months.

5. **Fleas** These bites are typically grouped urticarial papules, some with a central punctum.

IV. **ASSESSMENT** Patients with severe reactions should be cared for in facilities prepared to handle acute respiratory and cardiovascular emergencies.

V. **THERAPY**

A. **Spiders** Mild local reactions to black widow spider bites should be treated by cool compresses or application of an ice cube, calamine lotion, and/or a topical corticosteroid. When there is severe reaction to the black widow spider bites, treatment should be immediate and include a tight proximal tourniquet to occlude venous return, incision of the sting area, suction to remove the venom, opiates for pain, and specific horse serum antivenom effective against all *Latrodectus* (Lyovac®, Merck Sharp & Dohme). With *Loxosceles* bites, and those from unidentified spiders, when a local lesion appears and progresses over 12–24 hr, the patient should be started on a 6–8-day course of high doses of systemic steroids (equivalent to 80 mg prednisone qd). Intralesional corticosteroid injection may also be useful. Early excision is recommended when the type of spider has not been identified, when a well-developed cutaneous lesion is present, and when the patient is seen within 8 hr of the bite. Tetanus prophylaxis is, of course, mandatory, as with all serious bites or stings.

B. **Snakes** The best first aid measures for snake bites are: (1) Immobilize the injured part. Tourniquets should not be used as they will not prevent death, can cause extensive necrosis, and loosening may produce shock. (2) Make an incision at each site of venom injection and apply suction from a rubber cup (not by mouth). Suction should be started within 3 min and discontinued in 15–20 min. As much as 44 percent of the venom can be removed with 30 min of suction started as long as 2 hr after subcutaneous injection of venom. If the interval between bite and treatment is going to be prolonged, apply ice to the bite. (3) Get the victim to a physician or hospital as soon as possible.

At that time start an IV in the contralateral arm; type and cross-match blood early, before venom action makes this impossible; and check for the presence of coagulopathy. (4) Most important in severely envenomized patients, administer horse-based antiserum. Other treatment methods as well as sources of antivenom are detailed in Arnold (1973).

C. **Insects**

1. Flick (do not squeeze) the insect off the skin. This should also remove the venom sac. If the stinger is left in the skin, remove it carefully with tweezers.

2. Cold applications (ice, cold compresses) at the sting site may retard absorption and reduce chemical activity of the venom.

3. *Local reactions*

   a. Cold open wet compresses 1 hr 3id.

   b. Calamine lotion alone or with 0.25% menthol and 1% phenol will be soothing.

   c. A topical corticosteroid may be useful for the pruritus and inflammation.

   d. Systemic antihistamines.

4. *Systemic allergic reactions and treatment for anaphylaxis*

   a. Inject epinephrine HCl 1:1000 0.3–0.5 ml IM and repeat every 15–30 min as needed. If symptoms are minimal, subcutaneous injection will suffice. Only with profound anaphylaxis should intravenous administration be necessary. Start an IV drip as soon as possible. A 10-mg sublingual isoproterenol tablet or epinephrine inhalation aerosol may at times be substituted for the injection as these medications may be more easily self-administered by patients.

   b. Apply a tourniquet proximal to the sting on an extremity. The tourniquet should not be so tight as to cut off arterial circulation. Relax the occlusion 1 min every 3 min. Inject epinephrine HCl 1:1000, 0.2 ml, subcutaneously into the reaction site. Carefully remove the stinger, if present, by scraping it out with a knife blade or fingernail, or use tweezers to grip the stinger stylet. Do not pinch the venom sac.

c.   Administer an antihistamine PO or IM (chlorpheniramine 10 mg, diphenhydramine 50 mg, repeat q6h prn) depending upon the severity of the reaction. If laryngeal edema, bronchospasm, or hypotension are present, give the initial dose intravenously.

d.   For severe laryngeal edema, also use ephedrine, 25 mg q6h, hydrocortisone 100 mg q6h IV, consider tracheotomy or insertion of endotracheal tube. If mild, use ephedrine, 25 mg q6h PO, or a combination of theophylline, ephedrine hydrochloride, and phenobarbital (Tedral®) 1 tab q6h PO.

e.   For severe bronchospasm, also use aminophylline 500 mg IV q6h, hydrocortisone 100 mg q6h IV.

f.   For severe hypotension, use metaraminol bitartrate 100 mg in 1000 ml of 5% dextrose in water, or norepinephrine 4.0 ml of 0.2% solution in 1000 ml of 5% dextrose by IV drip.

g.   With (d), (e), and (f) one should also administer oxygen; monitor blood gases, ECG, and urine output; and observe the patient for respiratory failure.

Reactions usually subside within 1–2 days.

5. *Prophylaxis*

a.   Sensitive patients should carry medications such as an epinephrine inhalation spray, ephedrine, and antihistamine tablets with them at all times. Commercial kits are available that contain a syringe loaded with epinephrine, and a tourniquet and antihistamine tablets (Ana-Kit®, Hollister–Stier Laboratories; "Personal" Insect Sting Kit®, International Medication Systems, South El Monte, Calif.) Patients should also always carry an aerosol insecticide spray and avoid walking without shoes. They should dress in protective clothing, and avoid wearing the following items, all of which attract flying insects:

(1) Perfumes and other scented preparations (hair spray, aftershave lotion, deodorant).

(2) Brightly colored objects such as clothing or jewelry (white is said to be the least insect-attracting color).

(3) Wool, suede, and leather-like apparel.

b. Desensitization (hyposensitization, immunotherapy) is effective and **should be considered mandatory** for patients who have had serious local reactions. Successful desensitization is accompanied by a decrease in basophil histamine release and an increase in blocking (IgG) antibody level. The material of choice for desensitization appears to be Hymenoptera venom alone, rather than whole-body extract. These venoms, however, are still in the investigational stage and are available only in some clinical immunology centers. The only materials commercially available are monovalent and polyvalent extracts of the whole bodies of bees, wasps, hornets, and yellow jackets. With current programs, 96 percent of patients subsequently stung again experience less severe reactions.

c. *Insect repellents*

(1) Repellents containing diethyltoluamide are the agents of choice for protection against mosquitoes, flies, fleas, mites, and ticks. Ethyl hexanediol and dimethyl phthalate are also effective. No product will protect against spiders, wasps, or bees.

(2) Factors that attract mosquitoes to skin include warmth, sweat, moisture, carbon dioxide, and other body emanations found in the convection air currents above or downwind of man.

(3) Repellents do not mask these attractive stimuli but seem to form a barrier against penetration that extends to less than 4 cm away from the skin on which the repellent has been freshly applied. This means that nontreated areas only a few centimeters away from those protected may be bitten.

(4) At room temperature, protection time may last 10–12 hr. There are many factors that will decrease the protection time, including warmer temperatures, high wind velocities, loss of repellent from rubbing against clothing, and washoff with water or sweat.

(5) If mosquitoes are dense, a high dose of repellent must be applied. The volume will depend upon the amount of active ingredient in the repellent mixture. One should apply at least 1 mg/cm² of exposed skin, which means applying liberally and, under most outdoor conditions, frequently (q½ hr–2 hr).

(6) Repellent-treated nets and clothing not only prevent mosquitoes from biting through clothes, but also prevent them from biting adjacent areas. Repellents may remain effective for several days on fabric.

(7) Diethyltoluamide-containing products include Mosquitone® lotion, OFF® products, and Cutter® insect repellent. Ethyl hexanediol is present in 6–12® lotion, stick, or towelettes (see also p. 319).

REFERENCES

Arnold RE: What to do about bites and stings of venomous animals. New York, Macmillan, 1973, 122 pp

Barr SE: Allergy to Hymenoptera stings. JAMA 228:718–720, 1974

Barr SE: Insect sting allergy. Cutis 17:1069–1074, 1976

Berger RS, Adelstein EH, Anderson PC: Intravascular coagulation: the cause of necrotic arachnidism. J Invest Dermatol 61:142–150, 1973

Frazier CA: Insect Allergy: Allergic and Toxic Reactions to Insects and Other Arthropods. St. Louis, WH Green, 1969, 493 pp

Frazier CA: Cutaneous manifestations of insect allergy. Cutis 13:1038–1047, 1974

Harves AD, Millikan LE: Current concepts of therapy and pathophysiology in arthropod bites and stings. I. Arthropods. II. Insects. Int J Dermatol 14:543–562, 621–634, 1975

Jansen GT, Morgan PN, McQueen JN, Bennett WE: The brown recluse spider bite. Controlled evaluation of treatment using the white rabbit as an animal model. South Med J 64:1194–1202, 1971

Kelly JF, Patterson R: Anaphylaxis. Course, mechanisms and treatment. JAMA 227:1431–1436, 1974

Lichtenstein LM, Valentine MD, Sobotka AK: A case for venom treatment in anaphylactic sensitivity to Hymenoptera sting. N Engl J
Med 290:1223–1227, 1974

Maibach HI, Khan AA, Akers W: Use of insect repellents for maximum
efficacy. Arch Dermatol 109:32–35, 1974

Parrish HM, Wiechmann GH: Rattlesnake bites in the Eastern United
States. South Med J 61:118–126, 1968

Reisman RE, Arbesman CE: Stinging insect allergy. Current concepts
and problems. Pediatr Clin North Am 22:185–192, 1975

Sobotka AK, Valentine MD, Benton AW, Lichtenstein LM: Allergy to
insect stings. I. Diagnosis of IgE-mediated Hymenoptera sensitivity
by venom-induced histamine release. J Allergy Clin Immunol 53:
170–184, 1974

6
Burns

I. **DEFINITION AND PATHOPHYSIOLOGY** More than two million individuals in the United States suffer burns each year, of which 100,000 require hospitalization and 10,000 die. The incidence of burns is high among the very young and very old, among nonwhites and members of lower socioeconomic groups, and in rural areas where space heaters or fireplaces are used for heat. The degree of cutaneous damage caused by thermal injury to the skin is related directly to the duration and intensity of exposure to heat. The types of burns may be summarized as follows:

A. **First-degree burn**

   1. Histopathology

      a. Epidermis: loss of intercellular cohesiveness with cleft formation.

      b. Dermis: vasodilatation and edema.

   2. Clinical condition: red, swollen skin.

3. Course: heals within 3–4 days without scarring.

B. Second-degree burn (partial-thickness burn)

1. Histopathology

   a. Epidermis: coagulative necrosis with retained integrity of intercellular attachments; bulla formation at dermo-epidermal junction.

   b. Dermis: marked vasodilatation and edema.

2. Clinical condition: red, blistered skin with maintenance of epidermal integrity.

3. Course: reepithelialization takes place from epidermal appendages and, if left undisturbed, will heal within 2–3 weeks without scarring.

C. Third-degree burn (full-thickness burn)

1. Histopathology: necrosis of variable amounts of epidermis, dermis, and subcutaneous tissue.

2. Clinical condition: ulcerated wound with extensive tissue necrosis.

3. Course: heals slowly (in months) with scarring.

The depth of the burn may be related to its cause. Scalds from hot liquids are usually partial thickness, while injuries from contact with flames, hot metal, or electrical current are usually full thickness in depth. Chemical burn damage depends upon the agent, and injury may progress for several days. In practice, it is often difficult to determine the depth of injury during the first 2 weeks of healing.

II. SUBJECTIVE DATA   First- and second-degree burns are extremely painful, whereas deeper damage destroys nerves and renders the tissues insensitive to pain.

III. OBJECTIVE DATA

A. First-degree burns are erythematous and edematous and heal rapidly; there is mild epidermal desquamation and postinflammatory hyperpigmentation.

B. Second-degree burns demonstrate blistering; evidence of continued capillary circulation may be observed.

C. With deeper burns, coagulated blood vessels are present, and the skin appears dry and mahogany-colored. In damaged skin that appears marble-white, the depth of damage is difficult to assess. These wounds may be full thickness, but at times they heal spontaneously and are then best termed deep, partial-thickness injury.

IV. ASSESSMENT Partial-thickness burns that involve less than 15% of the body surface and spare the face, hands, feet, and perineum, and full-thickness burns of less than 2% of the body surface are classified as minor burns. Such burns can almost always be managed on an ambulatory basis.

V. THERAPY The pathophysiology and therapy of moderate and severe burns will not be discussed here. Such burns require intensive specialized care in hospitals for expert management of the wound and of the severe fluid and electrolyte changes associated with extensive cutaneous damage.

A. Immediate therapy Apply wet towels soaked in ice water or cold water, or ice itself, or immerse the burned area in static cold tap water (72–77°F). This is effective because burned skin retains enough heat to extend coagulation to surrounding tissues. Treatment should be started as soon as possible (within the first hour after injury) after the area has been cleansed with soap and water. Application of cold relieves pain, reduces edema and reactive hyperemia, and probably diminishes the extent of injury. The burned area should be kept in water until it is free of pain both in and out of water; this may take up to 45 min. Warm blankets should be put on uninvolved areas to prevent systemic hypothermia.

B. Postemergency therapy

   1. *Very superficial burns* require no dressing or medications, although the application of an emollient such as petrolatum may be soothing. Burn wounds should be washed gently with a bland soap and water and dirt removed. Patients should receive tetanus immunization and be given analgesics as required. Topical anesthetics containing more than 5% benzocaine base (e.g., Americaine® ointment) may dull the immediate discomfort but will add the risk of allergic contact sensitization. There are no clinical studies that demonstrate the efficacy of antibiotics after their topical application to the superficial burn and their use is contraindicated. A topical corticosteroid will inhibit inflammation and may also decrease pain.

2. *Second-degree burns* should be cleansed and a dressing applied. In general, it is best to remove blisters or dead tissue. Almost all burns treated on an ambulatory basis do better when treated with dressings. The dressing should occlude the wound, splint the part, be easily removed, and be comfortable. If oozing or weeping is present, application of a water-soluble ointment or ointment gauze next to the wound will keep the dressing from sticking. Absorptive material such as fluffed gauze pads should be placed over the initial gauze layer, and a final layer of elastic bandage should be put on with even compression. Dressings should remain in place for about 5 days unless there is much weeping, in which case they may need to be changed more often. If dressings are stuck, they should be moistened or the affected part soaked in warm water before the dressings are removed. If there is any question of infection, a topical antibacterial preparation, such as povidone-iodine ointment, solution, or spray (Betadine® products), silver sulfadiazine (Silvadene®), mafenide (Sulfamylon®), or gentamicin (Garamycin®), should be applied.

3. *Chemical burns* require immediate and prolonged irrigation with water. The depth of the injury may be reduced by 2–4 hr or more of washing. Do not rinse acid burns with alkali and vice versa; this causes an exothermic reaction, which leads to further tissue damage. Industrial toxicity texts should be consulted concerning any specific therapy for offending chemicals.

REFERENCES

Abston S: Burns in Children. Ciba Clinical Symposia 28, No 4, 1976, 36 pp

Artz CP, Moncrief JA: The Treatment of Burns (2nd Edition). Philadelphia, Saunders, 1969, 393 pp

Bloch M: Cold water for burns and scalds. Lancet 1:695, 1968

Bollin JC: Evaluation of a new topical agent for burn therapy. Silver sulfadiazine (Silvadene) JAMA 230:1184–1185, 1974

Dalili H, Adriani J: The efficacy of local anesthetics in blocking the sensations of itch, burning, and pain in normal and "sunburned" skin. Clin Pharmacol Ther 12:913–919, 1971

Moncrief JA: Burns. N Engl J Med 288:444–454, 1973

Moncrief J (ed): Topical antibacterial therapy of the burn wound. Clin Plast Surg 1:563–576, 1974

Nance FC, Lewis VL Jr, Hines JL, Barnett DP, O'Neill JA: Aggressive outpatient care of burns. J Trauma 12:144–146, 1972

Pearson RW: Response of human epidermis to graded thermal stress. A morphologic comparison of burns, cold-induced blisters and pemphigus vulgaris. Arch Environ Health 11:498–507, 1965

Sørensen B: First aid in burn injuries: treatment at home with cold water. Mod Treat 4:1199–1202, 1967

7
Corns and Calluses

I. **DEFINITION AND PATHOPHYSIOLOGY** Corns (clavi) and calluses are acquired areas of thickened skin that appear over sites of repeated or prolonged trauma to the epithelium. Neither soft corns nor hard corns occur in normal feet. These lesions arise as a result of pressure, friction, and perhaps shearing torque forces of bone, through the overlying skin, against soft tissues and bone of adjacent digits, metatarsal heads, or footwear. The severity and type of growth are related to the degree and chronicity of the local irritation. The formation of the center (nucleus, radix) of a corn is secondary to vascular changes and fibrosis underlying the point of maximum stress. In both conditions there is marked hyperkeratosis of the stratum corneum overlying an epidermis that is otherwise the same thickness as adjacent skin.

Some studies show that the structure of keratin in callus differs from that of the normal stratum corneum. The individual cells are thicker, much more highly interdigitated, and the intercellular spaces are occupied by a dense cement material. All signs of desquamation are absent. The keratin appears to be similar in structure to that of finger pad and nail.

Corns are more symptomatic and better demarcated than calluses. They appear most frequently over the dorsolateral aspect of the fifth toes, but may be seen commonly at any point under the metatarsal arch. Small "seed corns" may be found anywhere on the plantar surface. Poorly fitting shoes are the most frequent cause of corns. Soft corns that result from pressure of the head of the proximal phalanx of the fifth toe on the base of the proximal phalanx of the fourth toe, or those that result from interdigital maceration, are most often located in the fourth interdigital web.

Calluses are more diffuse hyperkeratotic areas present most commonly under the first and/or fifth metatarsal heads. They are seen also as occupational marks, e.g., the callused palms of a laborer or the callused fingers of a violinist.

II.　**SUBJECTIVE DATA**　Corns may cause a constant dull discomfort or a severe knifelike pain on downward pressure. Calluses are either asymptomatic or are painful on pressure, causing a feeling somewhat akin to walking with a pebble in one's shoe.

III.　**OBJECTIVE DATA**

　　A.　Corns are sharply delineated, hyperkeratotic, small (several millimeters in diameter or smaller) areas with a central translucent area. They are conical in shape, with the apex pointing into the tissue. Soft corns are less discrete, whitish thickenings found in the interdigital webs. If one palpates these lesions, an underlying bony prominence will always be found.

　　B.　Calluses are large (millimeters to centimeters in diameter) diffuse areas of thickened skin with indefinite borders.

IV.　**ASSESSMENT**　If a suspect lesion is pared down (debrided), a number of differential features become apparent.

　　A.　**Corns**　A central nucleus becomes evident; with continued debridement this clear area becomes smaller and eventually disappears, at which point the normal skin markings can again be followed through the lesion.

　　B.　**Soft corns**　These are often confused with simple maceration or an interdigital fungal infection. Paring the lesion will reveal a central nucleus and at times a small sinus tract at the base of the interdigital web. This sinus may close intermittently and result in recurrent bouts of bacterial infection.

C. **Calluses** The normal skin markings remain evident, and no nucleus is found.

D. **Plantar warts** (see also p. 212) A central area composed of red and black dots, punctate bleeding, and obliteration of skin marking will be revealed on debridement. The dots represent capillary thrombosis of vessels in the highly vascularized wart. A callus will commonly overlie a wart and be responsible for the discomfort associated with this lesion. Corns and calluses tend to be more tender on direct downward pressure, whereas warts are most uncomfortable when squeezed from the sides.

V. THERAPY

A. Therapy to allay symptoms

1. With both corns and calluses the cause of pain is thickened hyperkeratotic areas of skin. The pain caused by such a mass may be completely eradicated simply by reducing the lesion by debridement with a #15 blade or a #86 Beaver or #313 Gillette chisel blade. To insure satisfactory results with a corn, it is often advisable to anesthetize the area (to remove the entire central nucleus). The following instructions will enable the patient to carry out intermittent debridement:

   a. Cut out a piece of 40% salicylic acid plaster slightly larger than the lesion, apply it to the skin, sticky side down, and cover with adhesive tape.

   b. Leave overnight, or for as long as 5–7 days for very thick lesions.

   c. Remove the dressing and soak the foot in water.

   d. Remove whitened, soft, and macerated skin with a rough towel, pumice stone, or callus file.

   e. Reapply plaster as often as necessary to keep the lesion flat.

2. At times, injection of a small amount of corticosteroid (Aristocort®, Celestone®, Kenalog®) beneath a painful corn will result in dramatic relief of symptoms.

B. Definitive therapy Removal of the lesion treats only the result and not the cause of the difficulty. Poorly fitting footwear, anatomical malformations, faulty weight distribution, or similar factors must be corrected or the hyperkeratoses will rapidly recur. Both corns and calluses will disappear after the causative factors have been removed. Corrective shoe supports, x-ray studies for anatomical defects, and referral to a podiatrist or orthopedic surgeon are warranted in difficult cases.

REFERENCES

Carney RG: Confusing keratotic lesions of the sole. Cutis 7:32–34, 1971

Montgomery RM: Corns, calluses and warts. Differential diagnosis. NY State J Med 63:1532–1534, 1963

Orfanos CE, Mahrle G, Ruska H: Callus and its keratin before and after treatment with sodium thioglycolate. A study by scanning and conventional electron microscopy. Br J Dermatol 85:437–449, 1971

Potter GK: Histopathology of clavi. J Am Podiatry Assoc 63:57–66, 1973

Woodland LJ: Corns, callosities and footwear. Med J Aust 39:638–641, 1952

8
Dermatitis (Eczema)

DEFINITION AND PATHOPHYSIOLOGY The different forms of superficial inflammatory diseases of the skin represent the most common reaction pattern seen by the dermatologist. The morphologic and histopathologic changes in all forms of dermatitis and eczema, terms that are used interchangeably, are similar. The earliest and mildest changes are erythema and edema. These early changes may progress to vesiculation and oozing and then to crusting and scaling. Finally, if the process becomes chronic, the skin will become lichenified (thickened with prominent skin markings), excoriated, and either hypopigmented or hyperpigmented.

The microscopic changes in this process show: (a) early, intercellular and intracellular fluid accumulation, with resultant vesicle formation and associated dermal vasodilatation and infiltration with chronic inflammatory cells; and (b) later, thickening of the epidermis and altered keratinization patterns, with retention of nuclei in the stratum corneum.

The factors that may initiate dermatitis are numerous, and the patterns of the dermatitis will dictate both the clinical classification and therapy.

ATOPIC DERMATITIS

I. **DEFINITION AND PATHOPHYSIOLOGY** Atopic dermatitis is an intensely pruritic, chronic eruption. It is the most common type of infantile eczema and is also seen in characteristic patterns in children, adolescents, and adults. Approximately 70 percent of patients with atopic dermatitis have a family history of atopy, about 3 percent of infants have some evidence of atopic dermatitis during the first few months of life, and about 50 percent of children with atopic dermatitis develop either rhinitis or asthma. Severe, easily triggered itching is the outstanding feature of this entity. Many of the clinical signs seen are secondary to scratching and rubbing of the skin. Atopic dermatitis may be particularly devastating in its effects on the patient's mental well being and emotional development, as it is frequently present during the most critical periods of life; in infancy, it interferes with a healthy mother-child relationship; in adolescence and early adulthood, it plagues and disfigures patients during a crucial formative period. Emotional stress and altered family interactions play an important role in its course.

Patients with atopic dermatitis demonstrate elevated levels of IgE skin-sensitizing antibodies (reagin), and there is usually a correlation between IgE serum level and the severity, duration, and amount of body surface affected by dermatitis. There are, however, many facts that argue against IgE playing an important role in the causation of this entity. About 20 percent of adults with atopic dermatitis have normal or low IgE, and others have no IgE at all, while there are some patients with enormous elevations of IgE who have no dermatitis. Further, in infantile eczema IgE levels are consistently low or normal. Also, IgE does not mediate delayed hypersensitivity reactions of which eczema/dermatitis is considered an exemplary type. It has never been shown that reaginic antibodies, with their associated allergens, can actually incite clinical atopic skin disease. Skin testing, hyposensitization, and special diets are usually unrewarding.

A lower clinical incidence of allergic contact dermatitis is seen in patients with atopic dermatitis than in patients with some other dermatoses; it has been shown that the incidence of poison ivy allergy is 10 times less frequent in patients with atopic dermatitis than in the general population. Evidence of defective leukocyte phagocytosis, decreased absolute numbers of and percentage of T-lymphocytes, and depressed or absent T-cell response to *Candida*, phytohemagglutinin, and streptokinase-streptodornase in patients with atopic dermatitis suggests that this disorder may represent a state of cellular immunodeficiency rather than one of heightened allergy. There is also evidence that there is an abnormal balance between α (alpha) and β (beta) receptors in the skin, resulting, in a physiologic sense, in a blockade of the beta receptors on the surface of atopic epidermal cells. Atopic patients react in an aberrant fashion to many environmental and physiologic factors: they demonstrate heightened and prolonged pruritus in response to normally subthreshold stimuli and an altered vascular response to pressure and injections of histamine, serotonin, cholinergic and sympathomimetic agents, as well as abnormal reactions to heat and cold.

II.   SUBJECTIVE DATA   The primary and predominant symptom of atopic dermatitis is itching. This often sets up a vicious cycle: itching leads to scratching, scratching causes lichenification and other changes, and lichenification lowers the threshold for renewed itching.

III. OBJECTIVE DATA

A.   In the *infantile phase* of atopic dermatitis (age 2 months to 2 years) there is involvement primarily of the chest, face, scalp, neck, and extensor extremities with erythematous papulovesicles and oozing. Some infants also have very dry skin that predisposes them to itching and recurrent inflammation.

B.   In the *childhood phase,* between the ages of 4 and 10 years, the lesions are less acute and exudative, more scattered, and often localized in the flexor folds of the neck, elbows, wrists, and knees. Dry papules, excoriations, lichenification, and periorbital erythema and edema are common.

C.   In the *adolescent and adult phase,* from the early teens to the early twenties, the lesions are primarily dry, lichenified, hyperpigmented plaques in flexor areas and about the eyes. Persistent hand dermatitis may be the only remnant of an atopic diathesis.

D.   These three phases may imperceptibly blend together, or any of the changes may be seen at any time.

Although atopic dermatitis may disappear with time, it is estimated that between 30 to 80 percent of atopic patients will continue to have intermittent episodes of exacerbation throughout life, often when under physical or emotional stress.

IV. ASSESSMENT

A. A detailed personal, family, environmental, and psychological history is mandatory for delivering proper care.

B. Factors that often trigger pruritus include the following: extreme heat or cold, rapid changes in temperature, sweating, irritating or occlusive medications or clothing (especially wool and silk), greases, oils, soaps and detergents, and, at times, an inhalant or other environmental allergens.

C. Concomitants of atopic dermatitis include pathologic changes in the eye (posterior cataract, keratoconus, and retinal detachment) and lowered resistance to viral infections—especially with herpes simplex and vaccinia viruses—resulting in dissemination of usually localized infections. Patients with atopic dermatitis should not be vaccinated nor be near family or friends who have had recent vaccinations or have active herpes simplex infections. If vaccination is mandatory, it should take place immediately after administering vaccinia immune globulin (0.3 ml/kg IM), or should utilize newer strains of vaccinia virus that reduce the risk of eczema vaccinatum.

V. THERAPY
The aims of therapy are to decrease trigger factors and pruritus, suppress inflammation, lubricate the skin, and alleviate anxiety.

A. Preventive measures

1. The environment should be kept at a constant temperature, and excess humidity should be avoided. Clothing worn next to the skin should be absorbent and nonirritating (cotton), laundered with bland soaps, and thoroughly rinsed. A vacation in a warm, dry climate is often beneficial. Adequate rest and relaxation are important.

2. Eliminate excessive bathing and other factors that promote xerosis. Keep the skin moist and supple (see Dry Skin, p. 76). Use a bland nonirritating soap or just a bath oil.

3. Scratch and intradermal allergy tests are not useful. Patch tests for contact allergies may be productive. A decrease in environmental allergens and trial elimination diets might be considered if the more usual therapeutic measures fail, but these measures are usually not helpful.

4. The patient's emotional stability is essential. Continued contact with an optimistic and reassuring physician will allay much anxiety. Occasionally, formal psychiatric therapy will be of benefit.

5. Short-term hospitalization is often efficacious, and improvement in the skin may appear before medications are applied. This complete but temporary environmental and emotional rearrangement will often suffice to break the itch-scratch cycle.

B. Treatment for active dermatitis

1. Exudative areas should be compressed with *Burow's solution*, 20 min 4–6id, or the patient placed in a tub with antipruritic and/or emollient additives such as oatmeal (Aveeno® or Oilated Aveeno®) or lubricating bath additives (see p. 330).

2. The primary and most important therapeutic tool in eczema is the frequent use of *topical corticosteroids*. They should be applied in small amounts, but frequently (3–6id) and with occlusion if this is tolerated (see p. 295). This will suppress inflammation and stop pruritus, thus interrupting the inflammation - itch - scratch - inflammation cycle. Treatment should be initiated with a fluorinated steroid in order to quickly quell inflammation and pruritus. If maintenance therapy is needed, 1% hydrocortisone or a low-strength fluorinated steroid are more appropriate. Ointments are better lubricants for dry skin and are often the base of choice for chronic lesions.

3. *Tar compounds* (Estar® gel; Zetar® emulsion or ointment; liquor carbonis detergens, 5–10% in hydrophilic ointment; or others [see p. 324]) are useful as adjunctive therapy in patients with chronic dermatitis. Their use may be alternated with the corticosteroids (i.e., tars overnight, corticosteroids during the day), or they may be applied at the same time to affected skin, or used in the bath.

4. *Antihistamines* PO will often suppress pruritus and allay anxiety and allow sleep. These drugs are particularly useful in treating infants and children with widespread or very pruritic disease. The dose administered should be gradually increased to an effective level (see p. 266). In acute cases

these drugs should be given on a continuous basis. Hydroxyzine is often the drug of choice.

5. Long-term administration of systemic corticosteroids plays no part in the therapy of atopic dermatitis. Acute flare-ups may be suppressed by a short-term course of prednisone (40–60 mg PO qd to 0 in 10–14 days) or one injection of 6 mg betamethasone sodium phosphate and betamethasone acetate suspension (Celestone®), or 40–80 mg of methylprednisolone (Depo-Medrol®), or 40 mg triamcinolone acetonide (Kenalog®), or triamcinolone diacetate (Aristocort®). Occasionally the dermatitis will flare up after cessation of steroids, but usually the eczematous disease will not reappear for months after one such course.

REFERENCES

Blaylock WK: Atopic dermatitis: diagnosis and pathobiology. J Allergy Clin Immunol 57:62–79, 1976

Copeman PWM, Banatvala JE: The skin and vaccination against smallpox. Br J Dermatol 84:169–173, 1971

Jones HE, Lewis CW, McMarlin SL: Allergic contact sensitivity in atopic dermatitis. Arch Dermatol 107:217–222, 1973

Jordon JM, Whitlock FA: Emotions and the skin: the conditioning of scratch responses in cases of atopic dermatitis. Br J Dermatol 86: 574–585, 1972

Karel I, Myška V, Kuicalová E: Ophthalmological changes in atopic dermatitis. Acta Derm Venereol (Stockh) 45:381–386, 1965

Lobitz WC: Atopic dermatitis. J Dermatol 3:39–44, 1976

Luckasen JR, Sabad A, Goltz RW, Kersey JH: T and B lymphocytes in atopic eczema. Arch Dermatol 110:375–377, 1974

Michaelsson G: Decreased phagocytic capacity of neutrophil leukocytes in patients with atopic dermatitis. Acta Derm Venereol (Stockh) 53:279–282, 1973

Parish WE, Champion RH: Atopic Dermatitis, In Recent Advances in Dermatology. Edited by A Rook. London, Churchill, 1973, pp 193–217

Roth HL, Kierland RR: The natural history of atopic dermatitis. A 20-year follow-up study. Arch Dermatol 89:209–214, 1964

Winkelmann RK: Nonallergic factors in atopic dermatitis. J Allergy 37: 29–37, 1966

CIRCUMSCRIBED NEURODERMATITIS
(Lichen Simplex Chronicus)

I. **DEFINITION AND PATHOPHYSIOLOGY** Circumscribed neurodermatitis (lichen simplex chronicus) is a localized, chronic pruritic disorder resulting from repeated scratching and rubbing. Patients with neurodermatitis often have other atopic manifestations (asthma, allergic rhinitis) and frequently have a positive personal and family history of atopic disorders. The original pruritogenic stimulus usually remains undefined; it could have been an insect bite, constricting clothing, contact or seborrheic dermatitis, or psoriasis. Once the itch-scratch-lichenification cycle is established, it makes little difference what initially incited the problem. Scratching in these patients seems to be a learned (conditioned) response, one which becomes a fixed pattern and has a relative specificity for certain areas of skin, all in areas easily accessible to the patient. Lichenified skin tends to be more itchy than normal skin following minor stimuli, thus leading to further scratching. It must be emphasized that the scratching of these lichenified areas is not always unpleasant—it is sometimes almost erotic—and this secondary gain may interfere with conscientious application of therapy by the patient. Scratching is often vigorously accomplished with the heels, nails, combs, or other implements. This repeated trauma to the skin results in an increased number of cells undergoing mitosis, an increased transepidermal transit time, and hyperplasia involving all components of the epidermis. Within nodular lesions there may also be thickened nerve fibers, Schwann cell proliferation, neuroma-schwannoma formation, and axon swelling.

II. SUBJECTIVE DATA   Continuous, spasmodic, or paroxysmal pruritus is the only symptom.

III. OBJECTIVE DATA   These well-circumscribed, lichenified plaques, at times with psoriasiform scaling, are located most frequently on the ankles and anterior tibial and nuchal areas. The inner thighs, sides of the neck, extensor surfaces of the forearms, and anogenital areas may also be affected. Dry keratotic papules and giant "scratch papules" or prurigo nodules are also a response to repeated scratching. Patients will usually have only one area of involvement.

IV. ASSESSMENT   Detailed questioning regarding the itch stimulus is worthwhile but often fruitless. Psychogenic factors are important. Secondary infection or sensitization to topical therapeutic agents is not uncommon.

V. THERAPY   In spite of the chronicity of these lesions, effective therapy will usually induce remission of the pruritus and the lichenification within 1–2 weeks.

A. **Fluorinated topical corticosteroids,** usually applied under occlusion, are extremely effective. Cordran® tape applied repeatedly for 24-hr periods is also a most useful modality.

B. **Intralesional injection** of corticosteroids will induce involution most rapidly and is often the therapy of choice (see p. 294).

C. **Antihistamines** or ataractic agents occasionally are of value.

D. **Emollients** containing antipruritic agents (menthol, phenol) or tar can also be useful (see p. 306).

REFERENCES

Feuerman EJ, Sandbank M: Prurigo nodularis: histological and electron microscopical study. Arch Dermatol 111:1472–1477, 1975

Marks R, Wells GC: Lichen simplex: morphodynamic correlates. Br J Dermatol 88:249–256, 1973

Robertson IM, Jordon JM, Whitlock FA: Emotions and skin. II. The conditioning of scratch responses in cases of lichen simplex. Br J Dermatol 92:407–412, 1975

Shaffer B, Beerman H: Lichen simplex chronicus and its variants. A discussion of certain psychodynamic mechanisms and clinical and histopathologic correlations. Arch Dermatol Syphilol 64:340–351, 1951

Singh G: Atopy in lichen simplex (neurodermatitis circumscripta). Br J Dermatol 89:625–627, 1973

CONTACT DERMATITIS

I. **DEFINITION AND PATHOPHYSIOLOGY** Contact dermatitis may be produced by primary irritants or allergic sensitizers. **Primary irritant contact dermatitis** is a nonallergic reaction of the skin caused by exposure to irritating substances. Any substance can act as an irritant provided the concentration and duration of contact are sufficient. Most primary irritants are chemical substances, although physical and biological (infectious) agents may produce the same picture. Irritants account for 80 percent of occupational contact dermatitis and also cause the most frequent type of nonindustrial contact reaction. The two types of irritants are: (a) mild, relative, or marginal irritants, which require repeated and/or prolonged contact to produce inflammation and include soaps, detergents, and most solvents; and (b) strong or absolute irritants, which are such damaging substances that they will injure skin immediately on contact (strong acids and alkalis). If daily exposure to mild irritants is continued, normal skin may become "hardened" or tolerant to this trauma, and contact may be continued without further evidence of irritation.

Allergic contact dermatitis is a manifestation of delayed hypersensitivity and results from the exposure of sensitized individuals to contact allergens. The sequence leading to inflammation is initiated by the binding of relatively simple chemical group(s) to an epidermal protein to form a complete antigen, which then reacts with sensitized T-lymphocytes independent of free antibody or complement (type 4 reaction). These lymphocytes then release mediators that evoke the eczematous changes. Most contact allergens produce sensitization in only a small percentage of those exposed. Poison oak and ivy, which induce sensitization in more than 70 percent of the population, are marked exceptions to this rule. The incubation period after initial sensitization to an antigen is 5–21 days, while the reaction time after subsequent reexposure is 12–48 hr. Mild exposure of a sensitized person to poison oak or ivy, for example, will result in appearance of the rash in 2–3 days and clearing within the following 1–2 weeks; with massive exposure, lesions will appear more quickly (6–12 hr) and heal more slowly (2–3 weeks). Factors that contribute to the development of contact dermatitis include genetic predisposition, local concentration of antigen, duration of exposure, site variation in cutaneous permeability, and the development of immune tolerance. Other contributing factors may be friction, pressure, occlusion, maceration, heat and cold, and the presence of other skin diseases.

II.   **SUBJECTIVE DATA**   Primary irritants will cause an inelastic and stiff-feeling skin, discomfort related to dryness, pruritus secondary to inflammation, and pain related to fissures, blisters, and ulcers. As with other forms of acute and chronic dermatitis, the primary symptom of allergic contact dermatitis is pruritus.

III.   **OBJECTIVE DATA** (See color insert.)

    A.   **Mild irritants** produce erythema, microvesiculation, and oozing that may be indistinguishable from allergic contact dermatitis. Chronic exposure to mild irritants or allergens results in dry, thickened, and fissured skin.

    B.   **Strong irritants** cause blistering, erosion, and ulcers.

C. **Mild allergic contact dermatitis** is similar in appearance to the irritant eruption. A more typical allergic contact reaction will consist of grouped or linear tense vesicles and blisters. If involvement is severe, there may be marked edema, particularly on the face, and periorbital and genital areas. The allergen is frequently transferred from hands to other areas of the body, where the rash then appears. Palms, soles, and scalp, however, are relatively resistant to contact reactions because of thicker stratum corneum and greater barrier function. The gradual appearance of the allergic contact eruption over a period of several days reflects the amount of antigen deposited on the skin and the reactivity of the individual site. Vesicle fluid, as in poison ivy, is a transudate and will not spread the eruption elsewhere on the body or to other people.

It is not the specific morphology of lesions that clinically distinguishes contact dermatitis from other types of eczema, but their distribution and configuration. The eruption is in exposed or contact areas and typically has a bizarre or artificial pattern, with sharp, straight margins, acute angles, and straight lines. Any eruption with such an unusual appearance should suggest contact dermatitis.

IV. **ASSESSMENT** Exact diagnosis is very important, since successful therapy depends on avoidance of contact with irritants and elimination of contact with allergens. The patient must be questioned about his total environment: home, work, hobbies, medications, clothing, cosmetics, and any other contactants. Inquiry must be detailed, imaginative, and frequently repetitive if the necessary details are to be elicited. Sensitization to components of topical medications is not uncommon and must be considered when an eruption is slow to disappear while being treated with what appears to be appropriate therapy.

Patch testing for contact allergens is essential for specific identification of causative agents (see p. 243). This test, in effect, attempts to reproduce the disease in diminutive form. There are no clinically useful methods available to evaluate patients thought to have an irritant dermatitis.

V. **THERAPY**

A. **Preventive measures—for primary irritant or hand dermatitis**

1. *Decrease exposure to household and work irritants* such as soaps, detergents, solvents, bleaches, ammonia, and moist vegetables such as onions or garlic.

2. *Avoid abrasive soaps.* Remove all rings that occlude the underlying skin before doing any work. Waterless hand cleansers will remove stubborn soils and greases without significant damage to the skin. (Use of solvents to cleanse the skin is one of the most frequent predisposing factors.)

3. *Lubricate the skin* frequently with a bland cream or lotion such as Eucerin® (see p. 77).

4. If possible, *wear heavy-duty vinyl gloves* or plastic gloves while working. Lined rubber gloves (Bluettes® or Playtex®) are acceptable, but occasionally patients become allergic to the rubber. Gloves provide excellent protection against mild irritants, but some antigens such as nickel may penetrate rubber-base gloves. High concentrations of irritants such as 10% potassium hydroxide will also penetrate. Gloves should be carefully chosen and frequently changed. Tru-Touch® plastic gloves are very helpful, for they permit freer use of the hands while working. Thin white cotton liners (Dermal® gloves) should be worn next to the skin to absorb sweat and prevent maceration.

5. *Barrier protective creams* designed to be used against aqueous compounds (Kerodex® No. 71, West® No. 311), solvents (Kerodex® No. 51, West® No. 411), or dusts (West® No. 211) will be moderately useful. They should be applied in the morning and then reapplied at lunchtime and at work breaks.

B. **Preventive measures—for allergic contact dermatitis**

1. Wash thoroughly as soon as possible after exposure to antigens.

2. The results of hyposensitization to allergic contact antigens such as poison oak and ivy are usually of negligible to mild benefit. It is rarely worth recommending this prolonged therapy as it is now constituted.

C. **Treatment for active dermatitis**

1. *Acute, mild to moderate, exudative, and vesicular*

   a. Burow's solution (diluted 1:20) cold compresses 20–30 min 4–6id.

  b.   Soothing shake lotions, e.g., calamine.

  c.   After vesiculation subsides, a topical corticosteroid aerosol, cream, or lotion will help.

  d.   Antihistamines PO.

2.   *Acute, absolute irritant*

  a.   Forceful and prolonged irrigation with water.

  b.   Then treat as for a burn (see p. 42).

3.   *Acute, severe, marked edema and bullae*

  a.   Topical therapy as in C-1-a.

  b.   Tepid tub baths with Aveeno®, 1 cup to ½ tub, 2–3 id, or cornstarch (see p. 333).

  c.   Early and aggressive treatment with systemic corticosteroids: Initial prednisone dosage should be at least 60 mg qd; the course should be no shorter than 2–3 weeks. ACTH gel 80 units q12h × 2, 6 mg betamethasone sodium phosphate and betamethasone acetate suspension (Celestone®), 40–80 mg methylprednisolone (Depo-Medrol®), 40 mg triamcinolone acetonide (Kenalog®), or 40 mg triamcinolone diacetate (Aristocort®) is equally effective. Treatment with inadequate amounts of steroid for inadequate periods of time is unfortunately too common. Systemic corticosteroids should be withdrawn gradually to prevent a flare-up or rebound reaction. If the process is suppressed for too short a time, a generalized exacerbation of rash and symptoms may result when steroids are stopped. Inhibition of the rash and symptoms will be seen within 48 hr after therapy is initiated. It is essential that secondary infection such as impetigo, cellulitis or erysipelas be diagnosed and treated before corticosteroid therapy is initiated. The clinical picture of erysipelas can at times be quite similar to that of an allergic contact dermatitis.

4.   *Chronic contact or hand dermatitis*

  a.   Soak the hands or other affected area for 5 min in water; then immediately apply a hydrophobic emollient (e.g., petrolatum) and/or topical corticosteroid *ointment* with or without occlusion.

b. High-potency fluorinated corticosteroids are needed in the treatment of chronic hand dermatitis (fluocinonide [Lidex®, Topsyn®]; 0.5% triamcinolone [Aristocort®]; 0.2% fluocinolone [Synalar® HP]).

Occasionally a preparation more concentrated than those commercially available is needed. A pharmacist can prepare 1% triamcinolone acetonide in propylene glycol by pouring off the liquid from a 5-ml vial of triamcinolone acetonide 40 mg/ml (Kenalog® 40 injection) and then dissolving the sediment in 25 ml propylene glycol.

c. Tar and/or iodochlorhydroxyquin preparations (see pp. 290, 324) are useful adjuncts in chronic cases.

5. Bacterial superinfection is not uncommon and should be treated with topical and systemic antibiotics.

REFERENCES

Adams RM: Occupational Contact Dermatitis. Philadelphia, Lippincott, 1969, 262 pp

Bettley FR: Management and treatment of contact eczema. Br Med J 2:1245–1246, 1966

Epstein W: Poison oak hyposensitization. Arch Dermatol 109:356–360, 1974

Fisher AA: Contact Dermatitis (2nd Edit). Philadelphia, Lea & Febiger, 1973

Fregert S: Manual of Contact Dermatitis. Copenhagen, Munksgaard (distributed by Year Book), 1974, 107 pp

Hjorth N, Wilkinson DW: Contact dermatitis. Br J Dermatol 88:103–104, 1973

Kligman AM: Poison ivy (Rhus) dermatitis. Arch Dermatol 77:149–180, 1958

Rostenberg A Jr: Primary irritant and allergic eczematous reactions. Their interrelations. Arch Dermatol 75:547–558, 1957

Sax NI: Dangerous Properties of Industrial Materials (3rd Edit). New York, Van Nostrand-Reinhold, 1968, 1250 pp

Suskind RR, Ishihara M: The effects of wetting on cutaneous vulnerability. Arch Environ Health 11:529–537, 1965

HAND DERMATITIS

I. **DEFINITION AND PATHOPHYSIOLOGY** Hand dermatitis is a common, chronic pruritic disorder that is perplexing and frustrating to patient and physician alike. The clinical changes are not specific and may be a manifestation of one or several precipitating or predisposing factors. It is most commonly a reaction to repeated contact with mild primary irritants such as soap and water, detergents, and solvents. The eruption itself is common in housewives, food handlers, bartenders, nurses, dentists, and surgeons. It is often called "housewife's eczema," "dishpan hands," and other colorful names, and it is the most frequent dermatitis seen in industry.

Chronic hand dermatitis is often a remnant or part of **atopic** or **nummular dermatitis.**

Allergic contact dermatitis will tend to involve the sides of the fingers and the dorsa of the hands more than the palms and show a more bizarre configuration.

Primary fungal infection or ID reactions to *Tinea pedis* must always be considered in the differential diagnosis, and fungal scrapings and cultures obtained.

Dyshidrosiform eruptions involve the sides of fingers and palms preferentially and may also affect the soles of the feet as well. Hyperhidrosis may be seen in such patients, but no abnormality of sweating or of the eccrine apparatus is present.

Pustular psoriasis and hand involvement with other cutaneous eruptions, such as drug reactions, may also present as a hand dermatitis.

It is often impossible to find a specific etiology for chronic hand dermatitis.

II. **SUBJECTIVE DATA** Pruritus is the primary symptom, but dryness, fissuring, inelasticity, and superinfection often lead to inability to use the hands at all. Hand dermatitis is the cause of much social, personal, and financial grief.

III. **OBJECTIVE DATA**

A. Erythema, dryness, and chapping are the mildest changes.

B. The most characteristic lesions are myriads of small "bubbles" —intraepidermal spongiotic vesicles—scattered on the sides of the fingers and, less often, throughout the palms.

C. More severe changes include bulla formation and extreme hardening and inelasticity of the skin, with deep fissures.

D. Hyperhidrosis and secondary bacterial infections are common.

IV. **ASSESSMENT**   A detailed history and physical examination must include inquiry about a personal or family history of atopy or psoriasis or other cutaneous disease; factors that precipitate and alleviate the dermatitis; and occupational, household, and hobby contactants. Patch testing, using a screening tray as well as properly diluted occupational or other agents that the patient has supplied, may identify a causative agent.

V. **THERAPY**   See Contact Dermatitis, p. 59.

REFERENCES

Epstein E: Therapy of recalcitrant hand dermatitis. Cutis 15:346–376, 1975

Jordan WP: Allergic contact dermatitis in hand eczema. Arch Dermatol 110:567–569, 1974

Shelley WB: Dyshidrosis (pompholyx). Arch Dermatol Syphilogr (Paris) 68:314–319, 1953

Simons RDGPh: Eczema of the Hands. In Investigation into Dyshidrosiform Eruptions. St Louis, WH Green, 1966

NUMMULAR DERMATITIS

I. **DEFINITION AND PATHOPHYSIOLOGY**   Nummular dermatitis, characterized by coin-shaped eczematous plaques, is a chronic, often very pruritic, but nonspecific reaction pattern found most commonly in older patients. It may also be a manifestation of atopic dermatitis in children, a reaction to topical irritants, or a manifestation of xerosis, particularly in wintertime. IgE levels are usually not elevated. Emotional stress has been emphasized as a contributing factor. The course tends to be chronic, with remission occurring frequently during the summer.

II. **SUBJECTIVE DATA**   Pruritus is the primary symptom.

III. **OBJECTIVE DATA**   Dry to inflammatory papular, vesicular, exudative and/or crusted, round plaques 1–5 cm in diameter are located most commonly on the dorsa of the hands and forearms, lower legs, and buttocks.

IV. ASSESSMENT Questioning should be directed toward eliciting a history of predisposing environmental factors (i.e., dryness), occupational or household work habits, other cutaneous diseases, and any recent or chronic emotionally stressful situation.

V. THERAPY

A. Decrease exposure to irritants. If dryness is a factor, see the items outlined under Dry Skin, p. 76. Decrease amount of bathing and add bath oils and emollients.

B. For acute dermatitis, Burow's solution compresses 20 min 3id, followed by:

C. Topical corticosteroids 4–6id. Ointments are often preferable. Overnight application under occlusion is very effective.

D. Intralesional corticosteroid injection will rapidly eliminate lesions.

E. Tar compounds (Estar®; 10% liquor carbons detergens in hydrophilic ointment) and iodochlorhydroxyquin are occasionally useful. Daily application of topical corticosteroids and nightly use of the tar compounds and/or iodochlorhydroxyquin may work when either medication used alone is not wholly effective.

F. Antihistamines, particularly hydroxyzine (Atarax®, Vistaril®), will diminish itch and anxiety.

REFERENCES

Cowan MA: "Nummular eczema." A review, follow-up and analysis of 325 cases. Acta Derm Venereol (Stockh) 41:453–460, 1961

Hellgren L, Mobacken H: Nummular eczema—clinical and statistical data. Acta Derm Venereol (Stockh) 49:189–196, 1969

Krueger GG, Kahn G, Weston WL, Mandel MJ: IgE levels in nummular eczema and ichthyosis. Arch Dermatol 107:56–58, 1975

Weidman AI, Sawicky HH: Nummular eczema. Review of the literature: survey of 516 case records and follow-up of 125 patients. Arch Dermatol 73:58–65, 1956

9
Diaper Rash

I. **DEFINITION AND PATHOPHYSIOLOGY** Diaper rash is the end result of constant exposure to an adverse local environment. Multiple factors may initiate or aggravate this eruption but the most important is overhydration. Other factors include: constant dampness, irritant chemicals, intestinal enzymes, and stool; and contact reactions to rubber, plastic, diaper detergents, and disinfectants. Diarrhea, high environmental heat and humidity, infrequent change of diapers, inadequate skin cleansing, and occlusive, impermeable diapers also contribute to this primary irritant contact dermatitis. Once established, diaper dermatitis is colonized by many organisms (*Proteus, Pseudomonas, Streptococcus faecalis, Candida*) that induce secondary changes. Diaper rash is unusual during the first month of life and most common between the second and fourth months, but may continue until diapers are no longer needed. Underlying atopic, seborrheic, or psoriatic diathesis may predispose to this eruption.

II. **SUBJECTIVE DATA** The baby feels itchy and uncomfortable and is irritable.

III. OBJECTIVE DATA

A. The usual mild diaper rash is a primary irritant reaction and appears as simple erythema. The eruption is located over the convex contact areas, i.e., buttocks, genitalia, lower abdomen, and upper thighs, sparing the flexural folds. Legs and heels may be affected from contact with the wet diaper.

B. With more intense involvement there will be erythematous papules, vesicles or erosions, oozing, and ulceration.

C. An erosive and crusted urethral meatitis is often seen in males, and spots of blood may appear on the diaper.

D. A chronic eruption, or one that is slowly healing, appears as a glazed erythema.

E. Erythematous papules and pustules scattered within and outside the eruption suggest *Candida albicans* superinfection.

F. The explosive, widespread appearance of psoriasiform scaling papules and plaques, usually preceded by inflammation in the diaper area (or scalp), is not uncommon. These infants often have a family history of psoriasis and up to 25 percent later develop true psoriasis.

IV. ASSESSMENT

A. A detailed history concerning skin and diaper care is necessary to discover the immediate predisposing factors.

B. The entire child should be inspected to see if there is any evidence of infantile eczema or other skin disease.

C. Erosive lesions must be differentiated from congenital syphilis.

D. Pustule contents should be examined by gram stain and/or fungal stain and cultured on blood agar plates and/or fungal media for bacterial pathogens or *C. albicans*. Gram-negative rods may play a collaborative role with *C. albicans* in pustular eruptions; this is important to remember both in assessing the lesions and choosing therapeutic agents.

V. THERAPY

A. Preventive The primary aim of long-term management of diaper dermatitis is prevention. A number of measures must be kept in mind:

1. The area must be kept free of irritants and as dry as possible. This entails frequent diaper changes. Excessively bulky or multilayered diapers should not be used.

2. Cleanse the diaper area after each change with tepid to warm water, or with pledgets soaked in baby oil, mineral oil, Balneol® lotion, or Cetaphil® lotion. Avoid excessive use of soaps and water. Disposable paper diapers are useful.

3. Talcum or baby powder (not cornstarch, which may be metabolized by microorganisms) or a bland protective ointment (Desitin®, Diaparene®) or adherent paste (1 part Burow's solution, 2 parts Aquaphor®, 3 parts zinc oxide ointment) may prevent maceration and irritation.

4. Discontinue use of occlusive pants.

5. Try to keep the baby's room from becoming excessively hot and humid.

6. Thorough rinsing of diapers is necessary to reduce the alkalinity imparted by soap and detergent residues. A final rinse in dilute acetic acid (30 ml [1 oz] vinegar to 1 gallon water) will help.

B. Treatment of a preexisting inflammatory eruption

1. If mild, apply a topical corticosteroid, such as 1% hydrocortisone cream. This can be followed by application of zinc oxide ointment, adherent paste (as in A-3) or petrolatum, both of which may increase steroid penetration and keep the steroid from being washed off by urine.

2. If *C. albicans* infection is present, add an antiyeast agent to the steroid (1% hydrocortisone–3% iodochlorhydroxyquin [Vioform®-Hydrocortisone]; triamcinolone-neomycin-gramicidin-nystatin [Mycolog®]; corticosteroid cream plus antiyeast agent such as clotrimazole [Lotrimin®], or nystatin [Nilstat®, Mycostatin®]). An antiyeast medication may be used alone but the inflammation will subside very slowly. Take care to use the lowest potency corticosteroid cream that is effective, and for the shortest time possible. Nystatin powder is a convenient medication both for treating yeast infection and for decreasing maceration and friction. Oral nystatin suspension (1 ml [100,000 units] 4id)

should be given to infants with severe or recurrent eruptions.

3. Psoriasiform generalized lesions respond slowly (weeks to months) to topical corticosteroids and emollients. It is imperative to also treat any inflammatory lesions in the diaper area.

4. Local bacterial infection should be treated with an antibiotic or steroid-antibiotic cream: gentamicin (Garamycin®) cream, polymyxin B-neosporin-gramicidin (Neosporin-G®) cream, triamcinolone-neomycin-gramicidin-nystatin (Mycolog®) cream.

5. If more severe inflammation or vesiculation and oozing are present, Burow's solution compresses should also be used, 20 min 3id. Avoid greasy occlusive medications at this stage.

6. For urethral meatitis, remove crusts with water, saline, or Burow's compresses and apply topical antibiotic ointment.

REFERENCES

Andersen SL, Thomsen K: Psoriasiform napkin dermatitis. Br J Dermatol 84:316–319, 1971

Burgoon CF Jr, Urbach F, Grover WD: Diaper dermatitis. Pediatr Clin North Am 8:835–856, 1961

Dixon PN, Warin RP, English MP: Alimentary *Candida albicans* and napkin rashes. Br J Dermatol 86:458–462, 1972

Koblenzer PJ: Diaper dermatitis—an overview with emphasis on rational therapy based on etiology and pathogenesis. Clin Pediatr (Phila) 12:386–392, 1973

Neville E, Finn O: Psoriasiform napkin dermatitis—a follow-up study. Br J Dermatol 92:279–285, 1975

10
Drug Eruptions, Allergic

I. **DEFINITION AND PATHOPHYSIOLOGY** Drug reactions may take numerous forms. The commonest of these are hypersensitivity reactions, most frequently caused by mediators released after exposure to sensitizing molecules.

    A. **Immediate allergic reactions** occur within 1 hr and consist of pruritus, urticaria, flushing, or other manifestations of anaphylaxis.

    B. **Accelerated reactions** take place within 1–72 hr of drug administration and also consist primarily of itching and hives, but laryngeal edema may also be seen.

    C. **Late reactions** start more than 3 days after initiation of drug therapy and may be urticarial, serum-sickness-like, or exanthematous. In addition, drug reactions may be manifested as fever or as abnormal reactions of one or many organ systems (e.g., hemolysis, thrombocytopenia, renal damage).

D. **Exanthematous eruptions,** the most common type of reaction, usually appear within 1 week after the causative drug has been started; sensitization may occur after the first exposure or may develop to an antigen to which the patient has been intermittently exposed for years. Rash may also start within 4–7 days after the offending drug has been stopped. Whenever the eruption starts, whether it is while the patient is taking the drug or after its discontinuation, the cutaneous lesions will become more severe and widespread over the following several days to a week and then will clear over the following 7–14 days. This slow and constant evolution of the eruption makes it difficult to single out the offending agent from among numerous drugs, and whether or not the correct one has been stopped, the rash will go through its 2–3-week course.

II. **SUBJECTIVE DATA**   Mild to severe pruritus is the predominant symptom of late exanthematous eruptions.

III. **OBJECTIVE DATA**

A. The typical exanthematous eruption will begin as faint pink macules, which gradually enlarge to bright red macular areas or edematous plaques.

B. At times there is mild central clearing within an erythematous plaque.

C. The eruption may mimic the pinpoint redness of scarlet fever, the blotchy pattern of measles, or the generalized distribution of a viral exanthem.

D. Lesions most often start first and clear first from the head and upper extremities to the trunk and lower legs.

E. Palms, soles, and mucous membranes may be involved.

F. Mild petechiae or frank purpura on the lower extremities are commonly associated with a vigorous eruption, but this does not mean that vasculitis or thrombocytopenia is present.

G. More serious and violent reactions may include bullae, erosions, extensive purpura, or exfoliation.

H. Many types of drugs can produce the identical eruption; the morphology of the rash usually gives no clue as to the causative agent.

IV. ASSESSMENT Questioning about offending drugs must be detailed and direct. Any substance that enters any body orifice, with the exception of most foods and water, is suspect. Specific questioning concerning eye or ear drops, nasal sprays, suppositories, injections, immunization, nerve pills, vitamins, laxatives, sedatives, and analgesics, even including aspirin, must be pursued. Nonmedical items such as preservatives, tonics, toothpaste, and topical lotions must also be considered. Penicillin is present in small amounts in some biologic products (such as poliomyelitis vaccine) and in dairy products from cows treated for mastitis.

Penicillin drugs, sulfonamides, and blood products are the most common causes of cutaneous reactions to drugs. Ampicillin, for instance, can be expected to incite an eruption in approximately 5 percent of courses of drug therapy. Drug-specific quantitative data are now available to help evaluate which agents are the most likely causes of drug-induced rash, itching, or hives. This information gives reaction rates for all commonly used drugs and allows one to calculate which drug might (as well as might not) have caused an adverse reaction (see Arndt and Jick 1976).

Skin testing with penicilloyl-polylysine (PPL: Pre-Pen®) and a "minor determinant mixture" (usually diluted aqueous penicillin G) can accurately predict reactions to all penicillins. No other in vivo or in vitro tests are currently available or routinely used for ascertaining the cause of a drug eruption or screening potentially allergic individuals.

Table 1. Drugs with Reaction Rates > 1%

Drug	Reaction Rate (Reactions/1000 recipients)
Trimethoprim-sulfamethoxazole	59
Ampicillin	52
Semisynthetic penicillins	36
Whole blood	35
Corticotropin	28
Blood platelets	28
Erythromycin	23
Sulfisoxazole	17
Penicillin G	16
Gentamicin sulfate	16
Cephalosporins	13
Quinidine	12
Plasma protein fraction	12

FROM: Arndt and Jick 1976

V. THERAPY

A. Antihistamines PO.

B. Soothing tepid water baths with Aveeno® or cornstarch and/or cool compresses may be useful.

C. A drying antipruritic lotion (calamine with or without 0.25% menthol and/or 1% phenol) or lubricating antipruritic emollients (Eucerin® or Keri® lotion with 0.25% menthol and 1% phenol) applied prn will help relieve the pruritis.

D. If signs and symptoms are severe, a 2-week course of systemic corticosteroids (prednisone, starting at 60 mg) or injection of a repository corticosteroid preparation (see Contact Dermatitis, p. 61) will usually stop the symptoms and prevent further progression of the eruption within 48 hr of the onset of therapy.

REFERENCES

Arndt KA, Jick H: Rates of cutaneous reactions to drugs. JAMA 235: 918–923, 1976

Bruinsma W: A Guide to Drug Eruptions. Amsterdam, Excerpta Medica, 1973, 103 pp

Cluff LE, Caranasos GJ, Stewart RB: Clinical Problems with Drugs. Philadelphia, Saunders, 1975, pp 80–96

Demis JD: Allergy and drug sensitivity of skin. Annu Rev Pharmacol 9:457–482, 1969

Felix RH, Comaish JS: Value of patch and other skin tests in drug eruptions. Lancet 1:1017–1019, 1974

Levine BB: Immunochemical mechanisms of drug allergy. Annu Rev Med 17:23–38, 1966

Miller RR, Greenblatt DJ (Eds): Drug Effects in Hospitalized Patients. New York, Wiley, 1976, 346 pp

11
Dry Skin (Chapping, Xerosis) and Ichthyosis Vulgaris

I. **DEFINITION AND PATHOPHYSIOLOGY** Dry skin and ichthyosis vulgaris are often indistinguishable, and since the clinical findings blend together it is useful to discuss the two entities together. Dry skin, a dehydration of the stratum corneum, is a very common condition especially prevalent among the elderly. It is also found to be associated with diverse other developmental and acquired cutaneous conditions such as ichthyosis and atopic and contact dermatitis. When it is severe enough to be associated with inflammation and pruritus, it has also been termed *asteatotic eczema* and *winter itch.* The sequence leading to dry skin varies considerably from person to person and in many cases remains obscure. Some individuals will have always noticed a familial tendency to excessive dryness and chapping. Others will state that this problem appeared only with increasing age or illness and has tended to be seasonal.

Environmental factors are extremely important: repeated exposure to solvents, soaps, and disinfectants will remove lipid from the skin, thus damaging the cutaneous barrier and increasing water loss up to 75 times normal; decreasing relative humidity and exposure to dry, cold winds will lead to water loss from the stratum corneum and will literally "pull" water from the skin. Factors that act to decrease relative humidity include increasing room heat and ventilating with cold, dry, winter air, which holds little moisture when cool and thus becomes drier when warmed inside the house.

The typical patient is an elderly person who comes in with localized or generalized pruritus and dryness of the lower legs. These symptoms will have started in early winter soon after the heat went on. The relative humidity of his apartment decreased, and outdoors he began to be exposed to cold, dry winds. Rubbing and scratching caused increased irritation, thus leading to more pruritus and inflammation. If untreated, the symptoms would spontaneously subside the following spring.

Ichthyosis vulgaris is a dominantly inherited disorder of keratinization that is estimated to occur in 1:100 individuals. Skin changes, usually not present at birth, may be noted from early infancy to the teens; dry skin and prominant keratotic follicles are usually present by ages 5–10. Those with ichthyosis vulgaris also have a high incidence of atopic diseases (atopic dermatitis, rhinitis, asthma) and keratosis pilaris.

II. **SUBJECTIVE DATA**   Lesions are usually asymptomatic. If symptoms are present, the presenting complaint is always pruritus, at times severe.

III. **OBJECTIVE DATA**

   A. **Dry skin** covered with a fine scale is seen most often on the anterior tibial areas, dorsa of the hands, and on the forearms. The distribution may be both diffuse and in round patches. With more severe involvement the skin loses its suppleness, cracks, and becomes fissured. The superficial reticulated cracking takes on an uneven diamond pattern similar to cracked porcelain and erythema appears in and around involved areas (eczema or erythema craquelé). Nummular plaques of eczema also may be present.

   B. In **ichthyosis vulgaris** scaling is most prominent over the extensor aspects of the extremities. Flexural areas are spared. Milder forms appear as dryness present only during winter months. More severe lesions, particularly those seen on the lower legs in winter, may resemble the "fish skin" from which the term ichthyosis is derived. Follicular accentuation (keratosis pilaris) may be prominent over arms, thighs, and buttocks. The palms and soles have accentuation of the dermatoglyphic lines and appear to be wrinkled.

IV. **ASSESSMENT**   A detailed family history and history of the home and work environment are needed, both to help make an educated etiologic diagnosis and to outline a therapeutic program that will eliminate or counteract any causative factors. Hypothyroidism may be associated with xerosis, and this possibility should be investigated.

V. **THERAPY**   Skin is dry not because it lacks grease or skin oils, but because it lacks water. All therapeutic efforts are aimed at replacing the water in the skin and in the immediate environment.

A. **Preventive**

1. Room temperature should be kept as low as is consistent with comfort.

2. The use of humidifiers is to be encouraged. These may be either portable or installed in the ducts of forced-air heating systems. However, unless the house is relatively airtight with proper insulation, the moisture will either disperse rapidly to the outside or be caught within the walls and cause eventual damage to the house or paint.

3. Bathing should not be excessive (once every 1–2 days), and the bath water should be warm but not hot. Bath oils may be added (Alpha-Keri®, Domol®, Lubath®, or others [see p. 333]). These will, however, make the bathtub slippery and difficult to clean. An alternative instruction to the patient is to add 1 teaspoon of bath oil to ¼ cup warm water and to use the mixture as a rubdown either after the bath or as a substitute for a bath.

4. Excessive exposure to soap and water, solvents, or other drying compounds should be eliminated. It is the very mild irritants, often used casually and without thinking, that cause most of the trouble. Mechanical trauma from rough (often wool) or constricting clothing must be avoided.

5. Frequent use of emollients should be encouraged. The lubricating agents may range from lotions (Keri®, Lubriderm®) and creams (Keri®, Nivea®) to thicker preparations (Aquaphor®, Eucerin®, hydrated petrolatum, petrolatum [see

p. 314]). They are best applied when the skin is moist. Many elderly patients seem to tolerate petrolatum better than some of the more elegant preparations.

6. The patient should consider moving to a subtropical environment, especially for the winter.

B. Treatment of preexisting dryness

1. The primary means of correcting dryness is first to add water to the skin and then apply a hydrophobic substance to keep it there. In vitro, the stratum corneum can absorb as much as five to six times its own weight and increase its volume threefold when soaked in water. In vivo, this is accomplished by either soaking the affected area or bathing for 5–10 min and then immediately applying water-in-oil or fatty hydrophobic medications (Aquaphor®, Eucerin®, lanolin, petrolatum). Use of the latter ointments alone is only moderately effective; they would then hydrate the skin simply by preventing the normal transepidermal water loss.

2. Topical corticosteroid ointments used with occlusive dressings are the most effective and rapid therapy for symptomatic xerosis with associated eczematous changes.

3. Maximum hydration can be accomplished by the use of 40–60% propylene glycol in water applied under plastic occlusion overnight. If 6% salicylic acid is added to this formula (Keralyt® gel), an extremely effective keratolytic and hydrating gel is formed. Used overnight once or twice weekly initially and then only as often as needed thereafter, this product is the therapy of choice for the dry, scaly skin of ichthyosis vulgaris.

4. Urea-containing creams (Aquacare® [2% urea], Aquacare/HP® [10% urea], Calmurid® [10% urea], Carmol® [20% urea]) and those containing lactic acid (LactiCare®, Purpose® Dry Skin Cream) are claimed to produce good hydration and help remove scales and crusts.

REFERENCES

Anderson RL, Cassidy JM, Hansen JR, Yellin W: The effect of in vivo occlusion on human stratum corneum hydration-dehydration in vitro. J Invest Dermatol 61:375–379, 1973

Baden HP, Alper JC: A keratolytic gel containing salicylic acid in propylene glycol. J Invest Dermatol 61:330–333, 1973

Baden HP, Goldsmith LA: Current advances in the treatment of ichthyosis. Prog Dermatol 6:7–9, 1972

Blank IH: Action of emollient creams and their additives. JAMA 164: 412–415, 1959

Chernosky ME: Dry skin and its consequences. J Am Med Wom Assoc 27:133–135, 1972

Frost P: Ichthyosiform dermatoses. J Invest Dermatol 60:541–552, 1973

Middleton JO: The effects of temperature on extensibility of isolated corneum and its relation to skin chapping. Br J Dermatol 81:717–721, 1969

Warin AP: Eczema craquelé as the presenting feature of myxoedema. Br J Dermatol 89:289–291, 1973

12
Erythema Multiforme

I. **DEFINITION AND PATHOPHYSIOLOGY** Erythema multiforme is a reaction pattern of the skin that is characterized histologically first by a lymphohistiocytic infiltrate at the dermal-epidermal interface and later by subepidermal vesiculation and clinically by a variety of lesions, including the characteristic iris or target lesion. It is thought to be a hypersensitivity syndrome, but the exact immunologic mechanisms involved have not been identified. This acute, self-limited, frequently recurrent disorder occurs most commonly in winter and early spring in children and young adults.

Multiple precipitating factors have been found, including infections, drugs, endocrine changes, and underlying malignancy. Herpes simplex infections are the most frequent antecedent infectious cause, although many other viral, bacterial, and mycobacterial agents also have been implicated. Penicillin, barbiturates, sulfonamides, and many other drugs may initiate the same picture. In about 50 percent of cases, no provocative factor can be identified.

The mild form of erythema multiforme heals spontaneously in 2–3 weeks; the severe form, with widespread mucosal involvement, referred to by many as the Stevens-Johnson syndrome, may last 6–8 weeks and is a life-threatening disease.

II. SUBJECTIVE DATA   Mild prodromal symptoms of malaise and sore throat often precede the eruption, and drugs given for these symptoms are often inadvertently blamed for the erythema multiforme. Individual lesions may sting or burn, and large bullae may be painful. In severely ill patients there is high fever, malaise, and severe pain in mucosal areas with secondary photophobia and inability to ingest food or fluids.

III. OBJECTIVE DATA (See color insert.)

A. In the mild and typical case the patient will usually have lesions distributed symmetrically on extensor surfaces, distal limbs, palms and soles, and face and oral mucous membranes. Bright red-purple annular, macular, and papular areas and some urticarial-type lesions may be seen. The iris or target lesion is seen most often on the hands and consists of a central vesicle or livid erythema surrounded by a concentric pale and then red ring. Iris lesions need not be present in order to make a diagnosis of erythema multiforme. At times only mucous membrane lesions may be present.

B. With severe erythema multiforme there are usually generalized lesions (with and without bullae or hemorrhage) with severe involvement of ocular, oral, and other mucous membranes. A copious and often purulent discharge from the eyes and mouth may be present.

C. There are many variations in morphology and extent of the eruption.

IV. ASSESSMENT

A. **Workup**   Antecedent infection, drug administration, or illness for up to 3 weeks prior to the rash should be detailed. For a complete workup the following should be considered.

  1. Cultures for streptococci, *Mycoplasma*, and deep fungi (e.g., histoplasmosis, coccidioidomycosis).

  2. Serologic studies for Australian antigen, hepatitis, histoplasmosis, mononucleosis, *Mycoplasma* infection.

  3. Skin tests, chest film (to rule out *Mycoplasma* pneumonia, deep fungal infection, or tuberculosis).

4. Skin biopsy will demonstrate a characteristic histopatho-logic picture. This is worthwhile obtaining, particularly when the clinical presentation is not typical.

5. Has the patient been vaccinated recently, had a "cold sore," had x-ray therapy for a tumor? Is she pregnant or has she been taking birth control pills? The causes of erythema multiforme are so numerous that they cannot all be listed here, and the direct cause may escape detection.

B. **Differential diagnosis** includes: (1) other vascular reaction pattern diseases (urticaria, erythema nodosum, vasculitis); (2) blistering eruptions (pemphigus, bullous pemphigoid, toxic epidermal necrolysis); (3) mucocutaneous syndromes (Behçet's syndrome, hand-foot-and-mouth disease, acute herpetic gingivostomatitis); and (4) drug reactions.

V. THERAPY

A. Mild involvement

1. Antihistamines PO.

2. Antibiotics (tetracycline or erythromycin, 1 gm qd) if there is suspected *Mycoplasma* infection.

3. Open wet compresses for bullous or erosive lesions (see p. 330).

4. Mouth care:

   a. Hydrogen peroxide (3%) mouthwash for cleanliness 2–5id.

   b. Dyclone® solution applied directly to the lesions for pain prn.

   c. Chloroseptic® mouthwash may be utilized for both purposes as needed 3id.

5. Bland foods are preferable.

6. Analgesics (aspirin, 600 mg q4h).

B. Severe involvement

1. Immediate hospitalization and institution of intravenous fluid administration.

2. Prednisone PO or prednisolone IM 80–120 mg qd should be given until the disease responds, then tapered off over 2–3 weeks.

3. Local care as is previously described for mild involvement; bullae may be drained, but the blister roof is left intact.

REFERENCES

Ackerman AB, Pennys NS, Clark WH: Erythema multiforme exudativum: distinctive pathological process. Br J Dermatol 84:554–566, 1971

Bianchine JR, Macaraeg PUJ, Lasagna L, Azarnoff DL, Brunk SF, Hvidberg EF, Owen JA: Drugs as etiologic factors in the Stevens-Johnson syndrome. Am J Med 44:390–405, 1968

Leading article: Erythema multiforme. Br Med J 1:63–64, 1972

Lyell A: Erythema multiforme. Manifestations and management. Curr Med Drugs 8:3–14, 1968

Lyell A, Gordon A, Dick HM, Somerville RG: Mycoplasmas and erythema multiforme. Lancet 2:1116–1118, 1967

Orfanos LE, Schaumburg-Lever G, Lever W: Dermal and epidermal types of erythema multiforme. A histopathologic study of 24 cases. Arch Dermatol 109:682–688, 1974

Shelley WB: Herpes simplex virus as a cause of erythema multiforme. JAMA 201:153–156, 1967

13
Erythema Nodosum

I. **DEFINITION AND PATHOPHYSIOLOGY** Erythema nodosum, a cutaneous reaction pattern, consists of tender red nodules on the legs and occasionally elsewhere. It represents a hypersensitivity response, involving immune complex formation, to any of numerous factors. Erythema nodosum appears most commonly in young women, but may be seen in patients of any age. It indicates a need for an investigation of underlying precipitating disorders and should not be viewed as a disease in itself.

The most common cause of erythema nodosum in the United States is a preceding streptococcal infection. Reactions to medications, particularly sulfonamides and birth control pills, and concurrent sarcoidosis are also frequent causes. Other etiologic considerations should include primary infection tuberculosis, viral and deep fungal infections (coccidioidomycosis, histoplasmosis), and inflammatory bowel diseases (ulcerative colitis, regional enteritis).

Erythema nodosum usually will subside spontaneously in 3–6 weeks, temporarily leaving an area resembling a deep bruise.

II. **SUBJECTIVE DATA**   A 1–2-week period of malaise and arthralgias with or without fever may precede the outbreak of lesions. The overriding characteristic of these nodose lesions is their exquisite sensitivity, so severe that even contact with bed clothing or sheets may be intolerable.

III. **OBJECTIVE DATA (See color insert.)**   Single to numerous, bright red, hot, oval or round, slightly raised nodules, several centimeters in diameter, with diffuse borders and surrounding edema, are seen distributed unilaterally or bilaterally, although not necessarily symmetrically, on the pretibial surfaces. Other sites may include the thighs, arms, face, and neck. The extent of the lesions is easier to determine by palpation than by inspection. After 1–2 weeks the redness will become blue and then yellow-green as the nodules subside. Mild scaling will be seen as the lesions heal. Ulceration or scarring is never a part of the syndrome.

IV. **ASSESSMENT**

   A. Workup

   1. A detailed history concerning travel, present illness, and drug administration.

   2. A thorough physical examination.

   3. Laboratory studies should include a CBC, ESR, urinalysis, chest film, throat culture, antistreptolysin-O (ASLO) titer, and TB and deep fungal skin tests.

   B. Differential diagnosis   Other entities that may resemble the nodose lesions of erythema nodosum include erythema induratum, superficial thrombophlebitis, Weber-Christian disease, fungal granuloma, bite reactions, or fat necrosis produced by lipolytic enzymes liberated in acute or chronic pancreatic disease.

   C. Histopathology   Biopsy of erythema nodosum will reveal a lobular panniculitis. Although a specific histologic diagnosis may not be possible in all instances, many of the foregoing conditions have consistent clinicopathologic patterns. An adequate deep incisional biopsy should be considered part of a thorough investigation. Punch biopsies frequently provide insufficient information to make a diagnosis and should be avoided.

V. **THERAPY**

   A. Treat the underlying disease as indicated.

B. Bed rest with elevation of the patient's legs will gradually reduce pain and edema. A bed cradle will keep sheets and blankets from direct skin contact.

C. Analgesics (aspirin, 600 mg q4h)

D. Very symptomatic patients may be treated with potassium iodide 360–900 mg (or saturated solution of potassium iodide 0.36–0.90 ml [6–15 drops] in fruit juice) daily for 3–4 weeks. Decrease in pain and swelling should occur within 2 days and complete resolution within 2 weeks. Early cessation of therapy may result in relapse.

E. In chronic or recurrent cases unresponsive to these treatments, there is often a therapeutic dilemma. The most detailed investigation may not uncover the cause in the majority of cases, and yet some patients may be disabled, in pain, and unable to work. In such instances, the injection of small amounts of a corticosteroid suspension into the middle of each nodule will cause involution of the lesion within 48–72 hr. A 1–2-week course of oral corticosteroids is also effective; the possibility of an underlying primary tuberculous infection must never be overlooked.

REFERENCES

Blomgren SE: Conditions associated with erythema nodosum. NY State J Med 72:2302–2304, 1972

Editorial: "Nodules-on-the-leg" syndrome. N Engl J Med 274:463–464, 1966

Fine RM, Meltzer HD: Chronic erythema nodosum. Arch Dermatol 100: 33–38, 1969

Gordon H: Erythema nodosum: a review of 115 cases. Br J Dermatol 73: 393–409, 1969

Hughes PSH, Apisarnthanarax P, Mullins JF: Subcutaneous fat necrosis associated with pancreatic disease. Arch Dermatol 111:506–510, 1975

Medeiros AA, Marty SD, Tosh FE, Chin TD: Erythema nodosum and erythema multiforme as clinical manifestations of histoplasmosis in a community outbreak. N Engl J Med 274:415–420, 1966

Schulz EF, Whiting DA: Treatment of erythema nodosum and nodular vasculitis with potassium iodide. Br J Dermatol 94:75–78, 1976

Weinstein L: Erythema nodosum. DM, June 1969, 30 pp

Winkelmann RK, Forstrom L: New observations on the histopathology of erythema nodosum. J Invest Dermatol 65:441–446, 1975

14
Fungal Infections

CANDIDIASIS

I. **DEFINITION AND PATHOPHYSIOLOGY** The yeastlike fungus *Candida albicans* can normally be found on mucous membranes, skin, in the gastrointestinal tract, and in the vaginal vault. It can, under certain circumstances, change from a commensal organism to a pathogen and cause localized or generalized mucocutaneous disease.

Factors that predispose to infection include: (a) a local environment of moisture, warmth, maceration, and/or occlusion; (b) the systemic administration of antibiotics, corticosteroids, or birth control pills; (c) pregnancy; (d) diabetes; (e) Cushing's disease; and (f) debilitated states. Further, the normally circulating serum anticandidal components are reduced in infants up to 6 months of age and in patients with certain neoplastic diseases of the blood and reticuloendothelial systems, resulting in an increased incidence of *Candida* infections. The resident bacteria on skin, mainly cocci, presumably inhibit proliferation of *C. albicans*; it is often difficult to establish experimental *C. albicans* infection unless the bacterial population is reduced.

Much of the inflammation associated with *Candida* infection is mediated by a diffusible irritant endotoxin-like substance released by the organism.

II. **SUBJECTIVE DATA** In chronic paronychia the area surrounding the nail is tender on pressure, and the associated onychia is cosmetically and mechanically embarrassing. *Candida* intertrigo, perlèche, and vulvovaginitis are often pruritic and at times very uncomfortable. The lesions of thrush may be painful and may interfere with the normal ingestion of food.

III. **OBJECTIVE DATA**

A. **Paronychial lesions** show rounding and lifting of the posterior nail fold and erythema and swelling of the distal digit (usually without overt purulence). Often the nail becomes ridged and may have a green or brown discoloration.

B. **Intertriginous lesions** (inframammary, axillary, groin, perianal, interdigital) are moist and red, with occasional scaling, and are often macerated in the folds. Well-defined, peeling borders surrounded by *satellite erythematous papules or pustules* are characteristic of *Candida* infections.

C. **Thrush** appears as white plaques loosely attached to oral or vaginal mucous membrane. The underlying mucosa is bright red and moist. Lesions start as pinpoint spots and may extend to the corners of the mouth or into the esophagus.

D. **Perlèche** appears as a cracked and fissured erythematous and moist area in the corners of the mouth.

E. The lesions of **vulvovaginitis** are frequently, but not always, associated with a vaginal discharge. The degree of vulvar erythema and edema parallels the severity of the symptoms. Primary vulvar candidiasis appears similar to other intertriginous *Candida* involvement.

IV. **ASSESSMENT**

A. Direct examination with potassium hydroxide (KOH) or Swartz-Medrik stain (SMS) will reveal budding yeasts with or without hyphae or pseudohyphae. The presence of hyphal forms is pathognomonic of infection on mucous membranes, but they are usually not seen with infection on skin. On gram stain, fungi appear as gram-positive organisms larger than bacteria.

B. *C. albicans* grows readily within 48–72 hr on fungal or bacterial media. Specific identification is based on the presence of chlamydospores when the organism is subcultured on chlamydospore or cornmeal agar.

C. Gram-negative rods may play a synergistic role in infection of intertriginous areas; appropriate gram stain and culture are important.

D. A change in the predisposing environment, or evaluation and treatment of underlying medical conditions, is necessary for a successful and lasting cure. Diminution of factors which lead to accumulation of moisture is most important.

V. **THERAPY**   Three new agents have recently become available for the topical therapy of fungal infections. These are an alkylaryl ether, haloprogin (Halotex®), and two synthetic imidazole compounds, miconazole (MicaTin®) and clotrimazole (Lotrimin®) (see also pp. 280, 283). All three have the advantage of being effective both for dermatophyte fungi and *C. albicans*. The latter two compounds are at least as effective as nystatin for treating cutaneous candidiasis, and miconazole and clotrimazole vaginal creams may be more effective than nystatin in treatment of vulvovaginal candidiasis.

The polyene antifungal antibiotic nystatin is also a useful therapeutic agent for most forms of candidiasis (see p. 282). The use of nystatin tablets (500,000 units PO 3–4id) is beneficial in many circumstances. Recurrent or recalcitrant perianal, vulvar, or diaper-area involvement may represent reinfections from gut organisms and often can be controlled when oral medication is added to topical care. Often, women who have experienced vaginal candidiasis hesitate to take antibacterial antibiotics for control of conditions such as acne for fear of reactivation of disease. Recurrent infection can almost always be prevented by giving 1–2 weeks of oral nystatin and vaginal miconazole, clotrimazole, or nystatin therapy preceding antibiotic administration and continuing the PO nystatin along with the other antibiotic. This regimen appears to rid the gut and vagina of sufficient *Candida* organisms to prevent clinical symptoms and also keeps them inhibited during concurrent antibiotic therapy. Nystatin or amphotericin B PO is not otherwise needed along with broad-spectrum antibiotics in the therapy of young healthy women.

A. **Paronychia**

1. All wet work must be stopped. Gloves and cotton liners must be worn to protect the hands. If this is not possible, it is unlikely that any active therapy will be successful. Even successful treatment of a chronic paronychia is slow and requires weeks to months before remission occurs.

2. Apply clotrimazole (Lotrimin®) cream or solution or nystatin cream to nail folds frequently. If there is much associated pain or edema, a steroid-nystatin cream (e.g., Mycolog®) is useful. Overnight application of medication under a finger cot may increase effectiveness.

3. Amphotericin B (Fungizone®) lotion or cream or 1% alcoholic solution of gentian violet may also be of value.

4. The paradoxical approach of interdicting wet work yet applying aqueous medications may be circumvented by the use of 2–4% thymol in chloroform (or absolute alcohol). This nonaqueous preparation reaches the paronychial area by capillary action and should be applied 2–3id. It often works when other remedies have failed.

5. Nails will grow out normally within 3–6 months after the paronychial area has healed.

B. **Intertriginous lesions** (inframammary, axillary, groin, perianal, interdigital)

1. Conditions leading to moisture and maceration must be eliminated or countered. Inframammary or groin lesions should be exposed several times daily to the drying warmth of an electric light bulb or the drying breeze from a fan. Supportive clothing is useful, as is weight reduction. Air conditioning in warm environments may become a necessity. After lesions subside, continued application of a drying powder or nystatin powder should be emphasized.

2. Inflammatory lesions should be thoroughly soaked or compressed 3–4id with water or Burow's solution to cool and soothe as well as to remove the irritant endotoxin substance.

3. After compresses and thorough drying with a towel, bulb, or fan, apply clotrimazole (Lotrimin®), nystatin, or steroid-nystatin cream (or nystatin powder) to affected areas.

4. Amphotericin B (Fungizone®) lotion or cream also may be useful.

5. Resorcinol 5% in 1:2000 Zephiran Chloride Aqueous Solution® applied 3–4id also can be of value.

6. Gentian violet 0.25–2.0% or Castellani's paint (fuchsin, phenol, and resorcinol) are also effective but often sting and are messy, and they will stain clothing, linen, and skin.

C. Thrush

1. Nystatin oral suspension (4–6 ml [400,000–600,000 units] 4id) should be held in the mouth for several minutes before swallowing. The dosage for infants is 2 ml (200,000 units) 4id.

2. Amphotericin B (80 mg/ml) used as a rinse is also effective.

3. Gentian violet solution 1–2% is probably the most useful agent available, but is esthetically unappealing. With difficult or recurrent cases it is the therapy of choice.

D. Vulvovaginitis

1. Clotrimazole tablets (Gyne-Lotrimin®) should be inserted intravaginally once daily for 7 days.

2. Miconazole cream (Monistat®) may be instilled into the vagina once daily for 2 weeks.

3. Nystatin vaginal suppositories (100,000 units) may be slightly less effective; when used they should be inserted high into the vagina twice daily for 7–14 days, then nightly for an additional 2–3 weeks.

4. Canicidin (Candeptin®) tablets or chlordantoin (Sporostacin®) cream may be used in the same fashion.

REFERENCES

DeVillez RL, Lewis CW: Candidiasis seminar. Cutis 19:69–83, 1977

Kirkpatrick CH, Rich RR, Bennett SE: Chronic mucocutaneous candidiasis: model-building in cellular immunity. NIH Conference. Ann Intern Med 74:955–978, 1971

Maibach HI, Kligman AM: The biology of experimental human cutaneous moniliasis (*Candida albicans*). Arch Dermatol 85:233–257, 1962

Rebora A, Marples RR, Kligman AM: Erosio interdigitalis blastomy-cetica. Arch Dermatol 108:66–68, 1973

Rebora A, Marples RR, Kligman AM: Experimental infection with *Candida albicans*. Arch Dermatol 108:69–73, 1973

Stone OJ, Mullins FJ: Role of *Candida albicans* in chronic disease. Arch Dermatol 91:70–72, 1965

Witten VH, Katz SI: Nystatin. Med Clin North Am 54:1329–1337, 1970

DERMATOPHYTE INFECTIONS

I. **DEFINITION AND PATHOPHYSIOLOGY** The dermatophyte (or ringworm) fungi are a distinct and unique class of fungi, both botanically and pathologically. Man may acquire dermatophyte infection from three sources: organisms that live in soil, animal fungi, or, most commonly, pathogens that will infect only humans and cannot survive elsewhere. Dermatophyte fungi live in the superficial layers of the epidermis, in nails, and in hair. They do not invade living epidermis but will, however, grow readily on excised tissue from many organs, including skin. It has become apparent that dermatophyte fungi grow only within keratin layers because there is a serum fungal inhibitory factor that enters the extravascular space and protects living tissue against deep penetration of fungal elements.

Poor nutrition and hygiene, a tropical climate, debilitating diseases, and contact with infected animals, persons, or fomites all increase the likelihood of fungal infection. Pathogenic fungi of all kinds are common in our environment, yet the overall incidence of infection is low; host resistance factors would seem to be the most important determinants of susceptibility to clinical fungal infection. Acquired immunity occurs in the majority of infected patients; circulating antibody can be demonstrated in 50 percent of infected patients. Reinfection in such patients requires a greater inoculum, and lesions heal more rapidly. A protective cell-mediated immunity is acquired by 80 percent of patients after primary infection. Chronic infection develops in approximately 20 percent of those infected; these patients have been shown to have a less adequate cell-mediated immune response.

Although some species of dermatophyte tend to produce a specific clinical picture, it may be difficult to ascertain the causative organism from the clinical characteristics of the eruption.

II. **CLINICAL TYPES OF INFECTION**

A. **Tinea capitis,** or ringworm of the scalp, after affecting children for over 2000 years is now readily controlled by systemic antifungal antibiotics. Epidemic ringworm is transmitted by contact from child to child. Organisms have been cultured from such objects as barbers' instruments, hairbrushes, theater seats, and hats. Minor trauma with a break in the cutaneous barrier is necessary to initiate infection. Children up to puberty are more susceptible, and boys are infected more often than girls.

1. *Subjective data* Scalp ringworm is usually asymptomatic. A kerion, which is a deep, boggy swelling caused by infection with certain fungi, is painful.

2. *Objective data* Patchy hair loss, with broken hairs, inflammation, and scaling are characteristic. Such findings in children should be presumed to be ringworm until proved otherwise. A kerion appears as a pustular folliculitis within an area of purulence and swelling. The inflammation is often vigorous and scarring can result.

B. **Tinea barbae,** or ringworm infection of the beard and moustache, is confined to adult men and is much less common than it was years ago. Infections from barbers' instruments are now rare, and the organisms are usually acquired from animals.

1. *Subjective data* Pruritus or pain occurs.

2. *Objective data*

   a. The superficial type of infection looks like ringworm elsewhere (see C-2 below).

   b. The deeper type infection is associated with marked inflammation, pustular folliculitis, and kerion formation. Loss of facial hair is common. The angle of the jaw is the most usual location.

C. **Tinea corporis,** or infection of the nonhairy skin, may be seen in any age group, but children are most susceptible. It occurs in all parts of the world, but is most prevalent in hot, humid climates and rural areas.

1. *Subjective data* Tinea corporis may be either asymptomatic or mildly pruritic.

2. *Objective data* The typical lesions start as erythematous macules or papules that spread outward and develop into annular and arciform lesions with sharp scaling or vesicular advancing borders and healing centers. Tinea corporis is

most common on the exposed surfaces of the body, namely, the face, arms, and shoulders.

D. Tinea cruris, or ringworm of the groin ("jock itch"), is frequently found in obese men in the summertime. It is often associated with the simultaneous presence of tinea pedis. Heat, friction, and maceration predispose to this infection; it is most common in the tropics.

1. *Subjective data* Symptoms include pruritus, which may be intense, and discomfort due to the inflamed intertriginous tissues rubbing together. Many eruptions are asymptomatic, however.

2. *Objective data (See color insert.)* The eruption affects both the groin and upper inner thigh symmetrically and often has a butterfly appearance with clearly defined, raised borders. Lesions often extend into the gluteal folds and onto the buttocks.

E. Tinea of the hands (tinea manuum) and feet (tinea pedis) Tinea pedis is the most common of all fungal diseases; 30–70 percent of the population at some time have had a fungal infection of the feet. Unlike other ringworm, tinea pedis is generally a disease of adult life. This infection, too, is found most often in tropical climates and in the summertime.

The causative fungi may be found in shoes, flooring, and socks and have been recovered from clothing more than 5 months after laundering. Occlusive footwear is a strong predisposing factor. Simple contact with infected scales is not enough for infection; concomitant trauma to the feet is necessary for infection to take place.

1. *Subjective data* Pruritus is the most common symptom. Fissures may be painful and also are easy avenues for secondary local bacterial infection or lymphangitis. This is of particular importance in patients with diabetes, chronic lymphedema, and stasis syndromes.

2. *Objective data*

a. *Tinea pedis* may take several forms.

(1) Mild to severe interdigital scaling and maceration with fissures is the most common form.

(2) Widespread fine scaling in "moccasin-foot" distribution is very frequent. The scaling usually extends up onto the sides of the feet and lower heel, where it exhibits a characteristic clearly defined, fine polycyclic scaling border.

(3) Some fungi induce a vesicular or bullous eruption with large blisters.

b. *Tinea manuum* is usually seen as mild erythema with hyperkeratosis and scaling, mainly over the palmar surfaces. Hand infection is almost never found in the absence of foot involvement. Inflammatory lesions on the feet are often associated with a sterile vesicular "id" reaction on the hands, often misdiagnosed as a primary fungal infection. Unilateral involvement of either hands or feet is common and even helpful in making a clinical diagnosis.

F. **Onychomycosis,** or fungal infection of the nails, is seen in approximately 40 percent of patients with fungal infections in other locations. Fungi invade the nails by growing either into the ventral edge or extending from the distal lateral nail groove. The organisms become located in the soft keratin in the proximal nails; fungi carried to the distal nail may or may not be viable. Fingernails are less commonly involved than toenails.

1. *Subjective data* The nails become brittle, friable, and thickened. Patients often complain that the nails not only are cosmetically embarrassing but catch and pull on clothing.

2. *Objective data* Infection starts at the free margin or lateral borders of the nail as a white or yellow discoloration and progresses proximally. The nail may become thickened, distorted, and crumbly and may be lifted up by an accumulation of subungual keratin and debris. Destruction may be slight or very severe and leave only small remnants of keratinous material.

III. ASSESSMENT

A. Definitive diagnosis is made by the microscopic identification of hyphae and spores in scales or hair. In nails the presence of hyphae usually means dermatophyte infection; however, secondarily invading saprophytic fungi can also be seen at times. This procedure is discussed in detail on page 238.

B. Infection may be confirmed, or in some instances identified in the absence of a positive scraping, by fungal culture. This technique is discussed on page 240.

C. Examination of infected areas with longwave ultraviolet light (Wood's lamp) may be used to make a diagnosis, screen large populations of children, or follow the course of therapy for tinea capitis due to *Microsporum canis* or *M. audouini*. Scalp ringworm infection caused by many fungi does not fluoresce, however (see p. 241).

IV. THERAPY

A. Prophylactic measures

1. Development of fungal infections is enhanced by heat, moisture, and maceration. If these environmental factors cannot be changed, chances for cure are less and those for relapse are excellent. Intertriginous or interdigital areas should be dried thoroughly after bathing and a simple talcum powder or antifungal powder (Tinactin®) should be applied then and each morning.

2. Footwear should fit well and be nonocclusive (leather shoes or sandals are best; avoid plastic footwear or sneakers).

3. Patients with hyperhidrosis should wear absorbent cotton socks and avoid wool or synthetic fibers.

4. Clothing and towels should be changed frequently and be well laundered in hot water.

B. Local therapy
Infections of the body and groin, and superficial involvement of the bearded area, palms, and soles, usually can be treated by topical measures alone (see also p. 279).

1. Acute, inflammatory lesions with blistering and oozing should be treated with intermittent (4–6id) or continuous open wet compresses (see p. 330). Blisters should be decompressed but roofs left intact.

2. Clotrimazole (Lotrimin®), miconazole (MicaTin®), haloprogin (Halotex®), and tolnaftate (Tinactin®) solution or cream applied 3id will cause involution of most superficial

scaling lesions within 1–3 weeks. The first three are also effective against *C. albicans* infection. Overnight application of Keralyt® gel for 1–2 weeks is effective for toe-web infection, presumably by removing the stratum corneum in which the fungi are growing.

3. Thick, hyperkeratotic involvement, as on the palms or soles, may require local therapy with medications containing keratolytic agents such as salicylic acid, which will cause softening and exfoliation of the skin.

   a. The most useful means of combining keratolytic and antifungal therapy is to apply Keralyt® gel under occlusion overnight or for 2–3 hr in the evening, and to use an antifungal agent at other times. The use of Keralyt® alone may be sufficient to rid the skin of fungal organisms.

   b. Verdefam® solution, 3 or 6% sulfur and salicylic acid ointment, or half- or full-strength Whitfield's ointment are other keratolytic preparations which may be applied 2id or alternated with the preparations noted in B-2.

   c. Keratolytic preparations may irritate the skin and must be used with care.

4. Topical treatment of the nails rarely will, if ever, result in total cure of onychomycosis.

   a. 10% glutaraldehyde solutions buffered to pH 7.5 have been reported to be effective after application 2id for 1–4 months. Buffered glutaraldehyde has high bactericidal, sporicidal, fungicidal, and viricidal activity, but rapidly undergoes polymerization and loses activity after 2 weeks.

   b. Reduction of a thickened, crumbling nail mass with an emery board or electric rotary sandpaper drill will reduce complaints referable to cosmetic or mechanical difficulties.

   c. Local application of clotrimazole (Lotrimin®), miconazole (MicaTin®), haloprogin (Halotex®), or tolnaftate (Tinactin®), or Verdefam® solutions may be helpful occasionally.

d. Surgical avulsion of the toenails, concomitant with systemic griseofulvin therapy, is the only treatment that will often clear toenail onychomycosis.

C. **Griseofulvin** (see also p. 281), a fungistatic and fungicidal antibiotic derived from various species of *Penicillium*, is effective against all dermatophyte fungi but is of no value against bacteria, superficial fungal infections such as tinea versicolor, or yeast infections such as those caused by *C. albicans*. Griseofulvin causes stunting and curling of hyphae growing in vitro and was initially called the "curling factor." Griseofulvin resembles colchicine structurally and can cause metaphase arrest in rapidly dividing cells. It is absorbed by the GI tract more rapidly after a fatty meal, but total absorption after 24 hr is constant and is not affected by taking griseofulvin either with or between meals, or in single or divided doses. There is possibly greater absorption if the drug is taken during the middle of the day.

Griseofulvin enters the epidermis by diffusion forces from extracellular fluid (through transepidermal water loss) and from sweat and reaches higher concentrations in the horny layer than in serum. With excessive sweating in hot, humid climates the amount of griseofulvin in skin is likely to be reduced, and more of the drug should be taken. The response to therapy depends on the rate of keratinization and the time necessary for desquamation of infected keratinized structures. Its use is contraindicated in patients with porphyria.

Griseofulvin may cause a reversal of the hypoprothrombinemic effect of anticoagulants, necessitating an increase in the dose of anticoagulant to maintain a therapeutic range of anticoagulation. This effect occurs through increased synthesis of drug-metabolizing liver enzymes, leading to more rapid inactivation of anticoagulant. Phenobarbital has been postulated to decrease the gut absorption of griseofulvin, thus decreasing blood levels and presumably decreasing antifungal action.

1. *Infection of nonhairy skin* usually responds to the use of micronized griseofulvin, 1 gm qd for 3–4 weeks, but it is needed only for extensive, recalcitrant, or recurrent lesions. Avoid terminating therapy until there is definite evidence of a cure, complete clearing of lesions, negative fungal scrapings, and a negative culture.

2. ***Tinea capitis*** due to *M. canis* or *M. audouini* will respond to 1 gm of micronized griseofulvin qd for a period of 3–6 weeks. Alternatively, a single dose of 3–4 gm (which may be repeated, if necessary, in 3–4 weeks) will result in cure of most children so treated. *Trichophyton tonsurans,* now the most common cause of tinea capitis in the southern United States, requires griseofulvin administration for 6 weeks or longer. Approximately 5 mg per pound of body weight is the effective dose for children. In general, children weighing 30–50 lb may take up to 250 mg daily, and children weighing over 50 lb, up to 500 gm daily. Therapy should be continued for at least 2 weeks after clinical and mycologic cure.

There is no further justification for cutting or shaving the hair, having the patient wear a skullcap, or irradiating the scalp. Local antifungal remedies add little to the results obtained from griseofulvin alone.

3. ***Griseofulvin therapy of fungal disease of the nails*** should be approached with the realization that prolonged administration may not lead to cure and that, even if it does, relapse is not uncommon. Fingernails respond more readily than toenails; in fact, infection of the first toenail responds hardly at all unless the nail is first removed.

The starting dose of micronized griseofulvin should be 1.5–2 gm qd for the first month, with gradual lessening of the dose to 1 gm qd over the following several months. Duration of therapy for fingernails will be 5–6 months, for toenails, 6–18 months. Local therapy adds little. Side-effects at these higher antibiotic levels are most commonly headache or mild gastrointestinal discomfort. Photosensitization may become a problem also.

4. Dogs and cats infected with ringworm fungi also can be treated with griseofulvin.

REFERENCES

Arndt KA: Superficial fungal infections. In Infectious Diseases. Edited by L Sabath. Boston, Little, Brown, 1977 (in press)

Baden HP: Fungal infections: treatment with a keratolytic gel. Cutis 16:574–575, 1975

Baer RL, Rosenthal SA: The biology of fungous infections of the feet. JAMA 197:1017–1020, 1966

Epstein WL, Shak V, Riegelman S: Dermatopharmacology of griseofulvin. Cutis 15:271–275, 1975

Fulton JE: Miconazole therapy for endemic fungal disease. Arch Dermatol 111:596–598, 1975

Goldman L: Griseofulvin. Med Clin North Am 54:1339–1345, 1970

Grant LV: A further look at the treatment of onychomycosis with topical glutaraldehyde. J Am Podiatry Assoc 64:158–161, 1974

Hildick-Smith G, Blank H, Sarkany I: Fungus Diseases and Their Treatment. Boston, Little, Brown, 1964, 494 pp

Jones HG, Reinhardt JH, Rinaldi MG: Model dermatophytosis in naturally infected subjects. Arch Dermatol 110:369–374, 1974

Rebel G, Taplin D: Dermatophytes: Their Identification and Recognition. Second edition. Coral Gables, University of Miami Press, 1970

Smith EB: New topical agents for dermatophytosis. Cutis 17:54–58, 1976

Spiekermann PH, Young MD: Clinical evaluation of clotrimazole. A broad-spectrum antifungal agent. Arch Dermatol 112:350–352, 1976

Zaias N: Onychomycosis. Arch Dermatol 105:263–274, 1972

TINEA VERSICOLOR

I. **DEFINITION AND PATHOPHYSIOLOGY** Tinea versicolor is a chronic, asymptomatic, superficial fungal infection caused by the organism *Malassezia furfur*. This organism represents the pathogenic filamentous form of the yeastlike *Pityrosporun orbiculare*, a normal skin resident. The eruption is found worldwide, is seen most commonly in young adults in temperate zones, and accounts for about 5 percent of all fungal infections. Although the fine scales are teeming with hyphae and spores, the organisms cannot readily be cultured. They are found only in the stratum corneum, never penetrate deeper, and cause no inflammatory response.

Tinea versicolor develops either as a result of change in host resistance or because certain strains of *P. orbiculare* are capable of transforming into a more aggressive form. Factors predisposing to clinical infection include (a) pregnancy, (b) serious underlying diseases, (c) a genetic predisposition, or (d) high plasma cortisol, as in patients taking corticosteroids. Tinea versicolor often infects people for years, because of inadequate treatment, reinfection, or an inherent predisposition to infection.

The decreased or increased pigmentation in affected areas has long been considered to be secondary to a "sun screening" effect of infected keratin. The infected areas may be darker than surrounding skin in wintertime, but they do not tan after sun exposure and in summer become lighter than surrounding areas. Although this "fungus filter" perhaps plays some part in the pathogenesis of the hypopigmentation, it appears that the pigmentary changes are primarily related to fungus-induced effects on melanosome size and distribution. In hypopigmented tinea versicolor, the fungus initiates the production of abnormally small, occasionally packed melanosomes that are not transferred to keratinocytes properly. Conversely, in hyperpigmented tinea versicolor, melanosomes are larger and singly distributed within keratinocytes in a fashion similar to that of normal black pigmentation.

II. **SUBJECTIVE DATA**   The eruption is almost always asymptomatic and only of cosmetic significance.

III. **OBJECTIVE DATA**   Lesions vary in color from white and pink to brown, but usually consist of tan, desquamating, round or perifollicular, coalescing macular patches found primarily on the trunk. Involved untreated areas may be lighter than surrounding skin in the summer and become relatively darker during the winter.

IV. **ASSESSMENT**

A. Examination of scales under the microscope with potassium hydroxide (KOH) Swartz-Medrik stain (SMS) will reveal numerous short, straight, and angular hyphae and clusters of thick-walled, round and budding yeasts (see p. 238). A negative microscopic examination virtually excludes the diagnosis, unlike dermatophyte infections.

B. The causative organism of tinea versicolor cannot be cultured on artificial media.

C. Wood's light examination will intensify the pigmentary changes and allow the extent and margins of involvement to be seen more readily. Infected areas may show a gold-to-orange fluorescence.

V. **THERAPY**

A. Tinea versicolor may be treated with many therapeutic agents, all of which will be successful if used for an adequate length of time. The evening application of medication should follow a bath. Most treatments will remove any evidence of active infection (scaling) within several days, but to insure cure these regimens should be continued for several weeks. The pigmentary changes resolve much more slowly (months). In spite of seemingly adequate therapy, relapse or reinfection is common, but it always responds to retreatment. Tinea versicolor does not respond to griseofulvin.

B. The frequency of relapse has led some to recommend that therapy be continued for 2 consecutive nights each month for 1 year in order to insure a cure.

C. Useful agents

1. *Selenium sulfide suspension* (Exsel®, Selsun®, Iosel®) should be applied to the affected areas, allowed to dry, and then allowed to remain for 15 min for 7–14 consecutive days. As little as a 5–20-min application on alternate days for 2 weeks may be effective in some instances.

2. *25% sodium hyposulfite* should be applied to lesions 2id for several weeks. Tinver® lotion (25% sodium thiosulfate, 1% salicylic acid, and 10% alcohol) is used in the same fashion.

3. *Keratolytic creams,* ointments, lotions, or soaps containing 3–6% salicylic acid (Keralyt® gel; Sebulex® shampoo; 3–6% sulfur and salicylic acid ointment; 6% salicylic acid cream; 3% salicylic acid in 70% alcohol; salicylic acid soap) applied overnight for 1–2 weeks are also effective.

4. *Akrinol®* cream contains the hexylresorcinol salt of 9-amino-acridine and should be applied 2id for 6 weeks to prevent relapse.

5. *Clotrimazole (Lotrimin®), miconazole (MicaTin®), haloprogin (Halotex®), or tolnaftate (Tinactin®)* preparations will eradicate tinea versicolor, but they are more expensive and no more effective than any of the foregoing.

6. *Retinoic acid cream (Retin-A® cream)* applied twice daily for 2 weeks will cure the tinea versicolor and may be accompanied by lightening of pigmentation in the areas to which it is applied. It may therefore be more useful in those particularly embarrassed by the hyperpigmentation of infected skin.

REFERENCES

Allen HB, Charles CR, Johnson BL: Hyperpigmented tinea versicolor. Arch Dermatol 112:1110–1112, 1976

Bamford JTM: Tinea versicolor treatment. Arch Dermatol 110:956, 1974

Barnes WG, Sauer GC, Arnold JD: Scanning electron microscopy of tinea versicolor organisms. Arch Dermatol 107:392–394, 1973

Boardman CR, Malkinson FD: Tinea versicolor in steroid-treated patients. Incidence in patients with chronic ulcerative colitis and regional enteritis treated with corticotropin and corticosteroids. Arch Dermatol 85:44–52, 1962

Burke RC: Tinea versicolor: susceptibility factors and experimental infection in human beings. J Invest Dermatol 36:389–402, 1961

El Gothamy Z, Abdel-Fattah A, Ghaly AF: Tinea versicolor hypopigmentation: histochemical and therapeutic studies. Int J Dermatol 14:510–515, 1975

McGinley KJ, Lantis LR, Marples RR: Microbiology of tinea versicolor. Arch Dermatol 102:168–170, 1970

Mills OH Jr, Kligman AM: Tretinoin in tinea versicolor. Arch Dermatol 110:638, 1974

Roberts SOB: Pityriasis versicolor: a clinical and mycological investigation. Br J Dermatol 81:315–320, 1969

Tosti A, Villardita S, Fazzini ML: The parasitic colonization of the horny layer in the tinea versicolor. J Invest Dermatol 59:233–237, 1972

15
Herpes Simplex

I. DEFINITION AND PATHOPHYSIOLOGY Cutaneous herpes simplex infections take two distinct forms: (a) the painful and disabling primary infection, seen only in previously uninfected individuals without circulating antibody, and (b) the common, bothersome recurrent form of "cold sores" or "fever blisters," found at some time in approximately 75 percent of patients previously infected.

Herpes simplex is a DNA virus, infects man alone, and has an almost universal distribution. There are two types of herpes virus: type 1, which is usually responsible for nongenital herpetic infections; and type 2, which is usually the agent involved in genital infections in both males and females. Type 2 herpes virus exhibits biologic as well as morphologic differences from type 1. In addition to the potential threat to the fetus and neonate when the virus infects the reproductive tract during pregnancy, a possible etiologic role in cervical dysplasia and carcinoma has recently been documented. Women with genital herpes simplex infections appear to have 5–10 times greater likelihood of developing cervical carcinoma than do uninfected women.

Type 2 infection primarily involves persons beyond the age of puberty, is spread by sexual contact, and is one of the most common sexually transmitted diseases.

The majority of affected individuals probably have subclinical primary herpetic infections with both type 1 and 2 viruses; a few may subsequently excrete the virus in respiratory or other secretions and thus constitute a reservoir of infection. The primary infection runs a course of 1–3 weeks, while recurrent lesions heal more quickly (7–10 days).

After primary infection, the virus appears to remain latent in sensory ganglia. In patients with recurrent herpes, the virus is periodically reactivated and conducted to the epidermis via peripheral nerve fibers. It then replicates in the skin, producing the recurrent herpetic lesion. Trigger factors include emotional stress, physical trauma (including genital trauma for lesions in this area), sunburn, menses, fever, and systemic infections. Patients with atopic dermatitis risk the development of generalized lesions (eczema herpeticum) regardless of whether or not their eczema is active. Diseases that interfere with host response, such as leukemia and lymphoma, also predispose to widespread, slowly healing, and more destructive infections.

II. SUBJECTIVE DATA

A. Primary symptomatic oral or genital infections

1. Infections on mucosal surfaces are preceded by a day or two of local tenderness.

2. The lesions are accompanied by severe and disabling pain and tender lymphadenopathy, often making it impossible for those with gingivostomatitis to eat or drink, or women with vulvovaginitis to walk or urinate.

3. High fever and purulent malodorous secretions accompany oral or vaginal infections.

4. Primary infection in men usually results in painful penile lesions, but it may also cause urethritis, with dysuria and discharge.

B. Recurrent lesions are preceded by several hours of a burning or tingling sensation. They are uncomfortable, but much less so than the lesions of the primary infection.

III. OBJECTIVE DATA (See color insert.)

A. Primary infection

1. *Gingivostomatitis* is the most frequent manifestation of primary infection.

   a. Vesicles, erosions, and maceration are seen over the entire buccal mucosa.

   b. Marked erythema and edema of the gingiva are typical.

   c. Submandibular adenopathy usually is present.

2. *Vulvovaginitis* is seen most frequently in girls and young women.

   a. It consists of widespread vesicles, erosions, and edema in the vulva, labia, and surrounding skin.

   b. These areas become very edematous, erythematous, and extremely tender.

   c. A profuse vaginal discharge is present and some women develop urinary retention.

   d. Bilateral, tender, inguinal adenopathy is usually present.

3. *Urethritis* in men is accompanied by a watery discharge and the occasional presence of vesicles around the urethral meatus.

4. *Inoculation herpes* is commonly found on the paronychial area ("herpetic whitlow") of nurses and physicians, particularly those involved with mouth care, and may also be found on previously traumatized or burned skin. The lesions are characterized by the sudden appearance of vesicles and are accompanied by extreme local pain, sometimes a sterile lymphangitis, and a systemic reaction. Herpetic whitlow is often misdiagnosed as a bacterial paronychia and mistreated with incision and drainage of lesions, with subsequent implantation of the virus into the incised tissue.

5. *Cervicitis* is often asymptomatic but nevertheless important to recognize in pregnant women because of the associated risk of fetal infection and spontaneous abortion. Preg-

nant women who acquire genital herpes during the first 20 weeks of pregnancy have an increased risk of abortions, whereas the infants of those who acquire infection after 20 weeks have an increased incidence of prematurity.

B. Recurrent infection

  1. Multiple small vesicles, clustered together, appear at the site of premonitory symptoms.

  a. The vesicles may arise from normal skin or from an area that has a slight erythematous blush.

  b. Vesicles are initially clear, then become cloudy and purulent, dry and crust, and heal within 7–10 days.

  c. The mature lesion consists of grouped vesicles and/or pustules on an erythematous edematous base.

  2. The presence of a yellow or golden crust on older lesions indicates bacterial superinfection.

  3. Regional, often tender, adenopathy is almost always present.

  4. The most common sites for lesions are on the face (perioral area, cheeks, and nose) and neck. Next is the anogenital area, then the sacrum and buttocks. However, recurrent herpes can be seen anywhere on the skin. It is uncommon for recurrent lesions to be located inside the oral cavity except in the immunocompromised host.

IV. ASSESSMENT Any doubt concerning the presence of a herpes simplex infection may be clarified by any of several diagnostic procedures:

A. Skin biopsy of a typical viral vesicle will reveal a characteristic picture: (1) an intraepidermal lesion in the mid-to-upper epidermis, (2) ballooning degeneration of cells, (3) acantholytic cells floating free, and (4) large, multinucleated viral giant cells. Intranuclear inclusions may be seen in the giant cells as well as in other infected epidermal cells.

B. A cytologic smear of the vesicle, for the purpose of looking for giant cells and inclusion bodies, is easily and quickly done (see p. 237). It is important that the earliest vesicle be chosen for biopsy or cytologic smears. Lesions of herpes simplex, herpes zoster, and varicella will have the identical appearance on biopsy and tissue smear. Exfoliative cytology (Papanicolaou smear) is especially useful as a means of detecting asymptomatic cervical or vaginal infection in women.

C. The virus may be easily and rapidly grown from the vesicle fluid (48 hr).

D. Specific neutralizing antibody titers will rise after the first week of primary infection and peak at 2–3 weeks. Change in antibody titer cannot be used as a criterion for recurrent lesions.

E. If the appropriate facilities and reagents are available, the following procedures may be carried out if indicated:

    1. The virus may be easily identified under electron microscope.

    2. The virus can be demonstrated in tissue specimens using fluorescent antibody techniques.

    3. The virus may be typed by appropriate serologic tests.

V. THERAPY

A. **Prophylactic measures** There is no prophylactic therapy of proved value. Vaccines are being evaluated and may be useful in the future. The repeated use of smallpox inoculations has never been shown to reliably inhibit recurrent herpes simplex. If a consistent trigger factor can be identified after careful questioning, specific measures may be taken to counteract these stimuli (i.e., use of sunscreens or avoidance of sun or other specific trauma). Herpes progenitalis is a sexually transmitted disease, and primary infection can be prevented by avoiding sexual contact with an individual with active lesions.

Pregnant women with active herpetic vulvar lesions should be considered for cesarean section. Neonatal herpes, which may be acquired transplacentally or more often from direct inoculation in the birth canal, may be an overwhelming and fatal infection. If the virus is present in the canal at birth, the risk of infant involvement is 40 percent unless the infant is delivered abdominally before or within 4 hr of membrane rupture.

B. **Active therapy**

    1. *Primary infection*

        a. The primary infection is extremely painful, and adequate analgesia is important. If salicylates are inadequate, opiates may be needed for the first 7–10 days.

b. Healing time for primary stomatitis may possibly be decreased by application of 0.1% idoxuridine (IDUR). This topical antiviral agent inhibits the uptake of thymidine into viral DNA synthesis and/or is incorporated into fraudulent DNA. It may also inhibit DNA polymerase, an enzyme required for the production of viral DNA.

c. Cleansing mouthwashes (with benzalkonium chloride [Zephiran®] 1:1000 or tetracycline suspension 250 mg/60 ml H_2O) both clean and soothe involved mucous membranes as well as decrease secondary bacterial superinfections.

d. Vulvovaginitis and genital lesions may be aided by sitz baths in tepid water with or without Aveeno® colloidal oatmeal. Women unable to void may sometimes be able to do so while in a bath. If not, intermittent catheterization or a temporary indwelling Foley catheter is necessary.

e. This is one of the few instances in which topical anesthetics are justified (see p. 263). Dyclonine hydrochloride (Dyclone®), Benadryl® Elixir, or viscous Xylocaine® may be used for oral lesions (see Aphthous Stomatitis, p. 22), and benzocaine aerosol (Americaine®) may be beneficial symptomatically for the vulvar area. Application should be as frequent as is necessary to keep the patient comfortable. The benzocaine preparations may sensitize the skin and should not be used routinely.

f. Intravenous fluids and topical and/or systemic antibiotics should be used as needed.

2. *Recurrent infection*

a. There are no topical or systemic agents that have yet been shown to reliably shorten the healing time or lower the recurrence rate of herpes simplex infections. The methods listed below *may* provide some relief:

(1) Apply ethyl ether with a cotton swab or moistened pledget to the lesions until the skin blanches and local anesthesia is produced. Reapply prn during the next 24–48 hr whenever itching and

pain reappears. This therapy may be effective by acting on the lipid-containing membrane of herpes simplex, by acting as an anesthetic, and/or by altering or injuring epidermal cells so they cannot be infected. Ether is flammable and obviously should not be inhaled.

Other local drying and soothing agents (70% alcohol, 10% aluminum acetate, Blistex®, etc.) may be useful in the early vesicular stage.

(2) Early and aggressive use of topical IDUR or adenine arabinoside monophosphate is felt by some both to decrease the severity of the lesion and to shorten the healing time, but not all patients will benefit. IDUR solution or ointment (Herplex®, Stoxil®) or ARA-AMP (VIRA-A) should be applied hourly or even more frequently for the first day and then less so later.

(3) Photoactive dyes that bind to viral DNA and then destroy the virus when activated by light were postulated to prevent recurrence and shorten the course of infection. However, recent placebo-controlled studies have shown neutral-red photodynamic inactivation to be ineffective, and these dyes should not be used until shown to be efficacious by controlled clinical trials.

(4) Some physicians feel that early and repeated application of a potent fluorinated steroid to the lesion will decrease its severity by inhibiting the inflammatory response. If this modality is used, it is essential to avoid the immediate periorbital area.

(5) Topical antibiotics such as bacitracin ointment applied to healing lesions will prevent bacterial superinfection.

3. *Ocular infection* Patients with symptoms referable to corneal involvement (photophobia, pain) should be examined with a slit lamp. Herpes simplex keratitis is treated with IDUR (Herplex®, Stoxil®) or adenine arabinoside monophosphate (ARA-AMP); however, herpetic lesions of

the lids and the immediate periorbital area, in the absence of ocular involvement, need not be treated with intraocular medication.

REFERENCES

Baringer JR: Recovery of herpes simplex virus from human sacral ganglions. N Engl J Med 291:828–830, 1974

Corbett MD, Sidell CM, Zimmerman M: Idoxuridine in the treatment of cutaneous herpes simplex. JAMA 196:441–444, 1966

Douglas RG, Couch RB: A prospective study of chronic herpes simplex virus infection and recurrent herpes labialis in humans. J Immunol 104:289–295, 1970

Jaffee EC, Lehner T: Treatment of herpetic stomatitis with idoxuridine. Br Dent J 125:392–395, 1968

Juel-Jensen BE, MacCallum FO: Herpes Simplex, Varicella and Zoster. Philadelphia, Lippincott, 1972, 194 pp

Logan WS, Tindall JP, Elson ML: Chronic cutaneous herpes simplex. Arch Dermatol 103:606–614, 1971

Muller SA, Herrmann EC, Winkelmann RK: Herpes in hematologic malignancies. Am J Med 52:102–114, 1972

Myers MG, Oxman NM, Clark JE, Arndt KA: Failure of neutral-red photoinactivation in recurrent herpes simplex infections. N Engl J Med 293:945–949, 1975

Nahmias AJ, Roizman B: Infection with herpes simplex viruses 1 and 2. N Engl J Med 289:667–674, 719–725, 781–789, 1973

Rosato FE, Rosato EF, Plottan SA: Herpetic paronychia—an occupational hazard of medical personnel. N Engl J Med 283:804–805, 1970

Sabin AB: Misery of recurrent herpes: what to do? N Engl J Med 293:986–988, 1975

Wheeler CE Jr: Pathogenesis of recurrent herpes simplex infections. J Invest Dermatol 65:341–346, 1975

Wheeler CE Jr, Abele DC: Eczema herpeticum, primary and recurrent. Arch Dermatol 93:162–173, 1966

16
Herpes Zoster and Varicella

I. **DEFINITION AND PATHOPHYSIOLOGY** Infection with the zoster-varicella virus will produce one of two clinical entities. The generalized, highly contagious, and usually benign chickenpox will develop in the nonimmune host, while the localized and painful zoster (shingles) will develop in the partially immune host. The clinical manifestations reflect the interaction between this virus and the host immune mechanisms.

Chickenpox, usually acquired through droplets from a respiratory source, has an average incubation period of 2 weeks, begins abruptly, and the lesions heal or even disappear within 7–10 days. Ninety percent of reported cases occur in children less than 10 years of age. Subclinical infection is frequent. The disease is communicable from 1 day prior to the appearance of the exanthem to 6 days after, and crusts are noninfectious. Signs, symptoms, and complications often become more severe with age; adolescents and adults may become severely ill, particularly when there is pulmonary involvement.

Zoster results from reactivation of latent virus residing in dorsal root or cranial nerve ganglion cells. It is seen sporadically with no seasonal variation; two-thirds of patients are over 40 years old. Lesions erupt for several days and usually are gone within 2–3 weeks in children and 3–4 weeks in adults. Zoster is a self-limited, localized disease which causes discomfort for several days but usually heals without complications. Postherpetic neuralgia, however, is seen with increasing frequency in those over 60 years of age and can be an extremely painful, chronic, and, at times, unremitting plague.

In patients with serious underlying conditions that alter immunologic competence, much more severe disease develops. In children with lymphoma or leukemia, varicella is a life-threatening infection; adults with such diseases often acquire zoster, which may then disseminate. Approximately 1–2 percent of zoster cases, in normal hosts, will disseminate. However, of all cases of disseminated zoster, about two-thirds of the patients will be found to have lymphoma-leukemia or similar diseases; in Hodgkin's disease, dissemination may occur in 25 percent of cases with a mortality approaching 25 percent. In patients with any type of malignant disease, but particularly Hodgkin's disease, dermatomal zoster develops more frequently than in age-matched controls. The location of the dermatome affected is often related to a site of prior radiation therapy or to the presence of neoplastic lesions either centrally (lesions in or around the spinal column), causing neural irritation, or peripherally, as metastatic deposits. Immunosuppressive therapy for such diseases, or that used in transplantation programs, also predisposes to recurrence of zoster-varicella infection but not necessarily to dissemination.

II. SUBJECTIVE DATA

A. Varicella

1. Varicella in children is preceded by little or no prodrome; there may be only 24 hr of malaise and fever. In adolescents and adults, fever and constitutional symptoms almost always precede the exanthem by 24–48 hr.

2. The appearance of cough, dyspnea, and chest pain within 2–5 days after the onset of the rash is indicative of severe pulmonary involvement.

3. Pruritus is the primary and most annoying feature of chickenpox, and the patient's scratching contributes to secondary bacterial infection and scarring.

B. Zoster The appearance of zoster lesions is frequently preceded by a mild to severe preeruptive itch, tenderness, or pain; the last may be generalized over the entire nerve segment, localized to part of it, or referred. This pain may be confused with that of pleural or cardiac disease, cholecystitis or other abdominal catastrophe, renal or ureteral colic, sciatica, etc. Neurologic changes within the affected dermatome include hypesthesia, dyesthesia, or hyperesthesia. The interval between pain and eruption may be as long as 10 days, but averages 3–5 days. In some patients, particularly children, there are no sensory changes at all. The pain will usually subside within several weeks, but 73 percent of patients over 60 years of age have discomfort that persists over 8 weeks.

III. OBJECTIVE DATA (See color insert.)

A. Chickenpox begins abruptly with the appearance of discrete, erythematous macules and papules located primarily over the thorax, scalp, and mucous membranes; the face and distal extremities remain less involved. Lesions progress rapidly from erythematous macules to 2–3-mm, clear, tense, fragile vesicles surrounded by an erythematous areola. As the lesions progress, they first become umbilicated and then within hours become cloudy and purulent, with crusts forming in 2–4 days. Varicella lesions appear in 3–5 distinct crops for up to a 5-day period, and lesions in *all* stages of development may be seen within one area (an important difference from smallpox). Crusts fall off in 1–3 weeks.

B. Zoster lesions appear first posteriorly and progress to the anterior and peripheral distribution of the nerve involved (see endpaper figures for dermatome charts). Only rarely will the eruption be bilateral. Erythematous macules, papules, and plaques are seen first, and in most instances grouped vesicles appear within 24 hr, although blisters never develop in some patients. Plaques may be scattered irregularly along a dermatomal segment or may become confluent. Mucous membranes within the dermatomes are also affected. The vesicles become purulent, crust, and fall off within 1–2 weeks. The presence of a few vesicles (10–25) outside of the affected dermatome is usual and does not imply dissemination.

Zoster appears most often in thoracic and cervical segments. Lesions on the tip of the nose herald involvement of the nasociliary branch of the ophthalmic division of the trigeminal nerve, implying a strong possibility of concomitant keratoconjunctivitis. Paresis and permanent motor damage are more common than previously thought and are found mostly with involvement of the trigeminal and upper cervical and thoracic nerves.

C. Those predisposed to more severe disease may show hemorrhagic, bullous, and infarctive-gangrenous lesions, which will heal slowly with scarring.

IV. ASSESSMENT

A. Infection may be confirmed by a cytologic smear of the vesicle, by biopsy, or by serologic methods (see Herpes Simplex, p. 106).

B. Patients more at risk for severe varicella or those with disseminated zoster should be hospitalized and kept under strict precautions, in private rooms and away from seriously ill patients and those with lymphoproliferative disease or on immunosuppressive therapy. All patients with disseminated zoster or those severely ill with varicella should be investigated for underlying neoplastic or immunologic disease.

C. Approximately 50 percent of adults with varicella show nodular pulmonary infiltrates, but not all will manifest clinical respiratory disease. A chest x-ray is indicated for evaluation.

V. THERAPY

A. **Varicella** Most patients with varicella require only symptomatic therapy.

1. Localized itching may be alleviated by application of a drying antipruritic lotion (calamine alone or with 0.25% menthol and/or 1.0% phenol).

2. Antihistamines may help pruritus.

3. The patient should cut nails short and keep hands clean, and children should wear gloves, if necessary, to prevent excoriation.

4. Mouth and perineal lesions may be treated by rinses or compresses with hydrogen peroxide, saline, or other agents (see Herpes Simplex, p. 108).

5. Apply topical antibiotic ointments to locally infected lesions. If infection is widespread, it is most often due to Group A

beta-hemolytic streptococcus or staphylococcus and systemic antibiotics should be used.

6. High-risk susceptible patients (those with lymphoma-leukemia or immunodeficiency, those on immunosuppressive drugs, the newborn child of a mother with varicella) under 15 years of age with close exposure to varicella or zoster should be passively immunized by use of zoster-immune globulin (ZIG). This will effectively abort clinical infection if administered within 72 hr of exposure.

B. Zoster

1. Analgesics should be given as necessary. Opiates may be needed.

2. For the vesicular stages, one of the following may be effective:

   a. Application of cool compresses with 1:20 Burow's solution.

   b. Painting of lesions with equal parts of tincture of benzoin and flexible collodion, or with flexible collodion q12h.

   c. Application of a drying shake lotion containing alcohol, menthol, and/or phenol.

   d. Splinting the area with an occlusive dressing is often very useful in relieving pain. Lesions should be covered with cotton and then wrapped with an elastic bandage as for a fractured rib.

3. When lesions are crusted and/or secondarily infected, a topical antibiotic cream or ointment should be applied.

4. Ocular involvement should be evaluated by an ophthalmologist. Herpes zoster keratoconjunctivitis is treated with topical ophthalmic corticosteroids.

5. In patients over 60 years of age it is possible to decrease the incidence of postherpetic neuralgia by the use of systemic corticosteroids (presumably by inhibiting perineural inflammation and fibrosis). Prednisone or its equivalent should be administered at a dose of 60 mg qd for 1 week,

30 mg qd for the second week, and finally, 15 mg qd for the third week. Unless this regimen is started within the first 5–7 days of the eruption, however, it is unlikely to help. The risk-benefit pattern ratio must be determined for each patient; often it is too high. Usually, systemic corticosteroids do not influence either the symptoms or the healing time of the acute eruption and do not increase the risk of dissemination, although they will decrease the severity of edema and are useful in patients with severe facial swelling either with or without ocular involvement.

6. ***Postherpetic neuralgia*** Already existing postherpetic pain is extremely difficult to alleviate. There are several approaches that have been suggested.

   a. Chlorprothixene (Taractan®) was effective in bringing relief to 29 of 30 patients in one study. Patients with severe neuralgia should receive 50–100 mg IM followed by 50 mg PO q6h for 7–10 days. Patients with moderate neuralgia should take 50-mg tablets PO q6h for 4–10 days. Some improvement should be noted within 72 hr.

   b. The use of a combination of a tricyclic antidepressant and a substituted phenothiazine medication may lead to almost complete relief of pain within 1–2 weeks after institution of therapy. Amitriptyline (Elavil®) 75–100 mg qd should be used in combination with either perphenazine (Trilafon®) 4 mg 3–4id, fluphenazine hydrochloride (Permitil®) 1 mg 3–4id, or thioridazine (Mellaril®) 25 mg 4id. It may be necessary to continue medication for months.

   c. Pain relief in patients with acute herpes zoster and in many patients with post-zoster neuralgia has been claimed to follow daily intralesional or subcutaneous injection of triamcinolone 0.2 mg/ml into the affected dermatome. Up to 30 ml of the drug diluted in saline or 60 mg of triamcinolone can be administered at each session.

   d. Transcutaneous electrical stimulation has brought pain relief to a high percentage of patients treated in this fashion.

    e. Neurosurgical intervention is occasionally necessary in patients with intractable pain.

REFERENCES

Varicella

Gershon AA, Stanberg S, Brunell PA: Zoster immune globulin. A further assessment. N Engl J Med 290:243–245, 1974

Gordon JE: Chickenpox: an epidemiological review. Am J Med Sci 244: 362–389, 1962

Luby JP: Varicella-zoster virus. J Invest Dermatol 61:212–222, 1973

Zoster

Blank H, Eaglstein WH, Goldfaden GH: Zoster, a recrudescence of VZ virus infection. Postgrad Med J 46:653–658, 1970

Devriese PP: Facial paralysis in cephalic herpes zoster. Ann Otol Rhinol Laryngol 77:1101–1119, 1968

Eaglstein WH, Katz R, Brown JA: The effects of early corticosteroid therapy on the skin eruption and pain of herpes zoster. JAMA 211: 1681–1683, 1970

Farber GA, Burks JW: Chlorprothixene therapy for herpes zoster neuralgia. South Med J 67:808–812, 1974

Hope-Simpson RE: The nature of herpes zoster: a long-term study and a new hypothesis. Proc R Soc Med 58:9–20, 1965

Juel-Jensen BE, MacCallum FO: Herpes Simplex, Varicella and Zoster. Philadelphia, Lippincott, 1972, 194 pp

Miller LH, Brunell PA: Zoster, reinfection or activation of latent virus? Observations on the antibody response. Am J Med 49:480–483, 1970

Molin L: Aspects of the natural history of herpes zoster. A follow-up investigation of outpatient material. Acta Derm Venereol (Stockh) 49:569–581, 1969

Rogers RS, Tindall JP: Herpes zoster in children. Arch Dermatol 106: 204–207, 1972

Schimpff S, Serpick A, Stoler B, Rumack B, Mellin H, Joseph JM, Block J: Varicella-zoster infections in patients with cancer. Ann Intern Med 76:241–254, 1972

Taub A: Relief of postherpetic neuralgia with psychotropic drugs. J Neurosurg 39:235–239, 1973

17
Hyperpigmentation and Hypopigmentation

I. **DEFINITION AND PATHOPHYSIOLOGY** Patients with pigmentary changes on their skin seek advice primarily for cosmetic reasons; they complain of having either too much or too little pigmentation, or they are unhappy with its distribution. Although pigment changes are usually asymptomatic and of no medical consequence, they may signify systemic disease.

A. **Hyperpigmentation**

1. *Melasma* (*chloasma*) is found most often on the facial areas of women who either are taking anovulatory drugs or are pregnant, and has been called "mask of pregnancy." However, it may also be found in men or women with no endocrinologic abnormalities. Its cause remains unknown, but sun is necessary for its development. It is present more frequently in dark Caucasians (e.g., Puerto Ricans and those of Mediterranean background).

2. *Freckles* (*ephelides*), like melasma, are present only on light-exposed skin, and the pigment is found only in the

epidermis; neither are found on mucous membranes. Freckling is genetically determined, appears mostly by age 5–7, and is seen most in redheads, blondes, and other fair-skinned individuals. Paradoxically, there are fewer melanocytes in a freckle than in normal surrounding skin, but those that are present are large and able to form more melanin than usual. Freckles, like melasma, darken considerably in the summertime and may fade almost completely in the winter.

3. A *lentigo* is most often confused with a freckle. These hyperpigmented spots, which may appear at any age, are usually darker than freckles and are not induced by ultraviolet radiation. An increased number of melanocytes is present in the basal layer, and the epidermal rete ridges are elongated and clubbed. Lentigines are seen equally well in winter and summer and can be present on the palms, soles, and mucous membranes. The multiple lentigines ("leopard") syndrome is often associated with electrocardiographic changes. In the Peutz-Jeghers syndrome, lentigines on the lips and hands occur with small bowel polyposis. Such lentigines can be confused with the multiple, small, café-au-lait spots of neurofibromatosis. Solar ("senile") lentigines, commonly and incorrectly known as "liver spots," appear on the exposed surfaces of fair-skinned people long exposed to the sun, usually in association with other changes from sun damage, including wrinkling, dryness, and actinic keratoses.

4. *Postinflammatory hyperpigmentation* is common in more darkly pigmented persons and is more related to the nature of the insult than to the degree of previous inflammation; it is severe following some conditions such as thermal burns and mild after others. There is an increase in epidermal melanin, but there may also be melanin granules present in dermal macrophages. Postinflammatory hyperpigmentation may persist for months to years.

B. Hypopigmentation

1. *Vitiligo* is a disorder in which areas of the skin are completely lacking melanin pigmentation. Pigment cells (melanocytes) cannot be detected in depigmented areas, even on inspection by electron microscopy. This is in contrast to al-

binism, in which melanocytes are present, but there is little or no pigmentation because of faulty or absent tyrosinase. The cause of vitiligo is unknown, but abnormal neurogenic stimuli, an enzymatic self-destruct mechanism, and an autoimmune mechanism have been postulated as pathogenetic factors. It appears to be inherited in some kinships and is found with increased frequency in patients with hyperthyroidism, Addison's disease, and pernicious anemia. In vitiligo patients there is also an increased incidence of halo nevi and alopecia areata. Lesions rarely repigment spontaneously.

2. *Postinflammatory* or *posttraumatic hypopigmentation* may be profound enough to mimic vitiligo, but frequently appears as slightly scaly, slightly lighter areas of skin (*pityriasis alba*). It is often seen following cutaneous diseases such as psoriasis and atopic dermatitis and in those instances may be related to the inability of altered epidermal cells to accept melanin granules rather than to the decreased production of pigment in melanocytes. Pityriasis alba is found most frequently on exposed areas (e.g., face) in children with atopy in their backgrounds. Postinflammatory hypopigmentation slowly repigments but in rare instances may be permanent, especially if scarring has occurred.

II. **SUBJECTIVE DATA**   There are no symptoms associated with melasma, freckles, lentigines, or postinflammatory changes. The depigmented areas of vitiligo sunburn easily.

III. **OBJECTIVE DATA**

A. **Melasma** appears as large, tan macules with irregular borders in a reticulated pattern on the cheeks, upper lip, and forehead.

B. **Freckles** are small (usually 2–5 mm), pale to dark macules scattered irregularly on the face, shoulders, back, and other sun-exposed areas. There is usually a sharp line of demarcation between freckled and unexposed skin.

C. **Lentigines** may be the same size as freckles, or may be larger; they may be found anywhere on the cutaneous surface. **Solar ("senile") lentigines** are pale to dark brown macules found on the dorsum of the hand and on the face. They vary in color and size (from millimeters to centimeters in diameter) and may have indistinct borders.

D. **The lesions of vitiligo** are completely depigmented—pure white—except in the rare case of trichrome vitiligo, which has both depigmented and hypopigmented areas. They usually have sharp borders and are found symmetrically over bony prominences such as the wrists and around body orifices (lips, eyes, and anogenital areas). Injury to the skin of these patients will cause a temporary or permanent loss of pigment in that area. Scars, scratch marks, and bruises may thus heal with no pigment present. Hair growing from vitiliginous skin may or may not be white.

E. **Postinflammatory pigment changes** vary in size and are present only in the site of previous inflammation and trauma. The degree of hyper- or hypopigmentation may be mild or marked.

IV. **ASSESSMENT** It is useful to examine pigmentary lesions under Wood's light (see also p. 241). Pigmented skin absorbs the light, and hypopigmented skin reflects it; the result is heightened contrast between normal and abnormal pigmentation. Borders become distinct, and faint lesions become noticeable. Pigment located in the dermis becomes less visible, while epidermal pigment becomes more prominent.

Patients with generalized lentigines and those with vitiligo deserve a thorough history and physical examination to search for related systemic findings. Phenolic germicidal agents present in many household and industrial products may cause depigmentation indistinguishable from that of vitiligo.

V. **THERAPY**

A. **Treatment of hyperpigmentation**

1. Lentigo and senile lentigines may be removed or their intensity of pigmentation diminished by light cryosurgical freezing (10–15 sec) with liquid nitrogen. Melanocytes are more sensitive to cold injury than keratinocytes and may be selectively damaged by this technique.

2. The intensity of pigmentation in melasma, freckles, and senile lentigines and the epidermal component of postinflammatory hyperpigmentation may be decreased by the conscientious application of 2–5% hydroquinone cream (Artra®, Eldoquin®, Eldoquin Forte®) 2–3id for weeks to months. Hydroquinone is thought to act by inhibiting one

or more steps in the tyrosine-tyrosinase pathway of melanin synthesis. It also affects the formation, melanization, and degradation of melanosomes and eventually causes necrosis of whole melanocytes. The hyperpigmented areas fade more rapidly and completely than surrounding normal skin; 80 percent of patients with melasma will note some improvement within an 8-week period.

a. As the ability of the sun to darken these lesions is much greater than that of hydroquinone to "bleach" the pigment, strict avoidance of sunlight is imperative. Although sunscreens may help, even visible light will cause some pigment darkening and, to be totally adequate, sun protection must therefore be opaque (Reflecta®, RVPaque®, zinc oxide cream). Some hydroquinone products are available in an opaque base (Eldopaque®, Eldopaque Forte®). Monobenzyl ether of hydroquinone (Benoquin®) usually causes irreversible depigmentation and should be used only to eliminate residual areas of normally pigmented skin in patients with extensive vitiligo. It should not be used under any other circumstances.

b. A more effective formula for decreasing skin pigment consists of 0.1% tretinoin, 5.0% hydroquinone, and 0.1% dexamethasone in hydrophilic ointment, or in equal parts ethanol and propylene glycol. Twice daily application to hyperpigmented areas should induce considerable lessening of pigmentation within 6 weeks. Peeling and redness usually precede hypopigmentation.

B. **Treatment of vitiligo**   There are four methods that may be useful:

1. *Bleaching* the surrounding skin in order to blur the margins of the lesion, or removing all remaining pigmentation in extensive cases.

    Blurring of the margins of the lesion may be attempted with hydroquinone compounds (Artra®, Eldoquin®, Eldoquin Forte®). *Permanent* removal of pigment requires the use of monobenzyl ether of hydroquinone (Benoquin®) cream.

2. *Complete avoidance of the sun,* or conscientious use of broad-spectrum sunscreens, thus fading normal pigmentation

in the fair-skinned individual and making the vitiligo less noticeable. Vitiligo patients should routinely use sunscreens effective against UVB (see p. 195) when outside to prevent sunburn in nonpigmented areas.

3. *Attempting to repigment skin* with the topical or systemic use of psoralen compounds.

As a general guide, if the vitiliginous skin is less than 6 cm^2 (quarter or half-dollar size), topical psoralens may be used; if up to 40 percent of the body surface is involved, systemic psoralens and sunlight are indicated; if the area involved is greater, consider depigmentation with monobenzyl ether of hydroquinone.

Psoralen compounds, tricyclic furocoumarin-like molecules found naturally in a variety of plants throughout the world and also produced synthetically, radically increase the erythema response of skin to long-wave ultraviolet light (UVA) after either topical application or systemic administration. For this reason, therapy must be initiated gradually. There appears to be no toxicity associated with long-term psoralen administration. Systemic treatment is begun with 0.6 mg/kg (40 mg for a 70-kg patient) of trioxsalen (Trisoralen®) ingested 2 hr before 20 min of noonday sun exposure. Exposure is increased by 10–20 min per day, until redness, beginning about 12–18 hr after sunning and becoming maximal at 48 hr, is achieved after each exposure. If 1½ hr of exposure is reached without producing the desired results, the amount of trioxsalen may be gradually increased in 10-mg increments to a maximum of 80 mg. An alternative method for children or those who like to be outdoors utilizes longer exposures but specifies that the first treatment be late in the afternoon, i.e., 4:30 PM, the second treatment at 4, the third at 3:30, etc. In place of trioxsalen, 20–50 mg methoxsalen (8-methoxypsoralen) may be used. This will definitely produce more erythema; it is not yet clear whether or not it leads to greater repigmentation. The danger of a severe burn is much greater with methoxsalen. Treatment should be 2–3 times weekly, never two days in a row. Patients should be instructed to wear blue-grey plastic-lens sunglasses before and after exposure on treatment days (UVA passes through glass). On nontreatment days, sun exposure as tolerated is permitted for patients being treated with trioxsalen but not for those on methoxsalen. Cloudy weather does not interfere with treatment; ambient temperature also has no effect. Following treatment, a sunscreen effective against UVA such as Uval®, Solbar®, or Piz Buin Exclusiv Extrem Cream® should be applied to all exposed skin; this will provide partial protection. Those who sunburn easily may benefit from using a UVB sunscreen such as Pabanol® or PreSun® all day, even during treatment. Prolonged exposure to sunlight beyond the treatment period is to be avoided for 8 hr after the medication has been ingested. Nontender, minimal pink coloration of the patches of vitiligo is acceptable, but if increasing redness develops, discontinue treatments until only faint pinkness remains.

Pigment reappears first as dots around hair follicles and then slowly spreads, becoming confluent. To be successful, therapy must continue for 9–18 months and often through several summers, beginning in early April and continuing through September. It is estimated that it takes about 200 exposures to bring about significant improvement. The age of the patient and duration of vitiligo do not affect the response rate. Lesions on the face and neck repigment more easily than those over bony prominences such as the dorsa of the hands, the elbows, and the knees. If treatment is discontinued before an area has completely filled in, the lesion is likely to gradually become white again. Psoralen therapy also increases the tolerance of vitiligo skin to sunlight, perhaps through thickening of the stratum corneum.

Topical 1% methoxsalen solution (Oxsoralen®) should be used as follows:

a. Treatment should initially be administered once every 5 days and may be gradually increased to every 3 days.

b. Methoxsalen should be applied with a cotton swab, allowed to dry 1–2 min, and reapplied. The borders of the lesion should be protected with petrolatum and a sunscreen to prevent hyperpigmentation.

c. After a wait of 1 hr, the area should be exposed for 4 min to a black light source at 4 cm (1½ inches) or to 1 min of sunlight. A Wood's light, a small hand-held black light (e.g., UVL-21, UV Products, San Gabriel, Calif.), or fluorescent black light tubes (e.g., F-40BL [GE]) may be used.

d. After treatment the area should be washed with soap and water and, if clothing does not cover the lesions, a benzophenone sunscreen or opaque sunscreen (see pp. 196, 329) should be applied. Benzophenone products have broad absorption and will protect from 250 to 360 nm; however, they provide only partial protection. Do not allow the treated area to be exposed to direct sunlight for 12 hr.

e. If erythema does not appear (first appearance in 24 hr with maximum at 48 hr), increase the exposure to black light during the next treatment by 2-min increments or exposure to sun by 1 min until an adequate response is achieved. Proceed cautiously, since even a small overexposure will result in blistering.

4. *To hide the lesion* with stains or cosmetics, use Covermark®, an excellent cosmetic makeup; Dy-o-Derm®, a stain that contains aniline dyes and dihydroxyacetone; or Vitadye®, a cosmetic cover containing FD and C dyes and dihydroxyacetone. These latter agents do *not* provide protection against sunburn, and psoralen phototherapy can take place through such stains.

REFERENCES

Arndt KA, Fitzpatrick TB: Topical use of hydroquinone as a depigmenting agent. JAMA 194:965–967, 1965

Belliboni N, Yagima ME: Epidemiology of pityriasis alba. Ann Brasileiros Dermatologica 50:135–140, 1975

Dawber RPR: Clinical associations of vitiligo. Postgrad Med J 46:276–277, 1970

Fitzpatrick TB, Arndt KA, El Mofty AM, Pathak MA: Hydroquinone and psoralens in the therapy of hypermelanosis and vitiligo. Arch Dermatol 93:589–600, 1966

Fitzpatrick TB, Quevedo W: Biological processes underlying melanin pigmentation and pigmentary disorders. Modern Trends in Dermatology, vol 4. Edited by P Borrie. Glasgow, Butterworth, 1971, pp 122–149

Gorlin RJ, Anderson RC, Blaw M: Multiple lentigines syndrome. Complex comprising multiple lentigines, electrocardiographic conduction abnormalities, ocular hypertelorism, pulmonary stenosis, abnormalities of genitalia, retardation of growth, sensorineural deafness and autosomal dominant hereditary pattern. Am J Dis Child 117: 652–662, 1969

Jimbow K, Obata H, Pathak MA, Fitzpatrick TB: Mechanism of depigmentation by hydroquinone. J Invest Dermatol 62:436–449, 1974

Kahn G: Depigmentation caused by phenolic detergent germicides. Arch Dermatol 102:177–187, 1970

Kligman AM, Willis I: A new formula for depigmenting human skin. Arch Dermatol 111:40–48, 1975

Lerner AB: On the etiology of vitiligo and gray hair. Am J Med 51:141–147, 1971

Mehregan AH: Lentigo senilis and its evolutions. J Invest Dermatol 65: 429–433, 1975

Newcomer VD, Lindberg MC, Sternberg TH: A melanosis of the face ("cholasma"). Arch Dermatol 83:284–299, 1961

Parrish JA, Fitzpatrick TB, Shea C, Pathak MA: Photochemotherapy of vitiligo. Arch Dermatol 112:1531–1534, 1976

18
Infestations:
Pediculosis, Scabies, and Ticks

I. DEFINITION AND PATHOPHYSIOLOGY

A. Pediculosis There are two species of blood-sucking lice specific for the human host: *Phthirus pubis* and *Pediculus humanus*. These wingless insects are obligate parasites and are host-specific for man. The lice that inhabit the head or body are both types of *P. humanus*. They look similar to one another and will interbreed; however, they do have different physiologic feeding habits. The head louse is transmitted through shared clothing and brushes; the body louse, by bedding or clothing; and the pubic louse, from person to person and not infrequently on clothing, bedding, or towels.

The adult *P. humanus* louse is 2–4 mm long, has 3 pairs of legs with delicate hooks at the tarsal extremities, and is gray-white in appearance. The crab louse (*P. pubis*), which inhabits the the genital region, is shorter (1–2 mm) and broader, and the first pair of legs is shorter than the clawlike second and third pair. The adult female louse has a lifespan of about 1 month and lays up to 10 eggs each day. As the lice feed, they inject their digestive juices and fecal material into the skin; it is this, plus the puncture wound itself, that causes pruritus. The ova (nits), which are oval, gray, and firmly attached to the hair, hatch in about 7–9 days and become mature in another week.

B. **Scabies** is caused by infestation with the mite *Sarcoptes scabiei*. *S. scabiei* has four pairs of legs and transverse corrugations and bristles on its dorsal aspect. The 0.3 mm × 0.4 mm female mite, just visible to the human eye, excavates a burrow in the stratum corneum and travels about 2 mm every day for 1–2 months before dying. Each female lays a total of 10–25 eggs. The eggs reach maturity in about 3 weeks and start a new cycle. Most infected adults will harbor 10–12 adult mites.

Scabies is acquired principally through close personal contact, but may be transmitted through clothing, linens, or towels. The female can survive for 2–3 days away from human beings. Incubation period is usually less than 1 month but can be as long as 2 months. The severe pruritus is probably caused by an acquired sensitivity to the organism and is first noted 2–4 weeks after primary infestation, but sooner in subsequent infections. Canine scabies (sarcoptic mange) causes crusting and hair loss over the ear margins, legs, and abdomen of dogs. This is highly communicable and may result in small epidemics in man.

C. **Ticks** are large mites covered by a tough integument. These ectoparasites live by sucking blood from mammals, birds, and reptiles. They are found in trees, grass, or bushes, or on animals (dogs, cattle); after attaching to human skin, the female tick feeds, becomes engorged after 7–14 days, and then drops off. Ticks are capable of transmitting several rickettsial (e.g., Rocky Mountain spotted fever) and viral (e.g., encephalitis) diseases.

II. SUBJECTIVE DATA

A. Extreme pruritus is the primary characteristic of pediculosis. In some sensitized patients, generalized pruritus, urticaria, and eczematous changes may develop.

B. Scabies is noted for severe itching, which becomes most marked shortly after the patient goes to bed. Early in the course only the sites of burrows are pruritic; later, the itching may become generalized.

C. Tick bites are painless; often they are discovered several days later when itching develops or the engorged tick is found. Occasionally symptoms of fever, headache, and abdominal pain may occur while the feeding tick remains attached. Children very rarely can develop a reversible flaccid paralysis that starts after the tick has been attached for several days.

III. OBJECTIVE DATA

A. Pediculosis

1. *Scalp*

a. Nits may be found most easily on the hairs on the occiput and above the ears.

b. Adult lice are often impossible to find, and, in the average case, there will be fewer than 10 mature insects present.

c. Secondary impetigo and furunculosis with associated cervical lymphadenopathy is a frequent complication.

2. *Body*

a. Scratch marks, eczematous changes, urticaria, and persistent erythematous papules may be seen. Lesions frequently are most noticeable on the back.

b. The lice will be found in the seams of clothing and only rarely on the skin.

3. *Pubic*

a. Pubic and thigh hair can be infested by only a few or by uncountable numbers of nits.

b. The yellow-gray adults may be difficult to find.

c. Small black dots present in infested areas represent either ingested blood in adult lice or their excreta.

d. Body and axillary hair as well as the eyelashes and beard also should be examined for nits.

B. Scabies

1. Multiple straight or S-shaped ridges or dotted lines, 5–20 mm long, that frequently resemble a black thread and end in a vesicle, represent the characteristic burrow, although this

need not be present. Mites are also in papules and vesicles, the most common presenting lesions.

2. Sites of involvement are chiefly the interdigital webs of the hands, wrists, antecubital fossae, points of the elbows, nipples, umbilicus, lower abdomen, genitalia, and gluteal cleft. Lesions of the glans penis are characteristic in males. Infants and small children often have lesions on the palms, soles, head, and neck.

3. Generalized urticarial papules, excoriations, and eczematous changes are secondary lesions caused by sensitization to the mite.

4. Indurated erythematous nodules are more common than discrete burrows and are slow to resolve after treatment.

5. Secondary bacterial infection with impetiginization and furunculosis are common.

6. Canine scabies lesions are papules or vesicles without burrows seen on the trunk, arms, or abdomen.

C. **Ticks** The engorged tick, often the size of a large pea, may resemble a vascular tumor or wart.

1. Previously sensitized hosts may develop a localized urticarial response.

2. The usual bite reaction shows small dermal nodules surmounted by necrotic centers.

3. Granulomatous response to tick bites causes lesions that resemble dermal fibromas (dermatofibroma, histiocytoma).

IV. ASSESSMENT

A. Unexplained pyoderma of the scalp, inflammatory cervical or occipital adenopathy, or itching with mild inflammation of the occipital scalp and nuchal area should be attributed to pediculosis until proved otherwise. It is necessary to be persistent in searching for nits. If suspicion is high, a therapeutic trial or reexamination in 2–3 days is indicated.

Unexplained pubic pruritus very frequently is a manifestation of pediculosis. In fastidious individuals few adult lice and nits will be found, and a careful search—ideally employing a hand lens—should be made, with special attention to the genital area.

B. The diagnosis of scabies is made by first removing the mite from the burrow: A drop of mineral or immersion oil is placed over the lesion, the superficial epidermis scraped off with the edge of a #15 scalpel blade and placed on a microscope slide, and examined under 10× or 25× magnification. Demonstration of the eggs or the oval, brown-black fecal concretions is also diagnostic. Burrows or papules are found most often between the fingers, on the flexor aspect of the wrists, or on the ulnar aspect of the hands. It may sometimes be difficult to find either the burrow or the mite, and in that case the clinical picture of intense pruritus and papular and excoriated lesions will lead one to the correct diagnosis. The mite of canine scabies is easily demonstrated in scrapings from the dog, but rarely seen in preparations taken from human lesions.

V. THERAPY

A. Gamma benzene hexachloride (GBH) (Gamene®, Kwell®), a pesticide also known as Lindane, is the treatment of choice for pediculosis and scabies (see p. 288). GBH is available as a shampoo for the treatment of pediculosis capitis and/or pubis, and in cream and lotion form for treating scabies and all forms of pediculosis. GBH also repels ticks and other arthropods and kills chiggers. Up to 10% of the topically applied drug may be absorbed percutaneously; alternative treatments should therefore be used in infants, young children, and pregnant women.

GBH and benzyl benzoate kill the lice, but the dead organisms do not fall off hairs or body spontaneously. Most patients regard the continuing presence of dead organisms as evidence of continuing infestation and it is necessary to clearly instruct them otherwise. Application of a 1:1 solution of white vinegar and water followed by a shower, or combing the hair with a comb dipped directly into vinegar, may help dissolve the dead nits cemented to the hairs and wash off their remains. The only certain way to remove dead nits is with a fine-toothed comb or forceps.

1. *For pediculosis capitis or pubis,* 1 oz of shampoo is worked into a lather and left on the scalp or genital area for 5 min. After thorough rinsing, the hair should be cleaned with a fine-toothed comb to remove nit shells. Although usually not necessary, shampooing may be repeated in 24 hr but not more than twice in one week. Pediculocides have not been shown to be ovicidal.

2. ***For pediculosis corporis*** the patient need only wash with soap and water and apply topical antipruritic lotions. If lice get on the body, GBH should be used. Lice in clothing may be killed by boiling, followed by ironing the seams, dry cleaning, or by applying dry heat at 140°F for 20 min. Alternatively, they may be eliminated by dusting with 1% malathion powder or 10% DDT powder.

3. ***Pediculosis pubis*** should be treated with application of GBH cream or lotion to infested and adjacent areas for 24 hr. Alternatively, the shampoo can be used as described above. Clothing, linens, and towels should be washed in very hot water or dry cleaned. Treatment may be repeated in 1 week if necessary.

   a. Eyelash infestation with pediculosis pubis may be treated by applying:

      (1) 0.025% physostigmine ophthalmic ointment with a cotton-tipped applicator.

      (2) Petrolatum applied thickly twice daily for 8 days; or

      (3) Yellow oxide of mercury

4. ***Scabies*** is treated by application of GBH cream or lotion to the entire body from the neck down, with particular attention to the interdigital webs, wrists, elbows, axillae, breasts, buttocks, and genitalia. Approximately 30–60 gm or 60–120 ml is required to cover the trunk and extremities of an average adult. Medication should be applied for 24 hr, and then washed off. At that point, clothing should be thoroughly washed in hot water or dry cleaned and linens and towels changed. Transmission of scabies is unlikely after 24 hr of treatment. A second application 1 week later would destroy any recently hatched larvae or nymphs, as none of the scabicides has been shown to be ovicidal.

B. **Alternative treatments for scabies** are necessary because there may be an increasing incidence of mites resistant to GBH.

   1. Persistent itching in treated scabies patients may be due to either continued infestation, a slowly subsiding hypersensitivity response, or irritation from overuse of GBH.

a. Lesions should again be examined for the presence of mites. If persistent infection is judged present, retreatment or more vigorous treatment with GBH, or the alternative methods noted below should be used.

b. Persistent pruritic nodules may remain in patients seemingly otherwise cured of scabies. These lesions are similar to prurigo (neurodermatitis) nodules and respond only to intralesional corticosteroid injection.

c. If itching is related to sensitization, treatment with topical corticosteroids or with a short (7–10-day) tapering course of oral corticosteroids will bring relief.

2. *Crotamiton (10% N-ethyl-o-crotonotoluide; Eurax®)* cream applied twice during a 48-hr period is effective against scabies and also acts as an antipruritic agent (see p. 289). It is the usual primary alternate therapy.

3. *6–10% precipitated sulfur* in a water-washable base (or in petrolatum, which is messier), applied nightly for 3 nights, remains a reliable treatment. Patients may complain of the sulfur odor. This is the treatment of choice for infants and pregnant women.

4. *20–25% benzyl benzoate* in an alcoholic vehicle or emulsion applied daily for 48–72 hr is also effective (see p. 288).

5. *10% thiabendazole* suspension applied twice daily for 5 days or 10-day courses of oral thiabendazole (25 mg/kg daily) also have been reported to be useful.

C. Alternative treatments for pediculosis are also available.

1. *Pyrithrins* (A-200 Pyrinate®, RID®), rapid-acting compounds derived from chrysanthemum plants, are the leading over-the-counter louse remedy. Medication is applied for 10 min and then rinsed off. It should not be used more than twice within a 24-hr period.

2. *Copper oleate-tetrahydronaphthalene lotion (Cuprex®)* applied for 15 min to infected areas may be used for the eradication of head and pubic lice.

3. The WHO Expert Committee (1970) recommends an emulsion concentrate designated Enbin® (68% benzyl benzoate,

6% DDT, 12% benzocaine, 14% polysorbate 80) and 1% gamma benzene hexachloride in alcohol, both requiring 1:5 dilution with water before application.

4. *A 2–5% DDT emulsion, 10% DDT powder, 0.5% malathion lotion, or 1% malathion powder* are all effective against mature lice and larvae but not against nits. However, these preparations remain on the skin and clothing long enough for the nits to mature and be destroyed at that time. These agents are particularly effective in epidemics and in mass delousing.

D. **Epidemiologic treatment** Family, close friends, sexual contacts, and those sharing quarters of patients with pediculosis or scabies all should be considered for treatment to prevent reinfection or a small epidemic.

E. **Protection against tick infestation** is best accomplished by applying repellents to clothing. The most efficient agent is diethyltoluamide (deet) (see p. 319).

F. **Tick removal methods** are multiple and each has its advocates. The important consideration is that the organism not be crushed while being taken off the skin.

1. The easiest and most efficient method entails grasping the tick near its mouth with forceps and lifting it gently upward and forward. A needle or other sharply pointed object should be inserted between the tick and skin to help pry it out.

2. If tightly adherent or deeply embedded, the tick may be induced to loosen its grasp by touching it with a hot object, such as a matchhead that has just been extinguished or a hot nail, or by applying a few drops of a solvent such as chloroform or gasoline.

REFERENCES

Ackerman AB: Crabs—the resurgence of *Phthirus pubis.* N Engl J Med 278:950–951, 1968

Carslow RW: Skin infestation. Practitioner 216:154–158, 1976

Charlesworth EN, Johnson JL: An epidemic of canine scabies in man. Arch Dermatol 110:572–574, 1974

Feldman RJ, Maibach HI: Percutaneous penetration of some pesticides and herbicides in man. Toxicol Appl Pharmacol 28:126–132, 1974

Hejazi N, Mehregan AH: Scabies—histological study of inflammatory lesions. Arch Dermatol 111:37–39, 1975

Hubler WR, Clabaugh W: Epidemic Norwegian scabies. Arch Dermatol 112:179–181, 1976

Marples MJ: The Ecology of the Human Skin. Springfield, Ill., Thomas, 1965, 970 pp

Mellanby K: Scabies (2nd Ed.). Hampton, EW Classey, 1943

Muller G, Jacobs PH, Moore NE: Scraping for human scabies. A better method for positive preparations. Arch Dermatol 107:70, 1973

Orkin M: Today's scabies. JAMA 233:882–885, 1975

Orkin M, Epstein E, Maibach HI: Treatment of today's scabies and pediculosis. JAMA 236:1136–1139, 1976

19
Intertrigo

I. **DEFINITION AND PATHOPHYSIOLOGY** Intertrigo is an inflammatory dermatosis involving the body folds. It is most common in obese individuals during hot weather and is found principally in the inframammary, axillary, and inguinal folds, but it may also affect the other similar areas (folds of the upper eyelids, neck creases, antecubital fossae, and umbilical, perineal, and interdigital areas). As a result of skin constantly rubbing on skin, the heat, moisture, and sweat retention lead to maceration, inflammation, and often secondary bacterial or *Candida albicans* infection.

Other eruptions that localize in the body folds and must therefore be differentiated from simple intertrigo include seborrheic dermatitis, psoriasis, dermatophyte infections, erythrasma, and miliaria.

II. **SUBJECTIVE DATA** Mild or early involvement is associated with soreness or itching. The more intense the inflammation, the more severe the discomfort.

III. **OBJECTIVE DATA** Mild erythema is seen initially. This may then progress to more intense inflammation with erosions, oozing, exudation, and crusting. Finally, vegetative changes, overt purulence, and surrounding cellulitis may arise in these areas.

IV. ASSESSMENT

A. Examine pustule contents or scales microscopically and by culture for evidence of bacterial, *Candida,* or dermatophyte infection.

B. Initiate investigation for and treatment of associated medical conditions such as diabetes and obesity.

V. THERAPY

A. **Environmental changes** to promote drying and to aerate the body folds are essential.

  1. The living and working areas should be cool and dry. Air conditioning or fans will help. Having the patient disrobe for at least 30 min 2id and expose the involved folds to a fan or electric bulb will promote drying.

  2. Clothing should be light, nonconstricting, and absorbent, avoiding wool, nylon, and synthetic fibers. Bras should provide good support. Prolonged sitting and driving are obviously harmful.

  3. Wash, rinse, and dry intertriginous areas at least twice daily and liberally apply a talc-containing powder.

  4. Occlusive, oily, or irritant ointments or cosmetics do more harm than good and should be avoided. Lotions, sprays, powders, creams or gels may be useful.

B. **Specific measures**

  1. Apply cooling tap water or Burow's solution compresses or soaks 3–4id to exudative areas.

  2. Separate folds with absorbent material, e.g., cotton sheeting well dusted with drying powders. Cornstarch should not be used, as it will encourage bacterial and fungal overgrowth.

  3. Initially, corticosteroid or steroid-antibiotic lotions, creams, or gels should be applied 4–6id, but prolonged use should be avoided, since continued application of fluorinated steroids may lead to intertriginous striae and cutaneous atrophy. Hydrocortisone (1%), with or without iodochlorhydroxyquin (Vioform® or Vioform®-hydrocortisone), will usually be effective and its use obviates concern about corticosteroid side-effects.

4. Bland lotions (calamine) are soothing and drying.

5. Some physicians apply drying antiseptic dye preparations to these areas and instruct patients to use them once daily thereafter. One-half or full strength Castellani's paint (fuchsin, phenol, and resorcinol [see p. 284]) or 0.5–1% gentian violet solution may be used. These dyes are very effective but messy and may sting or burn on application.

20
Keloids and Hypertrophic Scars

I. **DEFINITION AND PATHOPHYSIOLOGY** Keloids and hypertrophic scars both represent an excessive connective tissue response to cutaneous injury. These fibroblastic lesions may differ only slightly in clinical and histologic appearance, but they represent quite different types of tissue growth and require somewhat different treatments.

The circumstances that increase the likelihood of developing keloids or hypertrophic scars are similar. Excessive or poorly aligned tension on a wound, the introduction of foreign material into the skin, and certain types of trauma, such as burns, all are provocative factors. Some areas of the body—presternal, shoulders, back, chin, ears, lower legs—are much more at risk. Blacks and deeply pigmented individuals are affected more frequently, and young adults develop lesions much more commonly than do children or the elderly.

The excessive amount of collagen found in keloids or hypertrophic scars is not resistant to degradation. These lesions lack neither the ability to synthesize collagenase nor do they contain collagen resistant to this enzyme. A collagenase proenzyme recently has been found, and it is possible that its activation in vivo may be suppressed in certain types of scars. Some preliminary data suggest that the tendency to form keloids is transmitted as a single autosomal dominant gene and results in defective fibroblasts that synthesize collagen more rapidly than normal scars. The keloid-former's collagen may be abnormal as well.

II.   **SUBJECTIVE DATA**   Keloids are usually asymptomatic, although some are pruritic and others may be quite painful and tender.

III.   **OBJECTIVE DATA** (See color insert.)

A.   Hypertrophic scars appear as scars that are more elevated, wider, or thicker than expected. They correspond in size and shape to the inciting wound.

B.   Keloids start as pink or red, firm, well-defined, telangiectatic, rubbery plaques which for several months may be difficult to distinguish from hypertrophic scars. Later, uncontrolled overgrowth causes extension beyond the size of the original wound, and the tumor becomes smoother, irregularly shaped, hyperpigmented, harder, and more symptomatic. The tendency to send out clawlike prolongations is typical of keloids.

IV.   **THERAPY**

A.   **Hypertrophic scars** usually require no treatment and often spontaneously resolve in 6–12 months. However, they will respond to intralesional corticosteroid injections as noted below, or they may be managed by careful reexcision, as they tend to recur much less readily than keloids.

B.   **Keloids**

1.   Prophylactic considerations are of paramount importance. Clearly, optional elective surgical procedures should be avoided in keloid-formers. When surgery is necessary for cosmetic reasons, early childhood is the best time. Scalpel surgery with strict aseptic technique and avoidance of wound tension is mandatory. Electrosurgery and chemosurgery should be avoided; cryosurgical procedures are usually not followed by keloid formation.

2.   Intralesional corticosteroid injection by syringe or needleless jet injector often brings excellent results and is the treatment of choice.

a. In this instance one strives to achieve with corticosteroids the effect we most often try to avoid: atrophy. Therefore, use of high concentrations of medication (triamcinolone acetonide, 10 or 40 mg/ml) injected undiluted at 4-week intervals is warranted. Multiple injections over several months (to years) may be necessary.

b. Initially it may be difficult to force much medication into the tough collagenous mass. As the lesion softens and flattens, injection is more easily accomplished.

c. Injections at more frequent intervals may result in too marked a result, leading to a depressed atrophic lesion.

d. Perilesional atrophy and perilymphactic atrophy around draining vessels may be seen but will resolve over the subsequent 3–12 months.

3. Small lesions (less than 5 cm) may respond to cryosurgery with liquid nitrogen or CO_2 repeated q2–3 weeks.

4. Larger lesions or those in suitable areas may be reexcised or treated by radiation therapy, or both. When excising keloids it is desirable to dilute the local anesthetic 1:1 with a corticosteroid suspension and to reinject the healing wound with corticosteroids at 2–3 weekly intervals. Some also advocate postexcision x-ray therapy at 2-week intervals. Radiation therapy alone is often beneficial, particularly with lesions of less than 6 months' duration.

REFERENCES

Griffith BH, Monroe CW, McKinney P: A follow-up study on the treatment of keloids with triamcinolone acetonide. Plast Reconstr Surg 46:145–150, 1970

Ketchum LD, Smith J, Robinson DW, Masters FW: The treatment of hypertrophic scar, keloid and scar contracture by triamcinolone acetonide. Plast Reconstr Surg 38:209–218, 1966

Koonin AJ: The etiology of keloids: A review of the literature and a new hypothesis. S Afr Med J 38:913–916, 1964

Maguire HC Jr.: Treatment of keloids with triamcinolone acetonide injected intralesionally. JAMA 192:325–326, 1965

Mancini RE, Quaife JV: Histogenesis of experimentally produced keloids. J Invest Dermatol 38:143–181, 1962

Milsom JP, Craig RD: Collagen degradation in cultured keloid and hypertrophic scar tissue. Br J Dermatol 89:635–644, 1973

Peacock EE, Madden JW, Trier WC: Biologic basis for the treatment of keloids and hypertrophic scars. South Med J 63:755–760, 1970

Wilson WW: Prophylaxis against postsurgical keloids: results in 500 patients. South Med J 58:751–753, 1965

21
Keratoses

I. DEFINITION AND PATHOPHYSIOLOGY

A. **Seborrheic keratoses** are benign, noninvasive, hyperplastic epidermal lesions found most profusely on the face, shoulders, chest, and back. They are the most common skin tumor seen in the middle-aged and elderly population and are termed seborrheic only in relation to their greasy appearance and their location in areas that have many sebaceous glands. There is no known relationship to sebaceous gland function, seborrhea, or seborrheic dermatitis; their cause is unknown. In mature seborrheic keratoses, DNA synthesis is decreased while RNA and protein synthesis are increased. Concern about these lesions is primarily cosmetic; occasionally they cause anxiety because their dark color raises the question of melanoma.

B. **Actinic (solar, senile) keratoses** are premalignant lesions caused by the cumulative effects of solar radiation on the skin and are located solely on the exposed surfaces: face, ears, bald scalp, dorsa of the forearms, and hands. They may be seen in fair-skinned individuals in their twenties and thirties but are most common around age 50 and later. Without treatment up to one-eighth of patients may have one or more lesions that will invade as squamous cell carcinoma; however, progression to very aggressive lesions accompanied by metastasis rarely occurs.

II. SUBJECTIVE DATA

A. Seborrheic keratoses, particularly those in intertriginous areas, may itch intensely.

B. Actinic keratoses are usually asymptomatic.

III. OBJECTIVE DATA (See color insert.)

A. Seborrheic keratoses start as small, multiple, flesh-colored, yellow or tan, waxy papules, and slowly grow to become dark brown or black, greasy, verrucous lesions with a distinct border. The rough scale may sometimes flake or be rubbed off but will always regrow. A variant of seborrheic keratoses termed **dermatosis papulosa nigra** is seen primarily on the cheeks in blacks as multiple small, dark, pedunculated papules.

B. Actinic keratoses first appear as flesh-colored to pink, flat or slightly raised, well-defined, scaly lesions. They feel rough or like sandpaper on palpation and usually arise from obviously sun-damaged skin (dry, wrinkled, atrophic, telangiectatic). Whereas parts of seborrheic keratoses can easily be scraped off with the fingernail or a tongue blade, this is not at all true of actinic lesions. A horny, keratotic, conical protuberance, termed a **cutaneous horn,** may develop from an actinic keratosis. (Cutaneous horns may also form on verrucous epidermal nevi, warts, seborrheic keratoses, and squamous cell carcinomas.)

IV. ASSESSMENT
Any doubts concerning the exact diagnosis of the keratosis may be resolved by pathologic examination of a 4-mm punch biopsy, shave biopsy, or curettage specimen. The base of all cutaneous horns should be submitted for histologic diagnosis.

V. THERAPY

A. **Seborrheic keratoses** are benign lesions, and therapy should therefore be as simple, rapid, and cosmetically acceptable as possible. After treatment, a small area of hypopigmentation may be left at the site of the keratosis.

1. Simple curettage, with or without anesthesia, is the easiest method and leaves the best cosmetic result. Lesions lightly frozen with ethyl chloride, CO_2, or liquid nitrogen may sometimes be more easily scraped off. Monsel's solution (ferric subsulfate), Gelfoam®, Oxycel®, weak acids (30% trichloroacetic), or pressure alone may be used for hemostasis. Light electrodesiccation will accomplish the same end but adds the possibility of inducing a small scar. Lesions should remain uncovered or have only a light, non-occlusive dressing.

2. Application of liquid nitrogen (15–20 sec) or dry ice will also result in removal of lesions without a subsequent cicatrix. Multiple areas can be treated easily without anesthesia by this method.

3. Excision or radiotherapy is unwarranted.

4. Lesions of dermatosis papulosa nigra may be treated by light electrosurgery, cryosurgery, or curettage; it is particularly important not to treat too aggressively so as to avoid posttreatment hypopigmentation.

B. Actinic keratoses

1. ***Prophylactic measures*** Patients must first be told that these lesions are a result of damage from the sun and should be instructed to avoid further damage from solar radiation (see p. 195).

2. ***Single or isolated lesions*** may be treated by any of the following methods:

    a. *Cryotherapy* with liquid nitrogen (20–30 sec) or dry ice application.

    b. *Curettage and electrodesiccation* under local anesthesia. This is a simple and rapid procedure and the wound heals quickly; in addition, this method provides tissue for histologic diagnosis. Mild acids (30–50% trichloroacetic acid) or Monsel's solution (ferric subsulfate) may be used for hemostasis.

    c. *Shave excision* (scalpel skimming) followed by electrosurgery or chemosurgery (acids).

    d. *Excision and primary closure* is almost always a more extensive procedure than the lesion warrants.

3. *Multiple and/or extensive lesions* are best treated with application of topical 5-fluorouracil (5-FU). This has the advantage of easily treating large areas of involvement and also of eliminating subclinical keratoses. The primary disadvantage is the brisk inflammatory response that accompanies successful therapy. A small number of treated patients have been found to have developed an allergic contact sensitivity to 5-FU. Medications should be used as follows:

    a. *Sequential method*

      (1) 5-FU is available as a 1% (Fluoroplex®), a 2% (Efudex®), and 5% (Efudex®) solution in propylene glycol, and a 1% (Fluoroplex®) and 5% (Efudex®) cream (see p. 321). Alternatively, a 1% solution may be prepared by diluting a 10-ml ampule of 5-FU (Fluorouracil, Roche®) with 40 ml of propylene glycol. At equivalent concentrations the solutions are more effective than creams. Higher concentrations induce a more severe inflammatory response but may be followed by slightly more complete involution of lesions and a lower recurrence rate. The higher concentration should always be used on areas other than the head and neck. On the face, the 1 or 2% solution or 1% cream often is sufficient.

      (2) Medication should be applied twice daily with a nonmetal applicator, gloved hand, or fingers (followed by hand washing). Care should be taken to avoid the eyes, scrotum, and mucous membranes of the nose and mouth.

      (3) The sequence of response is erythema, vesiculation, erosion, superficial ulceration, necrosis, and reepithelialization. Medication should be continued until the inflammatory response is at the ulceration and necrosis stage, which is usually 2–4 weeks. Patients may complain of intense burning and pain.

(4) At the point of ulceration, 5-FU may be stopped and a topical corticosteroid cream applied to hasten involution of the inflammation.

(5) Complete healing will be evident within 1–2 months. The cosmetic results are usually excellent. Residual postinflammatory hyperpigmentation occasionally follows this therapy.

(6) Patients should avoid excessive exposure to sunlight during 5-FU treatment or the intensity of the reaction may be increased.

b. *Combined method* (for face)

(1) Apply 1% 5-FU solution, and after 15 min apply 0.5% triamcinolone acetonide cream. Repeat nightly for 3 weeks.

(2) This method appears to be equally effective and may decrease or eliminate the brisk inflammation associated with the sequential method.

c. The effectiveness of the medication may be increased by applying both 5% 5-FU and 0.05% retinoic acid solution (tretinoin; Retin-A® cream) together 2id until lesions exacerbate, and then continuing with 5-FU for another 2–3 weeks. The tretinoin may act to increase percutaneous penetration but may also possibly have a direct effect upon keratoses. This is most useful for resistant areas such as the forearms or trunk.

d. 5-FU treatment should be repeated at yearly intervals in patients with severely sun-damaged skin.

4. ***Dermabrasion*** may also be effective for treatment of widespread facial actinic keratoses.

REFERENCES

Arndt KA, Freedberg IM: Macromolecular metabolism in hyperplastic epidermal disease—a radio-autographic study. Br J Dermatol 91: 541–548, 1974

Becker SW: Seborrheic keratosis and verruca, with special reference to the melanotic variety. Arch Dermatol 63:358–372, 1951

Breza T, Taylor R, Eaglstein WH: Noninflammatory destruction of ac-
    tinic keratoses by fluorouracil. Arch Dermatol 112:1256–1258, 1976
Dillaha CJ, Jansen GT, Honeycutt WM, Holt GA: Further studies with
    topical 5-fluorouracil. Arch Dermatol 92:410–417, 1965
Graham JH: Precancerous lesions of the skin. Part I. Dermatol Digest
    16–22, March 1970
Pinkus H: Keratosis senilis: a biologic concept of its pathogenesis and
    diagnosis based on the study of normal epidermis and 1,730 sebor-
    rheic and senile keratoses. Am J Clin Pathol 29:193–207, 1958
Pinkus H: Epithelial and fibroepithelial tumors. Arch Dermatol 91:24–
    37, 1965
Robinson TA, Kligman AM: Treatment of solar keratoses of the ex-
    tremities with retinoic acid and 5-fluorouracil. Br J Dermatol 92:
    703–706, 1975
Sanderson KA: The structure of seborrhoeic keratoses. Br J Dermatol
    80:588–593, 1968
Spira M, Freeman R, Arfai P, Gerow FJ, Hardy SB: Clinical comparison
    of chemical peeling, dermabrasion and 5-FU for senile keratoses.
    Plast Reconstr Surg 46:61–66, 1970
Williams AC, Klein E: Experiences with local chemotherapy and im-
    munotherapy in premalignant and malignant skin lesions. Cancer
    25:450–462, 1970

22
Milia

I. **DEFINITION AND PATHOPHYSIOLOGY** Milia are asymptomatic, small, subepidermal, keratinous cysts found in individuals of all ages, most often on the face. Primary milia are noninflammatory collections of lamellated keratin most frequently found within the undifferentiated sebaceous cells that surround vellus hair follicles. Milia found in infants tend to disappear spontaneously in a few months, but lesions in adults are chronic. Most arise spontaneously, but others may be localized in areas of damaged skin associated with bullous disease (porphyria cutanea tarda, dermolytic bullous dermatosis) and in areas treated by dermabrasion. These secondary milia arise predominantly from eccrine duct epithelium.

II. **SUBJECTIVE DATA** Facial milia are of cosmetic significance only.

III. **OBJECTIVE DATA** Milia appear as tiny (1–2 mm), white, raised, round lesions covered by a thinned epidermis found primarily on the cheeks and eyelids. No orifice can be seen.

IV.   ASSESSMENT   Inquire regarding previous inflammatory or blistering skin disease, trauma, or photosensitivity.

V.   THERAPY

    A.   Milia are easily removed without anesthesia as follows:

        1.   Gently incise the thin epidermis covering the milium with a #11 scalpel blade.

        2.   Carefully sever and tease away any connection or adhesions between the cyst and the overlying skin.

        3.   Apply mild pressure with a comedone extractor, curet, tongue blades, or the dull edge of the scalpel blade. The small keratin kernel should pop out as an intact ball.

    B.   Light electrodesiccation with a fine needle is also an effective method.

REFERENCES

Epstein W, Kligman AM: The pathogenesis of milia and benign tumors of the skin. J Invest Dermatol 26:1–11, 1956

Tsuji T, Sugai T, Suzuki S: The mode of growth of eccrine duct milia. J Invest Dermatol 65:388–393, 1975

23
Molluscum Contagiosum

I. **DEFINITION AND PATHOPHYSIOLOGY** Molluscum contagiosum is a viral tumor limited to man and monkeys and caused by a DNA-containing poxvirus. It cannot be easily cultured. The disease is contracted from other people by direct contact, through fomites, and by autoinoculation. Children with atopic dermatitis may be more easily infected. Estimates of the incubation period range from 2 weeks to 2 months. Molluscum lesions formerly were found primarily in children on the face and trunk, but now they are also being seen very commonly in the pubic area and genitalia of sexually active young adults. Many lesions are self-limited in duration (9 months) but others will last for years.

II. **SUBJECTIVE DATA** Most lesions of molluscum are asymptomatic. Occasionally, large lesions become inflamed and look and feel like a furuncle. Chronic conjunctivitis or keratitis may accompany lesions located on or near the eyelids.

III. **OBJECTIVE DATA (See color insert.)** Molluscum lesions are discrete, skin-colored or pearly white, raised, waxy-appearing, firm papules 1–5 mm in diameter, with a central punctate umbilication. They are found alone or in clusters on the face, trunk, lower abdomen, pubis, inner thighs, and penis. Mucosal lesions may be present.

IV.   **ASSESSMENT**   Diagnosis may be confirmed by incising one of the papules, smearing the contents between two glass slides, staining (with Wright's, Giemsa, Gram, or the rose bengal stain #2 of the Swartz-Medrik fungal stain), and then viewing under low or high dry magnification. Molluscum bodies, which are cytoplasmic masses consisting of mature, immature, and incomplete virus and cellular debris, are ovoid, smooth-walled, and homogeneous, and are up to 25μ in diameter. The lesions most often confused with molluscum are warts.

V.   **THERAPY**   Molluscum can be successfully treated by any of the following methods:

A.   Cryotherapy with liquid nitrogen (10–15 sec) or dry ice is generally the best treatment.

B.   Removal of the lesion with a sharp curet. Anesthesia is often not necessary. Some recommend touching the base of the lesion with iodine or a mild acid (30% trichloroacetic acid).

C.   Light electrodessication.

D.   Application of a vesicant such as cantharidin (Cantharone®) alone, or covered with Blenderm® (3M Co.) tape overnight. This method, though effective, may cause a severe inflammatory reaction. A keratolytic paint (16.7% salicylic acid, 16.7% lactic acid in flexible collodion; Duofilm®) may be used in the same fashion and will not cause as much inflammation.

REFERENCES

Glickman FS, Silvers SH: Eczema and molluscum contagiosum. JAMA 223:1512, 1973

Henao M, Freeman RA: Inflammatory molluscum contagiosum: clinico-pathological study of seven cases. Arch Dermatol 90:479–482, 1964

Leading article: Molluscum contagiosum. Br Med J 1:459–460, 1968

Lynch PJ: Molluscum contagiosum venereum. Clin Obstet Gynecol 15:966–975, 1972

Mehregan AH: Molluscum contagiosum. A clinicopathologic study. Arch Dermatol 84:123–127, 1961

Postlethwaite R: Molluscum contagiosum. A review. Arch Environ Health 21:432–452, 1970

Sutton JS, Burnett JW: Ultrastructural changes in dermal and epidermal cells of skin infected with molluscum contagiosum virus. J Ultrastruct Res 26:177–196, 1969

24
Pityriasis Rosea

I. **DEFINITION AND PATHOPHYSIOLOGY** Pityriasis rosea is a mild scaling eruption seen predominantly in adolescents and young adults during the spring and fall. It is self-limited in duration and thought to be viral in origin, although this is unproved. The lesions usually disappear within 6–8 weeks, and recurrences are uncommon.

II. **SUBJECTIVE DATA** Pityriasis rosea may be asymptomatic or pruritic, at times intensely so. The onset of the eruption is sometimes coincident with mild malaise and symptoms similar to a viral upper respiratory tract infection.

III. **OBJECTIVE DATA** (See color insert.)

A. The initial lesion is frequently a 2–6 cm, round, erythematous, scaling plaque, which may appear anywhere on the body. This "herald patch" is not present, or at least not noticed, in 20–30 percent of cases.

B. Within several days to 2 weeks, small 1–2 cm pale, red, round to oval macular and papular lesions with a crinkly surface and a rim of fine scales appear in crops on the trunk and proximal extremities.

C. The face, hands, and feet usually are spared except in children.

D. The long axes of the lesions are oriented in the planes of cleavage running parallel to the ribs and classically are said to form a fir-tree-like pattern.

E. Lesions may be few or almost confluent, slowly enlarging by peripheral extension, and can continue to appear for 7–10 days.

F. Variants of pityriasis rosea at times seem to appear as commonly as the classic disease.

    1. In children the lesions are often papular.

    2. Vesicular and bullous lesions may be seen.

    3. Occasionally, eruptions may be limited to the shoulder or groin region.

    4. Urticarial, intensely inflammatory, and very symptomatic lesions are less common.

IV. ASSESSMENT

A. The eruption is usually easily diagnosed by its morphology and distribution.

B. A serologic test for syphilis should be drawn on all patients, since secondary syphilis may mimic pityriasis rosea almost exactly.

C. Other differential diagnostic considerations include tinea corporis, seborrheic dermatitis, acute psoriasis, and tinea versicolor.

D. Lesions that do not resolve in 8–12 weeks should suggest chronic parapsoriasis or pityriasis lichenoides et varioliformis acuta (PLEVA), and a punch biopsy is indicated.

V. THERAPY

A. Most patients require no treatment.

B. Erythema doses of ultraviolet light or sunlight will almost always provide relief of pruritus and hasten involution of lesions. One treatment may be sufficient but three to five are sometimes necessary.

C. Itching may also be somewhat alleviated with drying and antipruritic lotions, emollients, or antihistamines.

D. Topical corticosteroids or bursts of oral corticosteroids are of benefit only in more severe inflammatory variations. They are both ineffective and unwarranted in mild cases, and it is rarely necessary to use these medications.

REFERENCES

Annotation: Pityriasis rosea. Lancet 1:33, 1968

Björnberg A, Hellgren L: Pityriasis rosea. A statistical, clinical and laboratory investigation of 826 patients and matched healthy controls. Acta Derm Venereol (Stockh) 42[Suppl 50]:1–68, 1962

Bunch LW, Tilley JC: Pityriasis rosea. A histologic and serologic study. Arch Dermatol 84:79–86, 1961

Burch PRJ, Rowell NR: Pityriasis rosea—an autoagressive disease? Statistical studies in relation to aetiology and pathogenesis. Br J Dermatol 82:549–560, 1970

Lipman Cohan E: Pityriasis rosea. Br J Dermatol 79:533–539, 1967

Merchant M, Hammond R: Controlled study of ultraviolet light for pityriasis rosea. Cutis 14:548–549, 1974

Plemmons JA: Pityriasis rosea: an old therapy revisited. Cutis 16:120–121, 1975

25
Psoriasis

I. **DEFINITION AND PATHOPHYSIOLOGY** Psoriasis is a chronic proliferative epidermal disease that affects 2–8 million people in the United States and 1–3 percent of the world's population. Its average age of onset is 7 years, but it may make its initial appearance late in life as well. The lesions, usually discrete scaling plaques, may become very extensive or even generalized. Histocompatibility antigens HL-A13 and 17 are present in a markedly higher frequency in psoriatics. The 5–10 percent of patients with an associated arthritis are often HL-A W27 positive and 13–17 negative. The finding of these genetic markers implies that the HL-A chromosomal region includes loci that are part of the genotype resulting in susceptibility to psoriasis. However, there is considerable genetic heterogenicity and it seems likely that in any family two or more genes may be involved.

The time necessary for a psoriatic epidermal cell to travel from the basal cell layer of the epidermis to the surface and be cast off is 3–4 days, in marked contrast to the normal 26–28 days. The psoriatic cell cycle time of 37 hr is also markedly reduced from the normal

163 hr. As a result of the six- to ninefold rate increase and rapid cell cycle, the normal events of cell maturation and keratinization cannot take place. This is reflected clinically by profuse scaling; histologically by a greatly thickened epidermis with increased mitotic activity and by the presence of immature nucleated cells in the horny layer; under the electron microscope by reduced production of the intracellular filaments and granules seen with normal keratinization; and biochemically by increased synthesis and degradation of nucleoproteins. Beneath these plaques of proliferative epithelium lies an extremely vascular dermis.

The course of psoriasis is prolonged but unpredictable. In most patients the disease remains localized. In some, however, its severity is incompatible with a productive and happy life. Spontaneous clearing is quite rare, but unexplained exacerbation or improvement is common. Stress and anxiety frequently precede flare-ups of the disease.

II. SUBJECTIVE DATA

A. Most lesions are asymptomatic.

B. Pruritus may be noted in 20 percent of patients.

C. Those with generalized disease may demonstrate all the signs and symptoms of an exfoliative dermatitis (loss of thermoregulation with findings of warm skin, a feeling of chilliness and shivering, increased protein catabolism, and cardiovascular stress).

D. Monoarticular or polyarticular pain, tenderness, and morning stiffness, especially in the small joints of the hands and feet, are the early manifestations of psoriatic arthritis. Intense pain in larger joints and the cervical and/or lumbosacral spine also may be present.

III. OBJECTIVE DATA (See color insert.)

A. The psoriatic lesion is an erythematous, sharply circumscribed plaque covered by loosely adherent, silvery scales. Acute lesions tend to be small and guttate (drop-shaped).

B. Inapparent scaling can be made noticeable by scratching the surface of a psoriatic lesion.

C. Any body area may be involved, but lesions tend to occur most often on the elbows and knees, scalp, genitalia, and in the upper gluteal fold.

D. Lesions of active psoriasis often appear in areas of epidermal injury (Koebner reaction). Scratch marks, surgical wounds, or a sunburn may heal with psoriatic lesions in their place.

E. The nails may show punctate pitting or profuse collections of subungual keratotic material, clinically reflecting psoriatic involvement of the nail matrix or nail bed, respectively. A yellow-brown subungual discoloration ("oil spot") is characteristic. Patients with distal interphalangeal joint involvement or arthritis mutilans usually have adjacent nail involvement.

F. Exfoliative psoriasis is indistinguishable clinically from other exfoliative dermatoses. It may occur spontaneously, follow a systemic illness or drug reaction, or be a reaction to some antimalarial drugs or to steroid withdrawal.

G. In acute psoriatic arthritis, one or several joints are erythematous and swollen—the distal phalanx classically has a "sausage" appearance. Long-standing or rapidly progressive disease may lead to severe bone destruction. Sixty to seventy percent of patients with psoriatic arthritis present with this asymmetric arthritis and 20 percent of this group may also suffer from sacroiliitis or ankylosing spondylitis; 5 percent of patients show a destructive polyarthritis.

IV. ASSESSMENT

A. The medical history may reveal a cause for the onset or exacerbation of psoriatic lesions. For example, acute psoriasis or a flare-up in chronic lesions may follow streptococcal pharyngitis by 7–10 days.

B. Biopsy of lesions will reveal a psoriasiform epidermal thickening, but the histologic picture often is not diagnostic.

C. Hyperuricemia is proportional to the amount of cutaneous involvement and is related to the increased nucleic acid degradation associated with accelerated epidermopoiesis. It rarely causes symptoms or requires therapy.

D. Patients with psoriatic arthritis will typically have an elevated erythrocyte sedimentation rate and by definition will have negative tests for rheumatoid factor. X-ray films of the hands may show characteristic subcortical cystic changes with relative sparing of the articular cartilage.

V. THERAPY

A. It is important to emphasize that psoriasis is a treatable disease. Optimism and encouragement are justified and make it easier for the patient conscientiously to apply sometimes awkward and messy dressings. All agents that are effective are toxic to epidermal cells, although mechanisms vary. Pharmacologic data concerning the mode of action of most of these topical medications are unavailable.

B. **Treatment for mild to moderate cutaneous involvement** (for scalp care see p. 164; for nail care, p. 165)

1. *Repeated exposure to sunlight or middle-wavelength, sunburn spectrum, ultraviolet light* (UVB) from artificial sources to the point of mild erythema will induce flattening or clearing of many lesions. UVB inhibits epidermal mitosis and presumably acts by this mechanism.

2. *Potent fluorinated corticosteroids* applied 3–4id to local lesions are quite useful, especially in reducing scaling and thickness. Overnight or 24-hr occlusive therapy with these medications or with fluandrenolide tape (Cordran Tape®) will initiate involution in most lesions. Corticosteroids exert their beneficial effects in this setting as mitotic inhibitors.

    Instructions: Patients should apply corticosteroid (from potency group 1–4, p. 296) to lesions without occlusion during the day; in the evening, apply medication to plaques immediately after bath or shower, and occlude with plastic wrap or suit for 4 hr or overnight (see p. 295 for occlusion techniques). As lesions subside, decrease the use of occlusion and increase the use of a bland emollient (e.g., Eucerin®).

3. *Injection of intralesional corticosteroids* beneath isolated chronic plaques will cause involution within 7–10 days (triamcinolone acetonide, diluted to 2.5 mg/ml).

4. *Coal tar therapy* (see also p. 324) may be combined with or alternated with topical corticosteroids: tar gel (Estar® gel), which is nearly colorless, or 1–5% crude coal tar ointment, which is very messy, is applied overnight. This is

often followed by exposure to ultraviolet light (UVL) or sunlight. Tars sensitize the skin to long-wave UVL (UVA) and also have a direct beneficial effect on psoriasis.

Instructions: As directed in the instructions in B-2, but on alternate nights, the patient should apply Estar® gel overnight and be exposed to UVL the following morning; or apply corticosteroid cream with or without occlusion during the day, tar gel overnight, and UVL exposure in the morning. The latter regimen is the protocol sometimes used to treat hospitalized psoriatics.

5. *Other topical agents*

   a. *Keralyt® gel* (6% salicylic acid, 60% propylene glycol, 20% ethyl alcohol) applied under occlusion to hydrated skin overnight is the most effective way to remove thick, adherent scaling. It is sometimes useful to start therapy by alternating the use of Keralyt® overnight and corticosteroid during the day, and then to stop using the keratolytic gel as the psoriasis improves and the lesions become flat and less hyperkeratotic.

   b. *Salicylic acid,* 2–10%, in other formations might also help remove scales and crusts and may be used along with corticosteroid or anthralin therapy. Formulations commonly used include 3–10% salicylic acid cream, 3–6% sulfur and salicylic acid ointment, and 3% sulfur, 3% salicylic acid, 4% cetyl alcohol-coal tar distillate (Pragmatar®) cream.

   c. *Mercury compounds* are very allergenic and not commonly used, but they can be effective topical agents. Long-term use has been reported to cause renal tubular damage. Ammoniated mercury cream (5%) may be used alone but is often combined with other agents as follows and used 2–3id:

      (1) Tar solution 2–10%
          Salicylic acid 1–5%
          Ammoniated Hg 5–10%
          This cream may be compounded at various concentrations with or without the tar or salicylic acid. Higher concentrations may act as irritants.

(2)   Tar distillate 5%
      Ammoniated Hg 5%
      Methanamine sulfosalicylate 2%
      This is available as Unguentum Bossi®.

C.   **Treatment for more severe or widespread involvement**

1.   *The anthralin paste method* is very effective for wide-spread lesions consisting primarily of thick plaques. Its disadvantages are that anthralin may be a primary irritant, it stains clothing and skin, and it is difficult to apply. Anthralin paste can be used on an outpatient or inpatient basis and will clear up the lesions on most patients within 2–3 weeks. The patient should use anthralin as follows:

     a.   Bathe at bedtime in a coal tar bath (Balnetar®, liquor carbonis detergens, Polytar®, Zetar®) and scrub scales off.

     b.   Liberally apply 0.1% or 0.2% anthralin with 0.2% salicylic acid and 5.0% hard paraffin in zinc oxide paste (Anthera®, Anthra-Derm®, Lasan® Unguent; see Farber and Harris 1970 for details) to lesions with a tongue blade or gloved fingers. The anthralin concentration may be gradually increased to 0.4% or greater.

     c.   Cover paste with powder and gauze dressing or stockinette, or simply wear old pajamas, and leave on 8–12 hr.

     d.   Remove paste in the morning. Bath or mineral oil will aid removal.

     e.   Apply a low-strength corticosteroid cream (fluocinolone 0.01%, triamcinolone 0.025%) to all lesions during the day.

     f.   UVL treatment may be used but does not add appreciably to the final result.

     g.   Use old sheets and bed clothing, since anthralin will stain them a violet color. Treat intertriginous areas cautiously with a 1:10 dilution of the paste and with sheeting separating body folds. Anthralin stain may be removed from the skin with 3–6% salicylic acid cream or ointment, which may also be used to rim lesions to limit the paste margins.

2. ***Tar and UVL therapy (Goeckerman regimen)*** is best an inpatient treatment, since tars are messy to apply and potent ultraviolet hot-quartz or fluorescent lights are needed. Tars and middle-wavelength ultraviolet light (UVB) act as separate, effective antipsoriatic agents.

   a. Apply tar gel (Estar®), a heavy layer of 1–5% crude coal tar in Aquaphor® or petrolatum with 1% polysorbate 80 (Tween 20), or other tar preparation in the evening. If these are too irritating or drying, use 10% liquor carbonis detergens in hydrophilic ointment or Nivea® oil.

   b. In the morning, remove the tar by rubbing with a towel and cottonseed or mineral oil and then bathing. If a tar layer is present, UVL will not reach the skin.

   c. Expose the skin to minimal erythema doses of UVL — an amount that will produce slight redness 12 hr later. This is equivalent to 20–30 min of sunlight; exposure time for artificial light sources is usually determined by experience and may be 30 sec or many minutes. Production of a mild phototoxic effect (sunburn) is probably necessary for an effective response. Gradually increase the duration of light exposure daily.

   d. Bathe and remove scales with a stiff brush. Too vigorous brushing, however, may cause a Koebner reaction.

   e. After bathing, liberally rub tar onto involved areas. Alternatively, steroids with occlusion may be used during the day, being applied after UVL exposure, with tars applied only overnight. Using the latter method, lesions will flatten more quickly, but there will be no overall difference in the time necessary for total clearing or length of remission.

   f. After a 2–3-week in-hospital stay, most patients will clear and prolonged clinical remission of psoriasis will occur.

3. *Photochemotherapy* (see also p. 249) is potentially the least discomforting and most effective method available to put widespread psoriasis into remission. A photoactive drug (a psoralen) is administered orally, followed 2 hr later by exposure to long-wave UVL (UVA). Psoralens form photo-adducts with DNA in the presence of UVA and in this way probably reduce the increased epidermal turnover characteristic of psoriasis. Repeated PUVA (psoralen plus ultraviolet-A) exposure causes disappearance of lesions in almost all patients with 10–20 treatments over 4–8 weeks. Psoriasis often recurs weeks to months after PUVA ceases, and twice-monthly treatment seems to be necessary to keep patients free of their disease. Scalp, body folds, and other areas not exposed to UVA respond poorly to the therapy.

D. Scalp care

1. *Mild involvement* may be treated by the patient with a tar shampoo (10% liquor carbonis detergens in tincture of green soap, Pentrax®, Polytar®, Sebutone®, Zetar®) and steroid lotion or solution 2id (Synalar®, Valisone®).

2. *More severe involvement* should be treated as follows:

a. If scaling is thick, it is necessary to first remove the scales and then apply something to inhibit their refor-mation. This is best accomplished by having the patient apply a keratolytic gel (Keralyt® gel) to a hydrated scalp and then cover it with an occlusive plastic shower cap for several hours or overnight. This will effectively loosen the scales, after which a steroid lotion or solution (Synalar®, Valisone®) should be ap-plied under a shower cap for the rest of the night, or without occlusion during the day.

b. Alternatively, chronic thick plaques may also be treated by the patient as follows:

(1) Apply anthralin (Anthera® ointment, Lasan® unguent) or 3% sulfur, 3% salicylic acid, 4% tar distillate (Pragmatar®) cream, or phenol/saline lotion (Baker's® "P&S" liquid) or, in severe cases, 20% oil of cade, 10% sulfur, 5% salicylic acid ("20-10-5" ointment) in hydro-philic ointment to the scalp, leaving overnight.

    (2)   Use tar shampoo in the morning.

    (3)   Reapply the preparation as in b-1 during the day until scaling is decreased. At that point, substitute a steroid lotion or solution.

E. **Nail care** There is no consistently effective therapy for psoriatic involvement of the nails. The nails will often improve coincident with remission of cutaneous lesions and will almost always improve after systemic antimetabolite therapy.

  1. Removal of subungual debris and application of corticosteroids under occlusion may offer some benefit.

  2. Injection of small amounts of triamcinolone acetonide (about 0.3 mg; or 0.1 ml at 3 mg/ml) into the nail bed at 2–3-week intervals will result in cure or improvement in about 75% of treated nails, but it is painful and time-consuming. Onycholytic nails respond least well. There will be about a 50% recurrence rate when treatment is stopped.

  3. 1% 5-fluorouracil solution (Fluoroplex®) applied twice daily to nail margins has been reported to decrease the severity of involvement by 75% in two-thirds of patients within 3–6 months.

F. **Psoriatic arthritis** often responds to aspirin titered to near toxicity, splinting, and local heat. This is particularly useful in reducing pain, swelling, and stiffness. Whether any of the treatments affect the progression of the disease is unclear.

  1. ***Indomethacin,*** 25 mg 3–4id given with antacids, is particularly effective in patients with sacroiliac, spine, and large joint involvement, and in selected cases, also in patients with peripheral joint symptoms. Large doses up to 150 mg per day often can be very useful.

  2. Newer ***nonsteroidal anti-inflammatory agents*** such as fenoprofen (Nalfron®), ibuprofen (Motrin®), naproxin (Naprosyn®), and tolmetin (Tolectin®) are also effective in controlling the inflammation of psoriatic arthritis.

  3. ***Folic acid antagonists,*** particularly methotrexate, are very useful in intractable cases unresponsive to the more conventional therapies. 6-Mercaptopurine may be more effective against the arthritis component but is less useful for the cutaneous lesions.

G. Acute psoriasis should be treated gently with just emollients or topical steroids. Avoid tars, salicylic acid, and aggressive UVL therapy, since they may irritate the lesions and lead to a more widespread eruption and a chronic course.

H. Antimetabolite therapy with agents that inhibit DNA synthesis (hydroxyurea, methotrexate) is reserved for those patients unresponsive to other approaches and for whom the disease is an economic and social disaster. These agents have serious side-effects and should never be considered unless topical therapy has proved ineffectual.

REFERENCES

Baden H, Pugliese MM: Psoriasis. DM, September 1973, 47 pp

Blecker JJ: Intradermal triamcinolone acetonide treatment of psoriatic nail dystrophy with Port-O-Jet. Br J Dermatol 92:479, 1975

Cohen GL: Psoriatic arthritis. Prog Dermatol 10:5–8, 1976

Eisen A, Seegmiller J: Uric acid metabolism in psoriasis. J Clin Invest 40:1486–1494, 1961

Farber EM, Cox AJ (Eds): Psoriasis: Proceedings of the International Symposium, Stanford University, 1971. Stanford, Calif, Stanford University Press, 1971, 478 pp

Farber EM, Harris DR: Hospital treatment of psoriasis. A modified anthralin program. Arch Dermatol 101:381–389, 1970

Fisher LB, Maibach HI: Topical antipsoriatic agents and epidermal mitosis in man. Arch Dermatol 108:374–377, 1973

Lomholt G: Psoriasis: Prevalence, Spontaneous Course and Genetics. Copenhagen, GEC Gad, 1963

Marisco AR, Eaglstein WH, Weinstein GD: Ultraviolet light and tar in the Goeckerman treatment of psoriasis. Arch Dermatol 112:1249–1250, 1976

Pariser H, Murray PF: Intralesional injections of triamcinolone. Effects of different concentrations on psoriatic lesions. Arch Dermatol 87:183–187, 1963

Peachey RD, Pye RJ, Harman RPM: The treatment of psoriatic nail dystrophy with intradermal steroid injections. Br J Dermatol 95:75–78, 1976

Tanenbaum L, Parrish JA, Pathak MA, Anderson RR, Fitzpatrick TB: Tar phototoxicity and phototherapy for psoriasis. Arch Dermatol 111:467–470, 1975

Weinstein GD, Frost P: Abnormal cell proliferation of psoriasis. J Invest Dermatol 50:254–259, 1968

Whyte HJ, Baughman RD: Acute guttate psoriasis and streptococcal infection. Arch Dermatol 89:350–356, 1964

Wolff K, Fitzpatrick TB, Parrish JA, Gschnait F, Gilchrest B, Hönigsmann H, Pathak MA, Tanenbaum L: Photochemotherapy for psoriasis with orally administered methoxsalen. Arch Dermatol 112:943–950, 1976

Woodrow JC, Dove VK, Usher N, Anderson J: The HL-A system and psoriasis. Br J Dermatol 92:426–427, 1975

Zaias N: Psoriasis of the nail. A clinical-pathologic study. Arch Dermatol 99:567–579, 1969

26
Rosacea and
Periorificial (Perioral) Dermatitis

I. DEFINITION AND PATHOPHYSIOLOGY

A. **Rosacea** is a chronic disorder of unknown etiology that affects the central face and neck. It is characterized by two clinical components: a vascular change consisting of intermittent or persistent erythema and flushing, and an acneform eruption with papules, pustules, cysts, and sebaceous hyperplasia. There is no correlation between the sebum excretion rate and the severity of rosacea. Onset is most often between ages 30–50. Although women are affected three times as frequently, the disease may become more severe in men.

Ocular changes (blepharitis, conjunctivitis, and keratitis) and sebaceous hyperplasia of the nose (rhinophyma) may be associated with rosacea. Differential diagnostic considerations include (a) acne vulgaris, which is characterized by a wider distribution of lesions and the presence of comedones; (b) periorificial dermatitis; (c) seborrheic dermatitis; (d) the malignant carcinoid syndrome; and (e) lupus erythematosus.

B. **Periorificial dermatitis** is a distinct clinical entity that can be easily confused with rosacea, seborrheic dermatitis, or acne. It primarily affects young women, is usually found around the mouth but occasionally around the nose or eyes, and is of unknown cause. As with rosacea, prolonged use of fluorinated topical corticosteroids can cause an eruption with similar features and can perpetuate preexisting disease.

II. SUBJECTIVE DATA

A. The facial lesions of rosacea and periorificial dermatitis often cause justifiable concern about personal appearance.

B. Rosacea papules and cysts can be painful; periorificial dermatitis papules may itch or cause a burning sensation.

C. Patients with rosacea may complain of feelings of facial heat and congestion.

III. OBJECTIVE DATA

A. **Rosacea (See color insert.)**

1. Recurrent erythema, located in the middle third of the face (midforehead, nose, malar areas, and chin), may later lead to a persistent flush and telangiectasia.

2. Acneform papules, pustules, and cysts may be present; comedones are not.

3. Rhinophyma, which predominantly affects men, is associated with follicular dilatation, irregular thickening of the skin, and hypertrophic soft masses centered about the tip of the nose.

B. **Periorificial dermatitis**

1. Discrete 1–3-mm erythematous or flesh-colored papules and pustules are seen singly, in clusters, or in plaques around the mouth, sparing the vermilion border. Lesions may occasionally occur around the nose and on the malar areas below and lateral to the eyes.

2. There is often a persistent erythema of the nasolabial folds that may extend around the mouth onto the chin.

3. Long-standing lesions show a flatter, more confluent eruption, with superimposed dry scaling.

IV. THERAPY

A. Rosacea

1. ***Precipitating factors*** Patients who flush easily should avoid all food, drink, and activities that induce this change. These may include tea, coffee, other hot foods and liquids, alcoholic beverages, highly seasoned foods, sunlight, extremes of heat and cold, and emotional stress. If flushing is not caused by these factors, there is no evidence that avoidance will result in improvement in the disease.

2. ***Systemic antibiotics***

   a. The most effective treatment for rosacea is the administration of tetracycline. Therapy should be initiated at 250 mg 4id until symptoms subside, after which the dosage can be slowly decreased or discontinued. Occasionally it is necessary to use larger doses (1.5–2.0 gm qd) for short periods of time in order to induce remission. Long-term administration usually is needed. Tetracycline is most effective in decreasing the acneform component and clearing the keratitis but will also diminish erythema.

   After discontinuing tetracycline therapy 25 percent of patients can be expected to relapse within a few days; about 60 percent will have relapsed within 6 months. Keratitis seems always to recur quickly and requires continual treatment.

   b. Ampicillin (250 mg 2–3id) also has been shown to be effective.

3. ***Topical therapy*** for the acneform lesions is similar to that for acne vulgaris. Preparations containing benzoyl peroxide and sulfur in concentrations of up to 15% are useful (see pp. 8, 259). Topical antibiotics (see p. 8) may be tried.

   a. Ultraviolet light (UVL) therapy is of no benefit.

   b. Topical corticosteroids are occasionally used to decrease erythema and inflammation. The high-potency fluorinated steroid preparations should never be used, since they may induce more widespread and irreversible telangiectasia. 1% hydrocortisone cream is acceptable.

4. Large telangiectatic vessels may be destroyed by electrosurgery, using the epilating needle (see p. 231).

5. Surgical reduction of the soft tissue enlargement in rhinophyma may be accomplished by a surgical shave, dermabrasion, or electrosurgery.

B. Periorificial dermatitis

1. *Systemic antibiotics* used as described for rosacea are the only reliable therapy. Periorificial dermatitis usually clears within 3–8 weeks, and it is often then possible to taper off tetracycline. Some patients need longer term maintenance therapy.

2. *Topical therapy* is of little use. Fluorinated corticosteroids must be assiduously avoided. 1% hydrocortisone or other nonfluorinated corticosteroid cream may be of symptomatic benefit but will not cure the eruption. Other topical agents as used for rosacea may be tried.

REFERENCES

Rosacea

Goldsmith AJB: The ocular manifestations of rosacea. Br J Dermatol 65:448–457, 1953

Knight AG, Vickers CFH: A follow-up of tetracycline-treated rosacea. With special reference to rosacea keratitis. Br J Dermatol 93:577–580, 1975

Leydin JL, Thew M, Kligman AM: Steroid rosacea. Arch Dermatol 110:619–622, 1974

Marks R: Concepts in the pathogenesis of rosacea. Br J Dermatol 80:170–171, 1968

Marks R, Ellis J: Comparative effectiveness of tetracycline and ampicillin in rosacea. A controlled trial. Lancet 2:1049–1052, 1971

Pye RJ, Meyrick G, Burton JL: Skin surface composition in rosacea. Br J Dermatol 94:161–164, 1976

Sneddon IB: A clinical trial of tetracycline in rosacea. Br J Dermatol 78:649–652, 1966

Periorificial dermatitis

Bendyl BJ: Perioral dermatitis: etiology and treatment. Cutis 17:903–908, 1976

MacDonald A, Feiwal M: Perioral dermatitis: aetiology and treatment with tetracycline. Br J Dermatol 87:315–319, 1972

Sneddon IB: Perioral dermatitis. Br J Dermatol 87:430–434, 1972

27
Seborrheic Dermatitis and Dandruff

I. **DEFINITION AND PATHOPHYSIOLOGY**   Seborrheic dermatitis and dandruff each may cause a scaling on the scalp that is often
associated with itching. There are, however, distinctions that can be
found between the two disorders. Dandruff is noninflammatory, increased scaling on the scalp that represents the more active end of the
spectrum of the physiologic desquamation. On a normal scalp approximately 487,000 cells per sq cm can be found after a detergent
scrub; scalps affected with dandruff and seborrheic dermatitis lib-
erate up to 800,000 cells per sq cm. Although it has long been
thought that microorganisms caused or contributed to the production
of dandruff, it is now clear that no organism or combination of
organisms is in any way responsible. Neither is seborrhea a causative
factor: dandruff subjects produce no more sebum on their scalps
than do controls.

Seborrheic dermatitis is an inflammatory, erythematous, and scaling
eruption that occurs primarily in "seborrheic" areas, i.e., those with
a high number and activity of sebaceous glands such as the scalp,

face, and trunk. Although seborrheic dermatitis occurs in neonatal and postpubertal life—times during which sebaceous glands are most active—no direct relationship between the amount or composition of sebum and the presence of dermatitis has been documented. Reducing sebum excretion affects neither dandruff nor seborrheic dermatitis. This disease is one of accelerated epidermal growth resulting in retention of nuclei in stratum corneum cells that have not had sufficient time to completely mature. On a normal scalp there are approximately 3700 nucleated cells per sq cm; on scalps with dandruff there are 25,000, and on those with seborrheic dermatitis the count is 76,000. It has been postulated that prolonged retention of sebum on the skin may in some way act as an irritant or alter epidermal function following its percutaneous reentry. A constitutional predisposition to seborrheic dermatitis seems to exist, and emotional or physical stress also may be important. There is both increased sebum output and an increased incidence of seborrheic dermatitis in Parkinson's disease and some other neurologic conditions.

II. **SUBJECTIVE DATA**   The lesions of seborrheic dermatitis and dandruff are often asymptomatic, but pruritus is not uncommon and may at times be intense.

III. **OBJECTIVE DATA**

    A. Dandruff appears simply as noninflammatory, diffuse scaling on the scalp only.

    B. With seborrheic dermatitis, there is erythema, greasy scaling, and at times exudation; areas may have better-defined borders. Mild erythema and fine dry scaling may also be found on the eyebrows, eyelids, nasolabial and postauricular folds, moustache, beard, and presternal areas. Inframammary folds, the groin, gluteal crease, and umbilicus also are affected. Lesions may become thick, semiconfluent, yellow, and greasy. Secondary impetiginization and folliculitis may occur.

    C. Seborrheic marginal blepharitis, which consists of erythema and scaling of eyelid margins and cilia, is often associated with mild granular conjuctivitis. Seborrheic dermatitis in other sites is often not present.

IV. **THERAPY**

    A. Agents effective in eliminating the scaling of dandruff and seborrheic dermatitis inhibit mitotic activity and slow down epidermal proliferation.

1. The most effective antiseborrheic shampoos contain 2% *selenium sulfide* (Exsel®, Iosel®, Selsun®). They should be applied 2–3 times weekly for 5–10 min each time.

2. Preparations containing 1–2% *zinc pyrithione* (Danex®, Head and Shoulders®, Zincon®) work almost as well.

3. *Salicylic acid–sulfur* shampoos (Ionil®, Meted®, Sebulex®, Vanseb®) are less effective but show definite activity.

4. *Tar* shampoos (DHS-T®, Ionil T®, Pentrax®, Sebutone®, Zetar®) make dandruff less visible but fail to lower the count of desquamating cells.

5. Any nonmedicinal shampoo, particularly those containing *surfactants and detergents,* will remove scales and lead to subjective clinical improvement and decreased desquamation for about 4 days. These agents should be used every 2 days to control dandruff.

B. If the lesions are extensive or very inflammatory, also have the patient apply either a topical corticosteroid solution, lotion, or spray (Valisone® lotion is generally most effective; Synalar® solution and other corticosteroid lotions are also useful). Alternatively, a sodium sulfacetamide lotion (Sebizon®) 2–3id may be used.

C. Thick crusts may be more easily removed by overnight applications of a keratolytic gel (Keralyt® gel), with or without plastic cap occlusion; 3% sulfur, 3% salicylic acid, 4% cetyl alcohol-coal tar distillate (Pragmatar®) cream; Baker's "P&S" liquid®; "20-10-5" ointment (see Psoriasis, p. 164); or a 30-min compress with warm mineral oil, prior to shampooing.

D. Seborrheic dermatitis lesions on other areas respond rapidly to a corticosteroid cream such as 1% hydrocortisone applied 1–3id. Aerosols or lotions are easier to apply to hairy areas. Prolonged application of high-potency fluorinated corticosteroids may lead to disfiguring telangiectasia and atrophy. Other useful topical agents for glabrous skin include sulfur-containing medications such as 10% sulfacetamide lotion (Sebizon®); 3% sulfur, 3% salicylic acid, 4% cetyl alcohol-coal tar distillate (Pragmatar®) cream; or formulations such as precipitated sulfur 3–10%, salicylic acid 1–5%, and tar 2% in an ointment base or 1–3% sulfur in calamine lotion.

E. Seborrheic blepharitis is treated 1–3id with either 10% sulfacet-amide-0.2% prednisolone-0.12% phenylephrine suspension (Blephamide®) or similar preparations (Cetapred®, Meti-myd®). It is essential to monitor intraocular tension concurrent with intermittent or chronic steroid therapy in or around the eye.

REFERENCES

Kligman AM, Marples RR, Lantis LR, McGinley KJ: Appraisal of anti-dandruff formation. J Soc Cosmet Chem 25:73–91, 1974

Leyden JJ, McGinley KJ, Kligman AM: Role of microorganisms in dandruff. Arch Dermatol 112:333–338, 1976

Marks R, Bhogal B, Wilson L: The effect of betamethasone valerate on seborrhoeic dermatitis of the scalp. Acta Derm Venereol (Stockh) 54:373–375, 1974

McGinley KJ, Leyden JJ, Marples RR, Kligman AM: Quantitative micro-biology of the scalp in non-dandruff, dandruff, and seborrheic derma-titis. J Invest Dermatol 64:401–405, 1975

Parrish JA, Arndt KA: Seborrhoeic dermatitis of the beard. Br J Dermatol 87:241–244, 1972

Priestly GC, Savin JA: The microbiology of dandruff. Br J Dermatol 94:469–471, 1976

28
Sexually Transmitted Disorders

Syphilis, gonorrhea, chancroid, lymphogranuloma venereum, and granuloma inguinale have long been considered the five venereal diseases. However, it is now quite apparent that there are numerous disorders that can be transmitted through close personal contact, and the expanded list included herein more truly reflects the actual sexually transmitted and sexually acquired diseases.

Entities will be discussed in this section in order of the incidence of new cases per 100,000 population found in hospital clinics in England. Our experience seeing patients in ambulatory venereal disease and dermatology clinics would probably differ in order of incidence but the diseases are the same. Note that four of the five least common disorders are the "classic" venereal diseases. This does not diminish their importance as infectious diseases of general concern, but it does point out that the spectrum of this type of communicable disorder is broad and the number of people affected by more common sexually transmitted disorders is high. Although some of these conditions are uncommon or do not have dermatologic findings, they all enter into the differential diagnosis and consideration of therapy and hence all will be discussed.

NONGONOCOCCAL URETHRITIS (NGU; incidence 181/100,000)

I. DEFINITION AND PATHOPHYSIOLOGY NGU is an inflammation of the urethra not caused by *Neisseria gonorrhoeae*. A small proportion of cases is associated with trichomoniasis or candidiasis, but in about 90 percent of cases a pathogen cannot be identified by routine methods. *Chlamydia trachomatis*, an obligate intracellular bacteria that is cultured like a virus, can be isolated from almost half of the etiologically diagnosed cases if appropriate culture and antibody tests are available. The cause of *Chlamydia*-negative NGU is not known; T-strain mycoplasma and *Mycoplasma hominis* are possible pathogens but their exact role remains unresolved.

II. SUBJECTIVE DATA Patients with NGU have variable symptoms; dysuria, when present, is usually not severe.

III. OBJECTIVE DATA The urethral discharge in NGU is usually scant and is white or clear in appearance.

IV. ASSESSMENT The NGU discharge will demonstrate no organisms on microscopic examination or culture. Specifically there are no gonococci or *Candida albicans* on Gram stain; no *Candida* on KOH or SMS smear; no trichomonas on saline wet amount; no bacteria on methylene blue and/or Gram stain of a spun-down midstream urine. There will be no growth for these agents in the appropriate media: Thayer-Martin (gonococcus), Feinberg-Wittington or Bushby (*Trichomonas*), Sabouraud's (*Candida*), phenyl ethyl alcohol/Mac-Conkey (urinary tract bacteria).

V. THERAPY

    A. Tetracycline 1.5 gm PO initially, followed by 500 mg 4id for 7 days. Eighty percent of patients will be cured on initial treatment. Steady sexual partners should also be treated.

    Other tetracyclines are also effective, e.g., minocycline 200 mg PO initially, then 100 mg PO 2id for 6 days.

    B. A first relapse should again be treated with tetracycline but a 14- or 24-day course is then advisable.

C. Erythromycin in the same dosage is a good alternative medication.

D. Patients with multiple recurrences should be referred to a urologist to rule out structural abnormalities.

GONORRHEA (incidence 125/100,000)

I. **DEFINITION AND PATHOPHYSIOLOGY** Infection with *N. gonorrhoeae* presents most often as an anterior urethritis in man and as an asymptomatic or minimally symptomatic endocervical colonization in women. Transmission of the gonococcus is almost wholly by sexual practices and their variations, except for conjunctivitis in infants and at times vulvovaginitis in prepubescent girls. Gonorrhea is diagnosed more in the male and at least half of all reported cases are 25 years of age or younger. The majority of the 2–3 million Americans infected each year reside in urban areas.

Neisseria are gram-negative, nonmotile, non-spore-forming cocci that tend to grow in pairs with the adjacent sides flattened. Man is the only natural host of *Neisseria*. *N. gonorrhoeae* is differentiated from nonpathogenic *Neisseria* through growth on selective antibiotic-containing media (Thayer-Martin agar) and from the meningococcus by sugar fermentation patterns on appropriate media.

Pathogenic gonococci have tiny proteinaceous surface projections called pili, which cause the organisms to stick to each other as well as to mucosal cells. The gonococcus enters the body by penetrating through columnar epithelial cells of the genitourinary tract and produces an acute inflammation.

II. **SUBJECTIVE DATA**

A. **Males**

1. After an incubation period of 2–5 days 80–90 percent of men have the sudden onset of uncomfortable sensations along the urethra followed by frequent, painful urination.

2. After a variable period of time (10–14 days or longer) infection may spread to the posterior urethra, prostate, seminal vesicles, and epididymis, causing pain and a feeling of fullness in the perineum or scrotum.

B. Females

1. Seventy to eighty percent of infected women have gonococci present in the endocervical canal or urethra with no symptoms or with nonspecific symptoms such as vaginal discharge, urinary frequency, or dysuria.

2. Pelvic inflammatory disease (salpingitis, parametritis, and localized peritonitis) present as fever, nausea, vomiting, and abdominal pain and may follow an acute infection or occur months later.

III. OBJECTIVE DATA

A. Males A profuse mucopurulent discharge is present.

B. Females

1. A mild discharge may be seen.

2. Patients with pelvic inflammatory disease have acute abdominal pain and fever that simulates appendicitis or other acute surgical conditions.

IV. ASSESSMENT

A. Diagnosis

1. In men, the finding of intracellular gram-negative diplococci within polymorphonuclear leukocytes in a gram-stained smear of a urethral exudate allows the presumptive diagnosis of gonococcal urethritis to be made with at least 99 percent accuracy. A urethral culture should be obtained from men suspected of asymptomatic urethral colonization, or for confirmation of adequate treatment.

2. In women, a smear will show about 5 percent false positives and 50 percent false negatives and is therefore of no diagnostic use. Cervical culture on Thayer-Martin media will detect 80–85 percent of those infected, and the addition of a culture of the anus will increase the yield to over 90 percent.

B. Extragenital infections and complications

1. *Pharyngeal infections,* usually asymptomatic, are present in about 20 percent of patients with anogenital gonorrhea who practice fellatio.

2. *Anal infections* in men are usually the result of anal intercourse among homosexuals. Fifty percent of women with gonorrhea will also have anal infection presumably because of contiguity but not necessarily from intercourse. Anal infection is almost always asymptomatic.

3. *Disseminated infection (gonococcemia, arthritis-dermatitis syndrome)* presents initially as a triad of fever, migratory polyarthralgias and tenosynovitis, and characteristic skin lesions with later development of stationary large-joint septic arthritis. Women are more commonly affected, and pregnancy and menstruation appear to predispose to dissemination.

   a. The cutaneous lesions are countable in number and are usually distally located over joints.

   b. They start as minute erythematous papules resembling mosquito bites, then progress to become pustules or, later, hemorrhagic infarcts.

4. *Other much less common complications* include meningitis, endocarditis, and pericarditis.

V. THERAPY

A. Anogenital infection, urethritis

1. Procaine penicillin (4.8 million units) IM in 2 doses at one visit, preceded by 1 gm of probenecid PO just before injection.

2. Penicillin V and semisynthetic penicillins are much less effective and should not be used.

3. *Alternative treatments*

   a. *Ampicillin* 3.5 gm PO plus probenecid 1 gm PO.

   b. *Spectinomycin hydrochloride* (Trobicin®) 2 gm IM.

   c. *Tetracycline* 1.5 gm PO, then 500 mg 4id for 4 days.

   d. *Erythromycin* 1.5 gm PO, then 500 mg 4id for 4 days.

B. Pharyngitis
Treatment is as for anogenital disease but tetracycline should be considered the only effective alternate drug.

C. **Pelvic inflammatory disease**—ambulatory patients

    1. Penicillin as for anogenital infections, followed by ampicillin 500 mg 4id for 10 days.

    2. *Alternative treatments*

        a. *Ampicillin* as for anogenital infection followed by 500 mg 4id for 10 days.

        b. *Tetracycline* 1.5 gm PO, then 500 mg 4id for 10 days.

D. **Disseminated infection**

    1. *Crystalline penicillin G* 10 million units IV until improvement, followed by ampicillin 500 mg PO 4id to complete 7 days, *or*

    2. *Ampicillin* plus probenecid as for anogenital, then 500 mg 4id to complete at least 7 days, *or*

    3. *Tetracycline* 1.5 gm PO, then 500 mg PO 4id for at least 7 days.

    4. *Hospitalization* is indicated for patients who appear to have septic arthritis or other complications, have an uncertain diagnosis, or are unreliable.

E. **Treatment failures** All patients with a positive follow-up culture after initial treatment for anogenital or urethral infection with penicillin, ampicillin, or tetracycline should receive 2 gm of spectinomycin IM. The recent emergence of penicillinase-producing gonococci will lead to revision of the above treatment regimens. Consult the latest CDC recommendations periodically.

F. **Epidemiologic treatment**

    1. Those known to have been recently exposed to gonorrhea should be treated with the same treatment as those known to have the disease.

    2. Penicillin treatment of gonorrhea will cure incubating syphilis; if treated with other schedules, serologic tests for syphilis should be made at monthly intervals for 4 months.

    3. Topical silver nitrate solution is the recommended drug for the prevention of gonococcal ophthalmia in the newborn.

CANDIDA ALBICANS INFECTION (incidence 70/100,000)

Candida albicans organisms may cause eruptions by direct infection or through an irritant action. See p. 86 for more discussion.

TRICHOMONIASIS (incidence 41/100,000)

I. **DEFINITION AND PATHOPHYSIOLOGY** The protozoan flagellate *Trichomonas vaginalis* may infect as many as 10–20 percent of sexually active males and females; in women it causes an infection of the vagina and urethra that may extend to involve the adjacent skin. Transmission is by sexual intercourse as well as from contaminated material or instrumentation. Organisms can be cultured from the urethra in 80 percent of infected women and about 70 percent of their male sexual partners.

II. **SUBJECTIVE DATA**

   A. When symptoms are present, vulvar pruritus is the predominant problem.

   B. Dysuria and dyspareunia may be complaints.

   C. Men can have mild urethral pruritus associated with dysuria and frequency.

III. **OBJECTIVE DATA**

   A. The vaginal discharge is characteristically cream-colored, frothy, and purulent.

   B. Signs of secondary irritant inflammation—edema, erythema, and excoriation of external genitalia—are often seen.

IV. **ASSESSMENT**

   A. Diagnosis is made by visualizing motile trichomonads on a wet mount.

   1. Mix a drop of discharge with a drop of saline on a slide, apply cover slip, view at 100–400× with the condenser down.

   2. Wet mount will be positive in only 75–90 percent of patients from whom trichomonads can be cultured.

   B. Organisms may be cultured on Feinberg-Wittington media.

V. **THERAPY**

   A. Metronidazole (Flagyl®) 250 mg PO 3id for 7 days for men and women. A single oral dose of 2 gm may be equally effective.

   B. Recurrent discharge may represent relapse or reinfection with *Trichomonas*, but because metronidazole therapy alters the normal vaginal flora, *C. albicans* vaginitis must be considered.

C. Metronidazole should not be used during pregnancy.

    1. Acidifying douches may give adequate relief of symptoms.

    2. If not, metronidazole vaginal inserts, 500 mg, 1 daily for 10 days may be used during the second half of pregnancy.

WARTS AND CONDYLOMA ACUMINATA
(incidence 40/100,000)

These slow-growing viral lesions may be found on any area of the ano-genital region, and they have clearly been shown to be sexually transmitted. See p. 211 for more discussion.

HERPES SIMPLEX (incidence 11/100,000)

Approximately 90 percent of genital herpes infections are with the type 2 virus. Some authorities in the United States claim this to be the third most common sexually transmittable disease. See p. 103 for more discussion.

PEDICULOSIS PUBIS (incidence 10/100,000)
SCABIES (incidence 6/100,000)

Both of these disorders present as moderate to severe pruritus in the pubic area and often elsewhere. See p. 127 for more discussion.

SYPHILIS (incidence 3.5/100,000)

I. DEFINITION AND PATHOPHYSIOLOGY Syphilis is caused by a delicate spirilliform organism *Treponema pallidum*, character- ized by thinness, motility, and the closeness and regularity of its 6–14 corkscrew-like spirals. These spirochetes, 6–15 microns long and 0.25 micron thick, pass through intact mucous membranes or abraded skin and are disseminated by the bloodstream throughout the body within hours. Approximately 3 weeks later (10–40 days) the primary lesion appears at the site of infection. This chancre per- sists 1–5 weeks and then spontaneously disappears. It is followed about 6 weeks later (2 weeks to 6 months, average 9 weeks after inoculation) by the signs and symptoms of secondary syphilis, which also disappear without therapy within a month. Late (tertiary) syphilis is now not commonly seen. If left untreated, in about 33 percent of patients both the clinical disease and positive serologic tests will completely disappear. Thirty-three percent will continue to have positive serologic tests for syphilis but enjoy good health, and 33 percent will later develop signs of late syphilis. Of the latter, about 25 percent can be expected to die primarily as a result of the disease, and 80 percent of these deaths are related to cardiovascular problems.

II. SUBJECTIVE DATA

A. The lesions of primary syphilis are either painless or much less discomforting than would be expected. Extragenital lesions may hurt.

B. Secondary syphilis is usually asymptomatic; specifically, the lesions rarely itch. Patients often note a flulike syndrome with headache, malaise, sore throat, and arthralgias.

III. OBJECTIVE DATA (See color insert.)

A. **The primary chancre** is usually a single, firm erosion or ulcer covered with a crust. Occasionally, multiple chancres are present.

Bilateral nontender inguinal adenopathy may be palpated.

B. **The secondary rash** consists of generalized, faint, red-brown macules and papules.

  1. The palms and soles are characteristically involved.

  2. Lesions on mucous membranes appear as raised white "mucous patches."

  3. Other findings may include generalized lymphadenopathy, patchy hair loss, and smooth-surfaced yet warty intertriginous plaques termed *condyloma lata*.

IV. ASSESSMENT

A. Definitive diagnosis is made by viewing the causative spirochete by dark-field microscopy in specimens collected from primary and secondary lesions.

T. pallidum is not stained by ordinary reagents and is so narrow that it cannot be visualized under the normal light microscope.

B. Invasion of the human host by this spirochete leads to production of multiple antibodies of two basic types, reflected in the two kinds of serologic tests for syphilis (STS).

1. The nonspecific, nontreponemal antibodies (reagins), directed against a lipoidal antigen that results from interaction of host and parasite, are measured by flocculation tests (VDRL [Venereal Disease Research Laboratories] and RPR [rapid plasma reagin]).

   These tests are sensitive, easy to perform, and are the screening tests of choice.

2. The specific treponemal tests measure antibody directed against the treponemal organism.

   a. The fluorescent treponemal-antibody tests (FTA), the reference test at present, employs the Nichol-strain treponemes on the slide as antigen to which the patient's serum is added.

   b. This test is needed to confirm the presence or absence of true treponemal infection in those with a positive nontreponemal test but no history or knowledge of syphilis or other treponemal disease.

V. THERAPY

A. **Early syphilis: primary, secondary, latent syphilis of less than one year's duration**

   1. *Benzathine penicillin* 2.4 million units IM once, or *procaine penicillin* 600,000 units IM daily for 10 days.

      Alternatives are *tetracycline* 500 mg 4id or *erythromycin* 500 mg 4id, both taken for 15 days.

B. **Syphilis of more than one year's duration: latent neurosyphilis, cardiovascular, gummatous**

   1. *Benzathine penicillin* 2.4 million units IM weekly for 3 weeks, or 600,000 units *procaine penicillin* IM daily for 15 days.

      Alternatives are *tetracycline* or *erythromycin* as above for 30 days.

   2. *Cerebrospinal examination* is mandatory for patients with possible neurosyphilis and is suggested for all other patients in this group to rule out asymptomatic neurosyphilis.

C. **Pregnant patients** should be treated with penicillin, or, if allergic to penicillin, with erythromycin stearate, ethylsuccinate, or base.

D. **Retreatment** The STS generally returns to normal within 6–12 months after treatment of primary syphilis or 12–18 months after treatment of secondary syphilis. Retreatment (same treatment as for syphilis of more than one year's duration) should be considered if:

   1. Clinical disease continues or recurs.

   2. The quantitative STS titer measured at 3-month intervals does not decrease at least fourfold (2 tube dilutions) within 1 year.

   3. The quantitative STS titer increases fourfold (2 tube dilutions), representing either relapse or reinfection.

E. Penicillin treatment of gonorrhea is curative for *incubating* syphilis.

MOLLUSCUM CONTAGIOSUM (incidence 1.4/100,000)

Many adult patients with molluscum have lesions in the anogenital region. See p. 151 for more discussion.

LYMPHOGRANULOMA VENEREUM
(incidence 0.10/100,000)

I. **DEFINITION AND PATHOPHYSIOLOGY** Lymphogranuloma venereum is a systemic disease caused by a *Chlamydia* organism. A 7–12-day incubation period is followed by an evanescent primary lesion, then inflammatory lymphangitis and serious late sequelae.

II. **SUBJECTIVE DATA**

A. The primary lesion is painless.

B. The inguinal adenitis is tender and is accompanied by malaise, arthralgia, and fever.

III. **OBJECTIVE DATA**

A. The primary lesion, seen 1–3 weeks after inoculation but most often going unnoticed, may be a transient papule, vesicle, or, rarely, an ulceration.

B. Inguinal adenitis, present 2–3 weeks after the primary lesion and 3–6 weeks after inoculation, is unilateral in 66 percent of cases, is initially discrete and movable, and later firm, oval, and elongated. Overlying skin is adherent, edematous, and violaceous in color and may form grooves between the matted nodes; suppuration may occur.

C. Erythema nodosum is seen in 2–10 percent of cases.

D. Late changes of chronic disease may include proctitis, rectal stricture, perirectal abscesses and fistulae, and severe genital swelling. Malignant transformation occurs in about 2 percent of cases.

IV. ASSESSMENT

A. The Frei test, a 72-hr intradermal reaction performed with specific antigen grown on chick yolk sacs, becomes positive 2–3 weeks after the onset of adenopathy. This reagent, however, is generally unavailable.

B. The complement fixation test becomes positive within 1 month after onset of infection.

C. The organism can be cultured only with special media; this is not a clinically useful procedure.

D. The differential diagnosis includes pyogenic lymphadenitis, syphilis, chancroid, granuloma inguinale, and metastatic tumor.

V. THERAPY

A. **Tetracycline** 500 mg PO 4id for 3–4 weeks, *or*

B. **Sulfisoxazole** (Gantrisin®) 4 gm initially and then 1 gm daily for 3–4 weeks.

C. **Aspiration,** but not incision, of suppurating adenitis should be performed before spontaneous breakdown of tissue.

CHANCROID (incidence 0.09/100,000)

I. DEFINITION AND PATHOPHYSIOLOGY Chancroid, seen 20 times more commonly in men than in women, is an autoinoculable, localized, sexually transmitted disease caused by *Hemophilis ducreyi*. The incubation period is only 24–72 hr; some lesions may heal within a few days.

II. **SUBJECTIVE DATA**   Severe pain from both the genital lesion and lymph node is typical and helps differentiate the disease from syphilis.

III. **OBJECTIVE DATA**

A. The primary lesions consist of single or multiple (in about 50 percent of cases), round to oval, deep ulcers with irregular outlines, sharply defined but ragged and undermined borders, and a purulent base. The lesion is soft to palpation and is surrounded by an erythematous halo.

B. Balanitis, phimosis, and paraphimosis are frequent.

C. Inguinal lymphadenitis, present in about 33–50 percent of cases, develops 1–3 weeks after the primary lesion, is most often unilateral, and resembles an abscess (bubo). Suppuration, breakdown, and sinus tract formation can occur.

IV. **ASSESSMENT**

A. Definitive diagnosis is best made by viewing this small organism on Wright's, Giemsa, or Gram stain under the microscope. Tissue should be taken from under the undermined borders or from material aspirated from an unruptured lymph node.

1. *H. ducreyi* is a short, gram-negative rod with rounded ends, usually found outside of cells and in bands in parallel rows ("school of fish").

2. Under the best of conditions smears are positive in less than 50 percent of cases.

B. In practice, the diagnosis is made by exclusion, on the basis of negative dark-field examination and serologic tests for syphilis and negative smears for granuloma inguinale and herpes simplex.

C. Up to 15 percent of these patients may also be simultaneously infected with syphilis and have a "mixed chancre."

V. **THERAPY**

A. **Sulfonamides** are often the treatment of choice. Either sulfisoxazole (Gantrisin®) 2–4 gm initially followed by 1 gm 4id, or 80 mg trimethoprim/400 mg sulfamethoxazole (Bactrim®, Septra®) 4id for 10–20 days.

1. Pain should decrease within 24 hr, and concurrent syphilis is not masked.

2. These agents are relatively ineffective against lymphatic lesions.

3. A prophylactic dose of 2 gm within 3 hr of contact usually prevents infection.

B. **Streptomycin** 1 gm daily for 8–10 days also will not mask syphilis, but this drug is effective against lymphatic lesions. The possibility of vestibular drainage is minimized by the short length of treatment.

C. **Tetracycline** 500 mg PO 4id until healing is complete is effective in less than 50 percent of cases and may alter concurrent syphilitic infection.

GRANULOMA INGUINALE (incidence 0.02/100,000)

I. **DEFINITION AND PATHOPHYSIOLOGY** This mildly contagious, chronic, granulomatous disease involves the skin and lymphatics in the anogenital area and is usually considered a sexually transmittable disease. The organism, *Calymmatobacterium* (*Donovania*) *granulomatis*, is related to the *Klebsiella* species. The incubation period is probably 3–6 weeks.

II. **SUBJECTIVE DATA** Lesions cause no discomfort but are usually malodorous.

III. **OBJECTIVE DATA**

A. The insidious onset of tissue breakdown leads to an irregular ulcer with a soft, beefy red, friable, exuberant growth base.

B. Inguinal swellings are not lymphoadenitis but represent subcutaneous perilymphatic granulomatous lesions which may eventually break through the skin, causing sinus formation.

IV. **ASSESSMENT** Diagnosis is confirmed by finding the organisms (Donovan bodies) in the lesions.

A. Remove a piece of the lesion with a scalpel or punch.

B. Smear undersurface of tissue onto slides, or crush between two slides.

C. Fix with alcohol, stain with Wright's or Giemsa stain.

D. Donovan bodies will be found within mononuclear cells; they appear as straight or slightly curved rods with more deeply staining poles, thus creating a "safety pin" appearance. The organism is gram-negative and stains red with Giemsa and blue or purple with Wright's stain. The capsule appears pink on Wright's stain.

V. THERAPY

A. **Tetracycline** 500 mg PO 4id for 3 weeks.

B. **Streptomycin** is an alternative antibiotic administered as 3 gm IM q6h for 3 days in early cases, and for 10 days in extensive cases.

OTHER DISEASES

Other infections that may be sexually transmitted include those caused by cytomegalovirus, hepatitis B virus, and *Corynebacterium (Hemophilus) vaginalis.*

REFERENCES

Abrams AJ: Lymphogranuloma venereum. JAMA 205:199–202, 1968

Bergues JP, Laugier P: Chancroid. Dermatol Digest Aug 1976, 13–16

Holmes KK: Gonococcal infection: clinical, epidemiologic and laboratory perspectives. Adv Intern Med 19:259–285, 1974

Holmes KK, Handsfield HH, Wang SP, Wentworth BB, Turck M, Anderson JB, Alexander ER: Etiology of nongonococcal urethritis. N Engl J Med 292:1199–1205, 1975

Jacobs NF Jr, Kraus SJ: Gonococcal and nongonococcal urethritis in men: clinical and laboratory differentiation. Ann Intern Med 82: 7–12, 1975

King A, Nicol C: Venereal Diseases (3rd Edit). Baltimore, Williams & Wilkins, 1975, 369 pp

Riberio J: Granuloma inguinale. Practitioner 209:628–630, 1972

Sexually Transmitted Diseases. Extract from the Annual Report of the Chief Medical Officer of the Department of Health and Social Security for the Year 1974. Br J Vener Dis 52:351–354, 1976

Sparling PF: Diagnosis and treatment of syphilis. N Engl J Med 284: 642–653, 1971

29
Skin Tags

I. **DEFINITION AND PATHOPHYSIOLOGY** Skin tags (acrochordons) are small papillomas found commonly on the sides of the neck, axillae, upper trunk, and eyelids of the middle-aged and elderly. Obesity, pregnancy, menopause, and endocrine disorders such as acromegaly predispose to these benign epithelial hyperplastic lesions.

II. **SUBJECTIVE DATA** Skin tags are cosmetically bothersome but asymptomatic. Occasionally, a lesion will twist on its stalk and become painful, erythematous, and necrotic.

III. **OBJECTIVE DATA** The lesions are single or multiple, 1–3 mm in diameter, soft, flesh-colored or hyperpigmented papillomas, which are usually pedunculated.

IV. **ASSESSMENT** Treatment of obesity or an underlying endocrinologic abnormality will decrease the likelihood of new lesion formation. Lesions may be confused with seborrheic keratoses, dermal nevi, or warts.

V.   THERAPY   Treatment is easily accomplished with any of the following methods:

   A.   Grasp the tag with forceps and sever the base with a sharp scissors or a scalpel blade. Hemostasis may be secured by pressure, Monsel's solution (ferric subsulfate solution), mild acids (30% trichloroacetic acid), or an electrosurgical spark. The lesion may be anesthetized with ethyl chloride or refrigerant spray prior to excision, but this is rarely necessary. Never use electrosurgical apparatus around flammable ethyl chloride spray.

   B.   Touch each lesion with a light electrosurgical spark or remove it with the cutting current. Administration of local anesthesia is usually unnecessary and causes as much pain as the treatment itself. Multiple lesions may be treated at one time.

REFERENCE

Pinkus H: Epithelial and fibroepithelial tumors. Arch Dermatol 91:24–37, 1965

30
Sun Reactions and Sun Protection

I. **DEFINITION AND PATHOPHYSIOLOGY** The sun radiates a broad spectrum of energy which may be categorized in terms of the wavelength of the electromagnetic waves. That radiation reaching the earth's surface may be broadly subdivided into (a) infrared (range 700 nm–100 microns), felt as heat or a sensation of warmth; (b) visible (range 400 700 nm), the energy that stimulates the retina, and (c) ultraviolet (range 290–400 nm), wavelengths shorter than visible beginning next to the violet end of the color spectrum (see also p. 245).

The ultraviolet spectrum is subdivided into three bands. UVA radiation (320–400 nm, long wavelength) can cause immediate pigment darkening of preformed melanin, may play an additive role in assisting UVB (see below) in causing sunburn or aging, and in the presence of some drugs (psoralens, antibiotics such as Declomycin®, some diuretics, and others) may induce severe photosensitivity (sunburn and blistering). UVB radiation (280–320 nm, middle wavelength) causes erythema and sunburn, stimulates melanocytes to

193

make melanosomes and to make them more rapidly, causing the increased pigmentation seen as a tan; and after chronic exposure it induces the changes of aging and carcinogenesis. UVC radiation (range 200–280 nm) from sunlight is absorbed by the ozone layer in the atmosphere and does not reach the earth's surface. This radiation kills bacteria, can cause mild conjunctivitis or sunburn, and is used in operating-room germicidal lamps.

Sunburn is usually the result of excessive exposure to UVB ultraviolet light but may be a response to excessive UVC from artificial light sources or UVA in the presence of a topical or systemic photosensitizing agent. It is seen most commonly after exposure to the sun but may also follow exposure to sunlamps or occupational light sources (welding arcs [250–700 nm], photoengraving [250–700 nm], bactericidal or cold quartz lamps [254 nm]). UVB is not screened out by thin clouds on overcast days but is fully absorbed by window glass and is partially absorbed in the smoke and smog around large cities. Much UVL reaches the skin through reflection from snow, sand, or sidewalks; hats and umbrellas provide only moderate protection.

Those with less melanin pigment (blue-eyed persons, redheads, blondes, and frecklers) withstand actinic exposure poorly, burn easily, and suffer the chronic effects of light exposure earlier in life.

Sun exposure will cause immediate erythema, which then fades. A delayed erythema appears in 2–4 hr, becomes maximum in 14–20 hr, and lasts 24–72 hr. Mild erythema will develop in a fair-skinned person after 15–20 min of noonday sun at latitude 40°N (Philadelphia, Toledo, Denver, northern California, Lisbon, Naples, Peking.) Four to eight times that amount will produce a moderate to severe burn.

II. SUBJECTIVE DATA

A. A mild sunburn will be tender to the touch and cause a hot, taut, drawn feeling.

B. Severe burns are accompanied by intense pain, inability to tolerate contact with clothing and sheets, and constitutional symptoms, including nausea, tachycardia, chills, and fever.

III. OBJECTIVE DATA

A. The earliest sign of a burn is a pink to scarlet hue of the skin and mild edema. The more severe the burn, the earlier it will be evident.

B. This may progress to a vivid erythema, intense edema, and blistering.

C. Peeling follows as a consequence of increased epidermal turnover during the repair response, usually a week or more after the burn.

D. Hyperpigmentation is seen as a result of UVB-induced new pigment formation and protects against further sunburn. This is evident as immediate pigment darkening of preformed melanin (2–24 hr) and delayed tanning, reflective of new pigment formation (4–7 days).

E. UVA reactions follow a slower time course; erythema becomes evident as late as 48 hr, and the reaction may become more severe for several days (see p. 250).

F. UVC reactions are seldom severe; overexposure to short-wave ultraviolet light rarely leads to blistering.

IV. ASSESSMENT   The patient's history will usually be adequate to explain the clinical picture. It is important to be certain that there are no predisposing or underlying causes (drug administration, topical application of photosensitizers, or systemic illnesses such as lupus or porphyria).

V. THERAPY

A. Preventive measures   Sun-protective topical medications are available as sunscreens, which contain chemical substances that absorb UVL, or sunshades, which contain opaque materials that reflect the light. Most sunscreens have been designed to block or absorb UVB.

1. *UVB sunscreens*   *Para-aminobenzoic acid (PABA)* preparations (see p. 328) are the most useful sunscreens. PABA absorbs UVB and will decrease or prevent sunburn as well as new pigment formation. The most effective formulations contain 5% PABA in 50–70% alcohol (Pabanol®, Presun®). Approximately 18 times as much UVB radiation would be needed to produce minimal erythema after application of these sunscreens. The patient should be warned that these sunscreens may photooxidize and produce a semi-permanent yellow stain on light-colored fabrics (especially cotton and synthetic materials). PABA esters in alcohol (Blockout®, Pabafilm®) are slightly less effective and raise

the erythema threshold five- to sixfold but do not stain so
much. These sunscreens should be applied 1–2 hr before
exposure and, although they do not wash off the skin easily,
should be reapplied after swimming or profuse sweating.

2. ***Broad-spectrum sunscreens and sunshades*** These
   are the agents of choice for protection against UVC and
   UVA and should be used for those patients with photo-
   sensitive drug reactions, porphyria, and polymorphous light
   reaction.

   a. *Benzophenone-containing products* (Solbar®, Uval®)
      (see p. 329) Although these agents will protect against
      a wider spectrum of light (250–360 nm), their degree
      of effectiveness in the UVB erythema band is some-
      what less than that of PABA in alcohol (they raise the
      erythema threshold six- to sevenfold). Also, these prod-
      ucts generally wash off the skin easily and must be
      reapplied more frequently. Piz Buin Exclusiv Extrem
      Cream® contains both benzophenones and cinnamates
      and provides excellent protection against UVB and
      UVA.

   b. *Sunshades* contain titanium dioxide (TiO_2) or other
      opaque substances (A-Fil®, Reflecta®, RVPaque®, and
      RVPlus® contain TiO_2 in a tinted base. Covermark® or
      zinc oxide paste also gives good protection [see p.
      329]). These are the most effective sun-protective agents
      but are less cosmetically acceptable.

3. ***Lipstick sunscreens*** include RVPaba®, Uval®, SunStick®.
   All give best protection in the UVB range.

B. **A mild sunburn** should be treated as follows:

1. Apply cool tap water or Burow's solution compresses 20
   min 3–4id or more frequently.

2. A topical corticosteroid spray, lotion, cream, or gel may
   reduce inflammation and pain.

3. Use emollients (Eucerin®, Lubriderm®, Nivea®, petrolatum)
   to soothe and relieve dryness.

4. Most proprietary OTC burn remedies contain local anesthetics (benzocaine, dibucaine, or lidocaine), antiseptics,
   emollients, and fragrant materials. There is little need for

any of these ingredients in the care of a sunburn, and only 20% benzocaine (Americaine®) has been demonstrated to be at all effective. The vehicles of "anesthetic" sprays, creams, and lotions may be cooling and the ointments lubricating, thus lessening the symptoms, but this must be weighed against the hazard of becoming sensitized, especially to benzocaine. As burns are intrinsically self-healing, it is mandatory that the therapy be less noxious than the disease.

C. Severe sunburn

1. Instruct patients to call immediately if they are overexposed to sunlamps or to sunlight, since it is easier and more effective to abort severe inflammation than to treat an already established reaction. A short course of systemic corticosteroids will almost completely ablate a potentially severe sunburn; 40–60 mg of prednisone or its equivalent should be given daily for 3 days, then discontinued.

2. Topical care of established severe sunburns entails almost continuous cool compresses, topical steroids and emollients, a cradle for bed linens, analgesics as needed, and careful surveillance for bacterial superinfection.

3. Some fair-skinned individuals may increase their tolerance of UVL through systemic administration of psoralen compounds. These drugs will increase the capacity of the skin to produce melanin after sun exposure and also will result in retention of melanin granules in a thickened stratum corneum. Two hours prior to sun exposure, 30 mg of methoxsalen (Oxsoralen®) or preferably trioxsalen (Trisoralen®) should be taken, and exposure during the first week should be gradually increased (see p. 123 for more detailed treatment description). Use of medication without subsequent exposure to light will be ineffective.

REFERENCES

Cripps DJ, Hegedus S: Protection factor of sunscreens to monochromatic radiation. Arch Dermatol 109:202–204, 1974
Dalili H, Adriani J: The efficacy of local anesthetics in blocking the sensations of itch, burning and pain in normal and "sunburned" skin. Clin Pharmacol Ther 12:913–920, 1971

Epstein JH: Adverse cutaneous reactions to the sun, Year Book of Dermatology. Edited by FD Malkinson, RW Pearson. Chicago, Year Book, 1971, pp 5–35

Langner A, Kligman AM: Tanning without sunburn with aminobenzoic acid-type sunscreens. Arch Dermatol 106:338–343, 1972

Leading article: Unhealthy tan. Br Med J 2:494–495, 1970

Macleod TM, Frain-Bell W: A study of physical light screening agents. Br J Dermatol 92:149–156, 1975

Parrish JA: Sunscreens. Med Lett Drugs Ther 14:27–28, 1972

Pathak MA, Fitzpatrick TB, Frenk E: Evaluation of topical agents that prevent sunburn—superiority of para-aminobenzoic acid and its ester in ethyl alcohol. N Engl J Med 280:1459–1463, 1969

31
Urticaria

I. **DEFINITION AND PATHOPHYSIOLOGY** Urticaria (hives) affects 20 percent of the population at some time during their lives. The same reaction taking place in submucosa or deeper dermis and subcutaneous tissue is termed **angioedema.** The injection of histamine or a histamine-releasing chemical into the skin, or release of histamine from mast cells following antigen-antibody reaction results in vasodilatation, increased vascular permeability, and extravasation of protein and fluids. Urticaria seems to be mediated principally by histamine, but the precise role of other mast cell-related mediators such as slow-reacting substance of anaphylaxis, eosinophil chemotactic factor of anaphylaxis, platelet-activating factor, kinins, as well as prostaglandins remains to be elucidated.

Acute urticaria is most often mediated by B-lymphocyte-produced IgE and is seen in patients with anaphylaxis, serum sickness, or atopy, or as a reaction to insect bites, foods, infection, or drugs. Urticaria of more than 6 weeks' duration, termed **chronic urticaria,** may have a multiplicity of trigger factors; the exact cause remains in doubt in 80–90 percent of cases. Immunologic cases of chronic urticaria include reactions to drugs or, less frequently, to foods and food additives (especially salicylates, tartrazine, and benzoates), inhalants, or parasitic infestations. The mean duration of urticaria alone is 6 months, angioedema alone 1 year, and urticaria with angioedema about 5 years (See Champion et al, 1969).

Hives also may accompany infections, collagen vascular diseases, and malignant tumors. Hives with arthralgias or arthritis may be an early sign of anicteric hepatitis or a manifestation of an underlying necrotizing vasculitis. Stress and anxiety are often thought to be important etiologic factors. Urticaria induced by cold or ultraviolet light is uncommon.

There are two common types of nonimmunologic urticaria. **Cholinergic urticaria** is induced by acetylcholine, not histamine, and is triggered by emotion, heat, exercise, or change in temperature. The lesions are usually smaller than those of allergic urticaria and are more evanescent. **Dermatographic lesions** are hives induced by trauma (scratching) or pressure (standing, tight clothing or shoes). In some instances this tendency appears to be mediated by IgE and is transferable. In others, kinins, slow-reacting substance, or other vasodilatatory mediators may play a role in production of these lesions, which appear similar to those of typical urticaria but which have bizarre shapes and borders. Although everyone will respond to cutaneous trauma with a triple response of Lewis (erythema, flare, wheal), in dermatographism the response is excessive, even to stimuli of low intensity.

Aspirin makes urticaria worse in up to 33 percent of patients and should be prohibited in all patients with urticaria. The ubiquitous yellow dye tartrazine and other food additives may have a similar action. Agents known to cause degranulation of mast cells (morphine, codeine, reserpine, polymyxin B, alcohol) also should be avoided.

Hereditary angioedema is a dominantly inherited disorder in which a normal serum inhibitor of the activated first component of complement is either deficient or absent. These patients suffer recurrent episodes of cutaneous angioedema as well as attacks of laryngeal edema and gastrointestinal involvement, thought to be mediated by the complement cascade.

II.   **SUBJECTIVE DATA**   Intense pruritus is the typical symptom of urticaria. Stinging and prickling sensations are also described.

III. OBJECTIVE DATA

A. Urticarial wheals are raised, erythematous, and edematous plaques with sharply defined, serpiginous, or polycyclic borders surrounded by an erythematous halo. Intensely edematous lesions will have a blanched center. Their diameters may range from millimeters to several centimeters. Individual lesions last up to 8–12 hr; those staying in one location for more than 24 hr cannot be considered true urticaria but must be regarded as a more fixed eruption such as erythema multiforme or urticarial vasculitis. The continuous spectrum of urticarial-type lesions, ranging from the evanescent wheal of true urticaria to the relatively fixed edema of erythema multiforme, makes precise diagnosis difficult at times.

B. The lesions of cholinergic urticaria are small, 1–3 mm, punctate, papular wheals surrounded by a large macular erythematous flare. They disappear spontaneously in 30–60 min.

IV. ASSESSMENT

A detailed and perceptive history and thorough physical examination frequently will reveal the cause and type of urticaria. If this is not rewarding, then other types of investigation, though usually unproductive, must nevertheless be pursued in patients with chronic urticaria. Pertinent tests would include CBC, differential, ESR, urinalysis, liver function tests, T4, and also complement levels (C3 and CH50) if there is suspicion of collagen-vascular disease, cryoglobulinemia, or vasculitis. Occasionally a brief trial of a rigid elimination diet and examination of fresh stools for ova and parasites is undertaken. Biopsy of chronic urticaria lesions is warranted and will occasionally show perivascular inflammatory changes suggestive of lupus erythematosus or vasculitis. Skin testing is of no value.

V. THERAPY

A. **Anaphylactic** and **acute urticarial reactions:** therapy outlined on p. 36

B. **Chronic urticaria**

1. Identification and treatment or removal of the trigger factor is the most important and the only effective long-term therapy.

2. Local measures

a. Cool or ice water compresses or tepid baths with Aveeno® colloidal oatmeal may eliminate itching.

b. Antipruritic lotions or emulsions may help: 0.25% menthol ± 1% phenol in calamine lotion or Eucerin® (see p. 307 for other preparations).

3. Systemic measures

a. Antihistamine therapy is the therapy of choice (see p. 266 for method of action and how to choose the appropriate agent). Hydroxyzine (Atarax®, Vistaril®) is often the best drug for cholinergic urticaria and dermatographism and is equal to any others for chronic urticaria. It may be used alone or with other antihistamines, and *dosage should be pushed to the limit of tolerance* or to subsidence of symptoms. If hydroxyzine is ineffective, chlorpheniramine maleate (Chlor-Trimeton®) or cyproheptadine hydrochloride (Periactin®) should be used next, either alone or in combination (see p. 267).

b. If lesions are more acute or severe, or if angioedema is present, inject 0.3–0.5 ml epinephrine (1:1000) subcutaneously or IM q1–2h.

c. Ephedrine, 25 mg 4id or sublingual isoproterenol (Isuprel®) may also be useful.

d. It is rarely necessary or justified to use systemic corticosteroids. However, in some instances, when all diagnostic and therapeutic methods have been exhausted, a 2-week course of corticosteroids (starting at 40–60 mg prednisone or equivalent) will temporarily suppress the disease. Occasionally after this treatment, the urticaria will not recur.

REFERENCES

Brasher GW, Starr JC, Hall FF, Spiekerman AM: Complement component analysis in angioedema. Diagnostic value. Arch Dermatol 111: 1140–1142, 1975

Braverman IM: Urticaria as a sign of internal disease. Postgrad Med 41:450–454, 1967

Champion RH: Drug therapy of urticaria. Br Med J 4:730–732, 1973

Champion RH, Roberts SOB, Carpenter RE, Roger JH: Urticaria and angioedema: a review of 554 patients. Br J Dermatol 81:588–597, 1969

Leading article: Urticaria. Lancet 2:1344–1345, 1969

Mathews KP: A current view of urticaria. Med Clin North Am 58:185–205, 1974

Matthews NA, Kirby JD, James J, Warin RP: Dermatographism: reduction in wheal size by chlorpheniramine and hydroxyzine. Br J Dermatol 88:279–282, 1973

Moore-Robinson M, Warin RP: Some clinical aspects of cholinergic urticaria. Br J Dermatol 80:794–799, 1968

Newcomb RW, Nelson H: Dermographia mediated by immunoglobulin E. Am J Med 54:174–180, 1973

Ostrov MR: Dermographia: a critical review. Ann Allergy 25:591–597, 1967

Shumaker JB, Goldfinger SE, Alpert E, Isselbacher KJ: Arthritis and rash. Clues to anicteric hepatitis. Arch Intern Med 133:483–485, 1974

Soter NA, Austen KF, Gigli I: Urticaria and arthralgias as manifestations of necrotizing angiitis (vasculitis). J Invest Dermatol 63:485–490, 1974

32
Vascular Neoplasms

I. **DEFINITION AND PATHOPHYSIOLOGY** Cutaneous abnormalities consisting of new vessel growths or vascular dilatation are extremely common; probably no individual escapes acquiring one or several throughout a lifetime. Angiomas may be most easily classified on the basis of their predominant vascular channels.

A. **Capillary vessels**

1. *Strawberry nevus* This vascular malformation, present at birth or in neonates, grows for 3–12 months and begins to subside after 1 yr; and 75–95 percent have regressed by age 5–7. Lesions that grow most rapidly usually regress most completely.

2. *Cherry angioma* Cherry angiomas (senile angiomas) appear in early adult life and increase in number with advancing age. These asymptomatic lesions remain indefinitely.

3. ***Pyogenic granuloma*** This misnamed, rapidly growing, and friable angioma often is located at a site of previous injury. Infection usually plays no part in the initiation or course of the lesion.

B. **Cavernous vessels**

1. ***Cavernous angioma*** These vascular tumors appear first during childhood, are frequently larger and deeper than capillary angiomas, and do not subside spontaneously. They may appear as isolated lesions or may be a part of such syndromes as the Klippel-Trenaunay-Weber syndrome, blue rubber bleb nevus syndrome, or Maffucci's syndrome.

C. **Disorders with vascular dilatation**

1. ***Port-wine stain (nevus flammeus)*** These lesions, which are entirely flat and seen only as a change in skin color, are commonly found on the nuchal and eyelid areas of infants. When located in other areas, they usually occur in a unilateral or in a dermatomal distribution and may be associated with the Sturge-Weber or Klippel-Trenaunay-Weber syndrome. Most eyelid lesions disappear within the first year of life, whereas only half of those on the nuchal area (salmon patch) will have disappeared by that time. Lesions in other areas are stable and do not fade.

2. **Venous lake (venous varix)** This is a soft ectasia frequently seen on the face, lips, or ears of the elderly. The lesions persist indefinitely and occasionally thrombose and involute.

3. **Telangiectasia and spider ectasia (nevus araneus)** These lesions resemble a spider in appearance and are most commonly seen in women and children on the face and upper trunk. Acquired lesions may appear in relation to liver disease such as hepatitis or cirrhosis; changes in estrogen metabolism, as in pregnancy or in women on birth control pills; or as a part of hereditary hemorrhagic telangiectasia. Other causes of facial telangiectasia include actinic damage, the prolonged use of topical fluorinated corticosteroids, and rosacea. Ectatic vessels and vasodilatation are also seen commonly on the lower extremities of women.

II. SUBJECTIVE DATA

A. Capillary vessels

1. *Strawberry nevus* The lesions are not painful, but large lesions may spontaneously erode or become infected.

2. *Cherry angioma* There are no symptoms.

3. *Pyogenic granuloma* The lesions may be painful, but the most frequent complaint relates to their friability; these angiomas bleed easily and may become secondarily infected.

B. Cavernous vessels There are usually no symptoms.

C. Vascular dilatation There are usually no symptoms.

Note: All angiomatous vessels may be readily visible and a cosmetic nuisance.

III. OBJECTIVE DATA (See color insert.)

A. Capillary vessels

1. *Strawberry nevus*

    a. Bright red to purple-blue lesions, which are raised, dome-shaped, or polypoid, with sharp borders.

    b. Compressible, but will not totally blanch.

2. *Cherry angioma*

    a. Bright red, raised, pinpoint to several millimeters in diameter; usually multiple and present in most profusion on the upper trunk.

    b. Will not blanch on pressure.

3. *Pyogenic granuloma*

    a. Bright red to brown, elevated, polypoid, or sessile.

    b. Usually single and found most commonly on the extremities.

    c. May be eroded, crusted, ulcerated, or infected.

B. Cavernous vessels

1. *Cavernous angioma*

    a. Small to very large, ill-defined lesion that is spongy and compressible but will slowly refill.

    b. The portions elevated above the skin's surface may be red-blue to purple.

C. Disorders with vascular dilatation

    1. *Port-wine stain*

        a. Macular, pink to burgundy in color, variable in size, with distinct borders.

        b. In older lesions, small, deep blue, nodular, or warty capillary or cavernous angiomas may develop.

    2. *Venous lake*

        a. Deep blue in color.

        b. Soft and consists of compressible, slightly raised vessels.

    3. *Telangiectasia and spider ectasia*

        a. Bright red, discrete, usually with a central, elevated punctum and many radiating branches.

        b. A pulsating center, if this is not readily seen, will become apparent on gentle pressure with a glass slide.

        c. More intense pressure will obliterate the lesion entirely.

        d. Other types of facial telangiectasia are present mostly over the malar regions and consist of single red-blue, enlarged vessels accumulated into telangiectatic "mats."

IV. ASSESSMENT

A. Capillary vessels

    1. *Strawberry nevus* Measure and photograph the lesion in order to follow its evolution and subsidence.

    2. *Cherry angioma* How long have they been there? The most frequent lesions confused with cherry spots, particularly in the hospitalized patient, are petechiae. Small angiomas must at times be biopsied to prove their unimportant nature.

B. Cavernous vessels

    1. *Cavernous angioma* X-ray studies of underlying tissue may be indicated.

C. **Disorders with vascular dilatation**

　　1. *Port-wine stain*　Neurologic and x-ray examinations may be warranted for all but the eyelid and nuchal lesions.

　　2. *Venous lake*　No investigation needed.

　　3. *Telangiectasia*　Investigation into the underlying cause of acquired telangiectasia by history, physical examination, and serologic tests may reveal otherwise unsuspected systemic disease.

V. **THERAPY**

A. **Capillary vessels**

　　1. *Strawberry nevus*

　　　　a.　As almost all lesions will involute spontaneously, they should be allowed to do so. Aggressive forms of therapy most often will leave a significant cosmetic defect.

　　　　b.　Small lesions may be treated by cryosurgery with liquid nitrogen or dry ice, if warranted.

　　　　c.　Systemic corticosteroid administration may initiate involution in very large or awkward lesions (see B-1a).

　　　　d.　X-irradiation may hasten shrinking in lesions of large size or in those in awkward areas such as around orifices.

　　　　e.　Electrosurgery of small lesions or excision of large ones occasionally may be justified.

　　2. *Cherry angioma*　Light electrodesiccation will easily remove these lesions.

　　3. *Pyogenic granuloma*

　　　　a.　Curettage and electrodesiccation is the therapy of choice.

　　　　b.　Cryosurgery may work but is less effective than the foregoing.

　　　　c.　Chemical cauterants (silver nitrate stick, mono-, di-, or trichloroacetic acids) may also be efficacious.

B. Cavernous vessels

1. *Cavernous angioma*

a. Aggressive treatment of cavernous and capillary angiomas with systemic corticosteroids (prednisone 20 mg daily for several weeks, then tapered off) should be considered in the following situations:

(1) Involvement of a vital structure.

(2) Rapid growth with cosmetic destruction.

(3) Mechanical orificial obstruction.

(4) Hemorrhage with or without thrombocytopenia.

(5) Threatened cardiovascular decompensation.

b. Excision is occasionally necessary.

C. Disorders with vascular dilatation

1. *Port-wine stain*

a. Tattooing with flesh-colored pigments, the use of laser beams, and the application of liquid nitrogen have all been used on port-wine stains with variable but not outstanding success.

b. The best answer for this problem, as well as for those of other cosmetically disfiguring angiomas or other lesions, is the use of a skin-colored cosmetic that will effectively hide the lesion from public view. Covermark®, which is available in a variety of colors (except very deep black) at the cosmetic counters of many stores, does this particularly well. Erace® may also be useful.

2. *Venous lake* Electrosurgery may be useful (see 3 below).

3. *Telangiectasia* Spider ectasias are simply effaced by electrosurgery. If anesthesia is used, mark the "body" of the spider before injection.

a. Insert either a #30 needle or a fine electrosurgical (epilating) tip into the central punctum and deliver as small a current as possible in one or more short bursts.

b. Destruction of the punctum will result in blanching of the entire lesion, but at times some of the radiating spokes must also be destroyed.

c. Other ectasias may be treated in the same way, but the tip should be inserted into several areas along the vessel's course.

d. Delivery of too much current can leave small, pitted scars.

e. It is usually unnecessary to anesthetize the lesion; the procedure is relatively painless, and the anesthetic temporarily makes the vessels disappear, complicating the procedure.

f. Telangiectatic vessels may also be destroyed in the same fashion by electrolysis.

REFERENCES

Bean WB: Vascular Spiders and Related Lesions of the Skin. Springfield, Ill., Thomas, 1968

Bowers RE, Graham EA, Tomlinson KA: The natural history of the strawberry nevus. Arch Dermatol 82:667–680, 1960

Braverman IM: Telangiectasia as a sign of systemic disease. Conn Med 33:42–46, 1969

Fost NC, Esterly NB: Successful treatment of juvenile hemangiomas with prednisone. J Pediatr 72:351–357, 1968

Lasser AE, Stein AF: Steroid treatment of hemangiomas in children. Arch Dermatol 108:565–567, 1973

Margileth AM, Museles M: Current concepts in diagnosis and management of congenital cutaneous hemangiomas. Pediatrics 36:410–416, 1965

Rees TD, Conners D: Complications in the treatment of hemangiomas. J Dermatol Surg 1:29–32, 1975

Ronchese F: Granuloma pyogenicum. Am J Surg 109:430–431, 1965

Whiting DA, Kallmeyer JC, Simson JW: Widespread arterial spiders in a case of latent hepatitis, with resolution after therapy. Br J Dermatol 82:32–36, 1970

33
Warts

I. **DEFINITION AND PATHOPHYSIOLOGY** Warts are intraepidermal tumors of the skin caused by infection with the human papilloma virus. This DNA papova virus cannot be easily cultured, and thus little is known about its growth patterns, immunology, or metabolism. The virus is never found below the granular layer. It is initially within the nucleus of keratinocytes, eventually fills the entire nuclear space, and spills into the cytoplasm; in the stratum corneum, the virus lies free within the keratin mass. Virus concentration is greatest in warts of 6–12 months' duration; after that virus particles decrease and disappear. There is a higher incidence of these benign tumors in patients who are immunosuppressed or have other defects of cell-mediated hypersensitivity (CMI). It is presumed that the same virus is responsible for all the different morphologic forms. The incubation period after inoculation into human volunteers varies from 1–12 months.

Warts may be found in persons of any age but are most common between ages 12–16; in a school population in Britain the prevalence of common warts was 16.2 percent. They may be spread by contact or autoinoculation; about 20–30 percent of all lesions will spontaneously involute within 6 months, 50 percent within 1 year, and 66 percent within 2 years. New lesions may continue to appear during this period of time and are seen three times more frequently in children with warts than in those without. The high rate of spontaneous involution, probably a CMI response, makes it difficult to evaluate the effectiveness of suggestion or "charming," as well as the more direct methods of wart therapy.

II. **SUBJECTIVE DATA** Most warts induce symptoms only when they become awkward because of their size or appearance. Although wart tissue is not inherently painful, condyloma acuminata (see III E) may be discomforting and friable for mechanical reasons; periungual lesions may develop fissures that hurt; and plantar warts can become very painful during walking or running.

III. **OBJECTIVE DATA** (See color insert.) There are several morphologic variants of warts:

A. **Common warts** start as small, pinhead-sized, flesh-colored, translucent papules and grow over several weeks or months to larger, raised, papillary-surfaced, flesh-colored or darker, hyperkeratotic papules. Black specks of hemosiderin pigment may be seen in thrombosed capillary loops. Paring the lesion results in punctate bleeding points. Common warts are found most often on the hands, especially in children, or on other sites often subjected to trauma but may grow anywhere on the epidermis or mucous membranes.

B. **Filiform warts** are slender, soft, thin, fingerlike growths seen primarily on the face and neck.

C. **Flat, plane, or juvenile warts** are flesh-colored or tan, soft, 1–3 mm in diameter, discrete papules appearing primarily on the face, neck, extensor aspect of the forearms, and hands.

D. **Plantar or palmar warts** are hyperkeratotic, firm, elevated or flat lesions that interrupt the natural skin lines (as opposed to calluses). Red or black capillary dots may be seen. A mosaic wart consists of the confluence of multiple lesions into one large, usually flat lesion.

E. Warts that grow in warm, moist, intertriginous areas develop into soft, friable, vegetating clusters. These **condylomata acuminata** are frequently found on the foreskin and penis, particularly in uncircumcised men, on vaginal and labial mucosa, and in the urethral meatus and perianal area.

IV: THERAPY

A. Many therapeutic modalities are available for the treatment of warts. It is important to remember that warts are benign cutaneous growths and that the therapy should also be benign. Therapy should present no hazard to the patient, no scarring should result, and side-effects should be minimal. It is not difficult to cause considerable pain, as well as permanent scarring, by an overly enthusiastic approach. This curative zeal must be curbed, for it is neither necessary nor warranted to remove every wart. On the other hand, the therapist should be optimistic, for most lesions can be successfully treated if warranted.

B. Bunney et al's data (1976) from comparative treatment trials give some indication of what may be expected from different modes of therapy. They demonstrated that 70–80 percent of patients with hand warts can be cured with nonblistering liquid nitrogen cryosurgery within 12 weeks, providing the interval between treatments is not more than 3 weeks; most patients require three treatments. Home treatment with salicylic acid–lactic acid paint (SAL, see p. 214) will cure as many patients within the same time period as liquid nitrogen. With simple plantar warts, SAL treatment will cure 84 percent of patients within 12 weeks as compared to 81 percent for podophyllin therapy. Mosaic warts are difficult to cure with any therapy; SAL treatment eradicated 47 percent within 12 weeks and was as efficient as any other method used. Throughout Bunney et al's study 30 percent of patients with hand warts, 20 percent of those with simple plantar warts, and 50 percent of those with mosaic warts were found to be resistant to treatment.

C. **Common warts** are best treated as follows:

1. Destruction by *light electrodesiccation and curettage* (see p. 230), *or*

2. *Cryosurgery* with liquid nitrogen. This technique, as well as electrodesiccation, carefully executed, will remove the lesion and usually will leave no scar and little or no pigmentary change (see p. 234 for details of therapy). Nonblistering therapy (5–30 sec application) is effective. In general, cryosurgery is the best therapy.

3. *Keratolytic therapy* with paints such as 5–20% salicylic acid and 5–20% lactic acid in flexible collodion (SAL) may be self-administered at home and in 60–80 percent of patients will lead to cures within 12 weeks on all but mosaic plantar warts. Keratolytic agents may act by mechanical removal of infected cells and wart virus and also by providing a mild inflammatory reaction that renders the virus more available to immunologic stimulation or response. Duofilm® (16.7% salicylic acid, 16.7% lactic acid in flexible collodion) is a commercially available SAL preparation; patients should be instructed to use it or other keratolytic paints as follows:

a. Wash area thoroughly with soap and water.

b. Rub surface of wart gently with mild abrasive such as emery board, pumice stone, or callus file.

c. Apply keratolytic paint to the wart with a sharpened matchstick or orange stick.

d. Allow to dry.

e. Keep bottle tightly closed.

f. Repeat each night.

g. If area becomes red or tender, discontinue therapy until this subsides and then start again. Alternatively, a keratolytic paint with a lower concentration of salicylic and lactic acids may be prescribed.

h. Do not apply paint to warts previously treated with liquid nitrogen until the inflammation has subsided.

4. *Cantharidin* (Cantharone®), a mitochondrial poison that leads to changes in cell membranes, epidermal cell dyshesion, acantholysis, and blister formation, is also useful (see also p. 320). Thick hyperkeratotic lesions should be pared down before painting. The lesion should then be painted with cantharidin, allowed to dry, and covered with Blenderm® or other nonporous occlusive tape; 40% salicylic acid plaster may be used to achieve greater activity. The tape is left on for 24 hr, or until the area begins to hurt. A blister, often hemorrhagic, will form, break, crust, and fall off in 7–14 days; at this time the lesion is pared down, and any wart remnants retreated. Since the effect of cantharidin is entirely intraepidermal, no scarring ensues. Ringlike recurrences may be seen occasionally after treatment with cantharidin or, at times, following liquid nitrogen therapy. Verrusol® (C&M Pharmacol, 1519 East Eight Mile Drive, Hazel Park, Mich. 48030), which contains 30% salicylic acid, 5% podophyllin, and 1% cantharidin, may be used in the same manner.

5. ***Podophyllum resin*** (podophyllin), a cytotoxic agent which arrests mitosis in metaphase, is used primarily for treatment of condyloma acuminata but may also be used on all other types of warts (see also p. 322). A 25% preparation in compound tincture of benzoin, or 10% podophyllum, 10% salicylic acid resin (Ver-Var®) should be applied overnight. The effectiveness as well as the irritant potential of this medication may be increased by covering with adhesive tape or plastic tape (Blenderm®).

6. Lesions may be painted weekly or more frequently with ***acids*** such as 50–80% trichloroacetic acid, saturated dichloroacetic acid, or 80% monochloroacetic acid. After a necrotic crust forms, it should be removed and the lesion retreated. This method is relatively painless and somewhat slow, but it may be carried out at home. Both the effectiveness and rapidity of therapy may be increased by covering the acid-treated lesion with a small pad of 40% salicylic plaster and adhesive tape for 12–24 hr.

D. **Filiform warts** are best treated by light electrosurgery or cryosurgery, or with keratolytic paints.

E. **Flat warts** should be treated with a short (5–15 sec) application of liquid nitrogen; with keratolytic paints; or with tretinoin preparations. Electrosurgery may also be used, but it may leave small, hypopigmented scars. Lesions on the male face constitute a difficult problem, as autoinoculation takes place each time the patient shaves. To avoid cosmetically damaging results it is especially important to be conservative. Use of an electric shaver or of depilatories may decrease autoinoculation.

F. **Plantar warts** are sometimes best left untreated. Unless a wart is painful, rapidly growing, or small, it is wise to recommend no therapy or nonaggressive therapy. If treatment is necessary, the following approaches can be used:

1. Enucleation by blunt dissection technique is often the therapy of choice if there is one or only a few lesions (see Heinlein 1974; Ulbrich et al 1974). This method of removal is also excellent for removal of verrucae vulgaris in other areas.

2. Intermittent flattening of the lesion with a pumice stone, callus file, or scalpel is usually enough to keep plantar lesions entirely asymptomatic.

3. Keratolytic therapy with salicylic and lactic acid paint (see p. 214) is the most convenient and effective nontraumatic method. The patient should apply medication nightly as follows:

    a. Remove the adhesive tape from previous night's treatment.

    b. Rub the surface of the wart with an emery board, pumice stone, or callus file.

    c. Soak the foot in hot water or a bath for at least 5 min.

    d. Apply a drop of keratolytic paint to the wart. Allow to dry. If the wart is large, apply another drop.

    e. When dry, cover with a piece of adhesive tape. If the lesion is very thick or more aggressive treatment is desired, apply a piece of 40% salicylic acid plaster to the wart and then cover with adhesive tape.

    f. If soreness occurs, stop treatment and restart after it subsides. Use of "micropore" tape rather than adhesive tape may lead to less inflammation.

4. Bimonthly debridement of lesions followed by application of acids and salicylic acid plaster (see p. 323) or 60% salicylic acid paste plus ¼ inch felt padding will reduce most lesions in 2–4 treatments.

5. Bimonthly debridement and treatment with cantharidin (see p. 214) is also effective but may be painful.

6. Liquid nitrogen freezing may produce good results, but it does cause discomfort during application; in addition, the resultant blister makes walking uncomfortable for the next several days.

7. Application of 25% podophyllin in compound tincture of benzoin under tape occlusion overnight, or nightly 15-min soaks in 3% formalin, may also be of some benefit. Alternatively, the warts may be painted with 10% formalin and covered with 40% salicylic acid plaster for 3–4 days. The lesions are then debrided by patient or physician, and the formalin and dressing reapplied. This painless therapy may be continued for weeks until the lesion is gone.

8. Destructive electrosurgery, sharp scalpel excision, and radiotherapy should be avoided, because although they may remove the lesion, the resulting scar often becomes a more difficult and less easily treated problem than the wart itself.

9. It is important to correct orthopedic defects and prescribe correct footwear. Plantar warts most often occur in areas of pressure and callus, and unless the incorrect weight-bearing condition can be alleviated, it is frequently difficult either to cure the wart or to make the patient comfortable.

G. Condylomata acuminata

1. Weekly painting of the lesion with 25% podophyllum resin in compound tincture of benzoin is the most effective therapy. Medication should be kept off uninvolved surrounding skin; this may be accomplished by applying a thin covering of petrolatum around the lesion before therapy. After the benzoin dries, the area should be liberally powdered to prevent undue maceration and inadvertent transfer of podophyllin from the lesions to apposing normal skin. At the start of therapy, the medication should be left on for only 1 hr and then washed off, particularly in the vulvar area and the area under the foreskin. As therapy progresses, podophyllin should be left in place 4–6 hr before it is removed. Treated lesions may become inflamed and painful during the following 2–3 days. It is wise to treat only parts of a large condyloma to prevent disabling pain, but it is important to repeat treatment every 7–10 days until all lesions are gone. A topical anesthetic preparation is often useful during the period of pain.

   Podophyllin can cause severe irritation and if absorbed may produce systemic toxic effects. It is inadvisable to apply it in large amounts to mucous membranes, and it is unwise to use in pregnant women because of its possible cytotoxic action on the fetus.

2. Liquid nitrogen cryosurgery is also excellent for condylomata acuminata. The amount and intensity of therapy and the delineation of treatment margins can be better controlled than with podophyllin. Liquid nitrogen plus podophyllin (and anesthetic) may be better than either alone.

3. Occasionally it is necessary and useful to approach such lesions with electrosurgery and curettage. This is particularly true when there are large masses of warty tissue, which may then be removed in one procedure, or when painting of the lesions with podophyllin appears to lose its effectiveness. This is sometimes best carried out as an in-hospital operating room procedure.

4. Proctoscopy and treatment of rectal lesions with podophyllin or liquid nitrogen is necessary in all patients with perianal condylomata.

5. Intraurethral and meatal condylomata may be treated conservatively with podophyllin or liquid nitrogen. Alternatively, 2–5% 5-fluorouracil solution may also be effective. Therapy must not be overaggressive if urethral stricture is to be avoided.

H. Special comments

1. Therapy for children should be gentle and nonaggressive. Keratolytic solutions and applications of acids are useful and nonpainful. Cantharidin is effective and does not cause pain during application. Electrosurgery and cryosurgical procedures are often traumatic to all involved. In this age group, hypnosis appears to work well at times.

2. Treatment with keratolytic paints, liquid nitrogen, or cantharidin generally produces the best cosmetic results. Acids and electrosurgery have a greater potential for scarring.

3. Periungual lesions are best treated with either liquid nitrogen or cantharidin.

4. OTC wart remedies such as Compound W® and WartAway® are liquids that contain 13–14% salicylic acid (a keratolytic) and acetic acid (a caustic). The OTC corn and callus remedies are usually salicylic acid compounds.

REFERENCES

Almeida JD, Oriel JD: Wart viruses. Br J Dermatol 83:698–699, 1970

Bunney MH: Warts. Br J Hosp Med 11:565–572, 1975

Bunney MH, Nolan MW, Williams DA: An assessment of methods of treating viral warts by comparative treatment trials based on a standard design. Br J Dermatol 94:667–679, 1976

Clarke GHV: The charming of warts. J Invest Dermatol 45:15–21, 1965

DeVillez RL, Lewis CW (Eds): Verruca Vulgaris Seminar. J Assoc Mil Dermatol 1:47–54, 1975

Epstein WL, Kligman AM: Treatment of warts with cantharidin. Arch Dermatol 77:508–511, 1958

Heinlein JA: Blunt dissection (letter to the editor). Cutis 13:297–299, 1974

Massing AM, Epstein WL: Natural history of warts. A two-year study. Arch Dermatol 87:306–310, 1963

Oriel JD: Natural history of genital warts. Br J Vener Dis 47:1–13, 1971

Perez-Figaredo R, Baden H: The pharmacology of podophyllin. Prog Dermatol 10:1–4, 1976

Powell LC Jr: Condyloma acuminata. Clin Obstet Gynecol 15:948–965, 1972

Pringle WM, Helms DC: Treatment of plantar warts by blunt dissection. Arch Dermatol 108:79–82, 1973

Ulbrich AP, Koprince D, Arends NW: Warts: treatment by total enucleation. Cutis 14:582–586, 1974

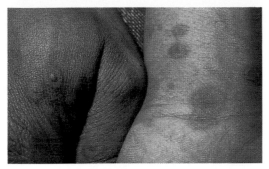

1. Erythema multiforme—iris (target) lesions

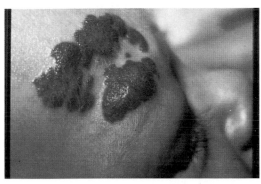

2. Strawberry nevus

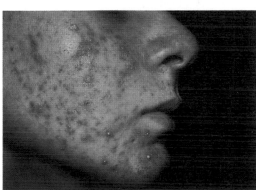

3. Acne—papules, pustules, and scarring

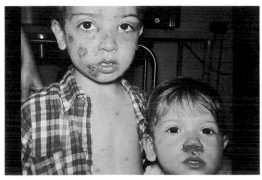

4. Impetigo

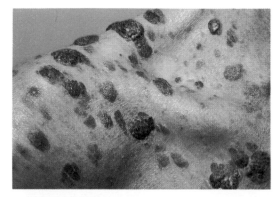

5. Seborrheic keratoses

6. Herpes simplex

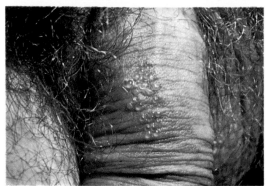

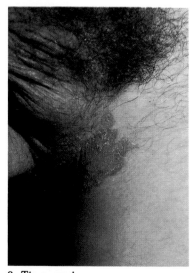

7. Pityriasis rosea

8. Tinea cruris

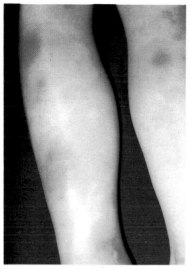

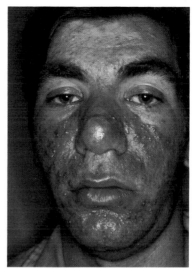

9. Erythema nodosum

10. Rosacea

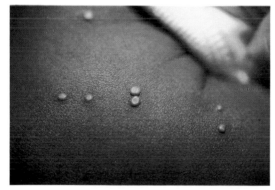

11. Molluscum
    contagiosum

12. Psoriasis

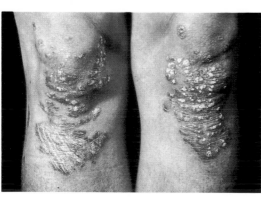

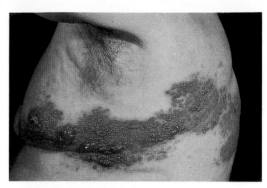

13. Herpes zoster

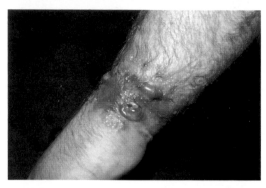

14. Contact dermatitis to leather (watchband)

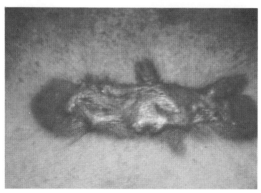

15. Keloid

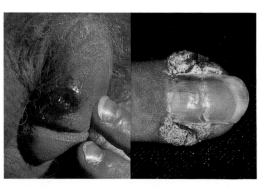

16. Primary syphilis—chancre

17. Periungual warts

II
Procedures and Techniques

34
Operative Procedures

Skin is uniquely available for diagnostic procedures as well as for the direct application of therapeutic agents. Single or multiple procedures can be performed within short periods of time with little discomfort to the patient. Most techniques are easily learned, easy to perform, and require only simple equipment.

BIOPSY

I. PROCEDURE

A. **The punch biopsy** is an extremely simple procedure which, in all but a very few cases, removes sufficient tissue for histo-pathologic study.

1. It is generally best to select a mature and well-developed lesion for biopsy. However, if blisters are present, choose the earliest lesion available and take care to keep the roof intact. Several biopsies should be obtained from evolving eruptions or those with various types of lesions (in this in-

stance, too, biopsy of early lesions may be especially rewarding). Lesions altered by trauma or treatment or old "burned-
out" areas will not yield useful information. Biopsies on the
legs and feet heal more slowly, especially if the circulation is
poor; if possible, choose a lesion above the knees. Choose a
site entirely within the lesion; avoid including normal skin
in the biopsy unless specifically desired, in which case the
pathologist should be informed of its inclusion and how the
specimen is to be oriented.

2. Clean the area gently with alcohol, taking care to leave
scales, crusts, and vesicles intact. It is often useful to outline
the small lesions before the swelling caused by injection of
local anesthesia or the effect of epinephrine distorts and
blanches the site.

3. Anesthetize the area by injecting into the deep dermis 0.2–
0.5 ml of 0.5–2% lidocaine or 1–2% lidocaine with 1:1000
epinephrine. Patients allergic to local anesthetic ether compounds (procaine, tetracaine) will tolerate use of amide
compounds (lidocaine, bupivacaine) without difficulty (i.e.,
procaine [Novocaine®] and lidocaine [Xylocaine®] do not
cross-react; see also p. 263). Warming the xylocaine before
use may lessen the burning discomfort noted on injection.
The epinephrine will inhibit bleeding, increase the duration
of anesthesia, and make the procedure much easier to perform. Local vasoconstriction will not become maximal before 15–20 min. Epinephrine-containing solutions should not
be used when anesthetizing the distal fingers or toes, or
when vasoconstriction will interfere with the histopathologic
findings such as with primarily vascular (angiomatous) lesions. It is probably preferable to ring an area with anesthesia, but intradermal injection directly into or below a
lesion appears to cause little or no perceptible microscopic
alteration.

a. To inject with the least trauma for both the physician
and the patient, a 1-ml syringe with a #25, #27, or
#30 needle should be used. The first two items are
available as prepackaged, sterile, disposable syringes.
The #30 needles must be purchased separately.

b. Ethyl chloride or other refrigerant spray is sometimes
useful for dulling the pain of injection or the discom-

fort associated with curettage, or incision and drainage of cysts or abscesses. *Ethyl chloride spray is flammable and must not be used during electrosurgical procedures.*

4. Biopsy punches, circular instruments with a sharp cutting edge and a handle, are available in sizes ranging from 2–8 mm in diameter; the 4-mm punch is generally the most useful. Removal of a specimen less than 4 mm in diameter may allow the histologic confirmation of a tumor, but it is inadequate for diagnosis of inflammatory processes. Sterile disposable 2-, 3-, 4-, and 6-mm punch biopsies are available through Chester A. Baker Laboratories, Inc. (Division of Key Pharmaceuticals, Inc.), 50 N.W. 176th St., Miami, Florida 33169.

   The skin surrounding the lesion should be stretched taut *perpendicular* to the wrinkle (relaxed skin tension) lines before the circular punch is inserted as demonstrated in Figure 1. See endpaper figures for a guide to the most common configuration of the relaxed skin tension lines. When the punch is removed, an ellipsoidal defect will be left (Fig. 1, insets). The biopsy punch is firmly pressed

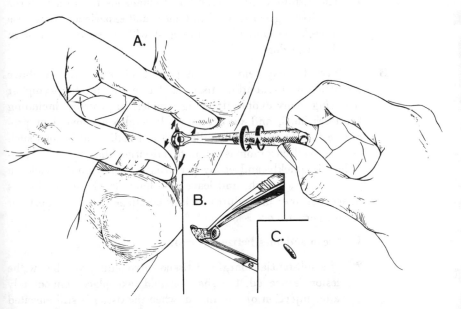

Figure 1. Punch biopsy technique. Note the oval (not round) defect left.

downward into the lesion with a rotary back-and-forth cutting motion until it is well into the subcutaneous tissue (Fig. 1).

5. The biopsied skin plug will either pop out or lie free within its circular margin. The specimen must be gently grasped and lifted out with either forceps or a needle without applying undue pressure, the base severed with scissors or scalpel blade as deep into the fat as possible, and the tissue placed in 10% neutral buffered formalin. The amount of formalin should be at least 20 times that of the specimen by volume. If the incision is made only to the middermis, tissue will be more difficult to remove, and the wound will heal less readily and with a poor cosmetic result.

6. Simple pressure is adequate for hemostasis, and use of caustics or Gelfoam® is rarely needed or warranted. Lesions will heal more rapidly and with a linear scar rather than a round defect if either a 4-0 or 5-0 nylon or silk suture is put in place (left for 3–5 days on the face, 7–14 days on the trunk) or adhesive strips are applied across the defect (left for 14–21 days).

7. The histologic interpretation of cutaneous reaction patterns requires a great deal of judgment and experience. It is wise to seek the help of a pathologist with a special interest in skin disorders.

B. **A shave biopsy** removes that portion of skin elevated above the plane of surrounding tissue and is useful for biopsying or removing many exophytic benign epidermal growths, including keratoses, nevi, and viral tumors. It is also a convenient procedure for obtaining tissue diagnoses of malignant lesions such as basal cell carcinomas prior to initiating therapy. This procedure is quickly and easily performed, heals rapidly, yields a good cosmetic result, and leaves the lower levels of the dermis intact if further procedures such as curettage, electrosurgery, or cryosurgery are necessary.

1. Clean and anesthetize the area.

2. If a substantial margin of tissue surrounding and below the lesion is needed, the shave should take place immediately after injection of anesthesia, when the tissue is still elevated

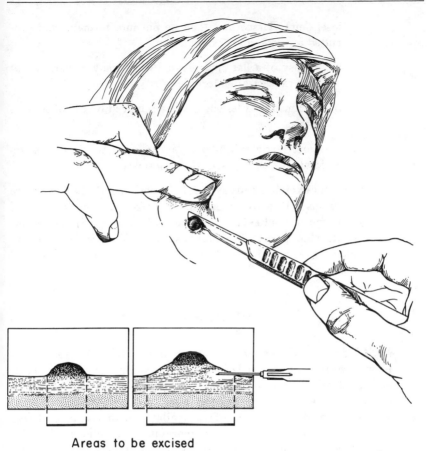

Areas to be excised

Figure 2. Shave biopsy technique.

from the injection fluid (Fig. 2, inset, right). Tissue is removed with a lateral (horizontal) "sawing" motion of a #15 scalpel blade or halved Gillette Super Blue Blade on the level of the surrounding skin (Fig. 2). The latter has the potential advantages of being thinner (cutting edge a millionth-inch thick), sharper, and more flexible. When hand-held, it can be used flat or bent to the precise arc desired to conform to the shape of the lesion and the depth of biopsy. Presuming the elevated lesion alone is being removed, it is necessary before proceeding to wait a few minutes until any sublesional swelling subsides (Fig. 2, inset, left). Tissue may then be put into formalin and submitted for pathologic examination.

   a. Biopsy of a flat or depressed lesion may be carried out by a saucerization technique.

   b. Pedunculated lesions may be removed by use of scissors alone.

  3. Pressure, ferric subsulfate (Monsel's solution), or electrodesiccation may be used for hemostasis.

C. **Surgical excision biopsy** should be considered when (1) there are lesions with active expanding borders; (2) the junction of lesion and normal skin is important to survey; (3) the lesions are atrophic, sclerotic, or bullous; and (4) it is important to acquire adequate full-thickness skin, e.g., in panniculitis and erythema nodosum.

CURETTAGE

I. **DISCUSSION** Curettage is a simple and useful technique for removing benign cutaneous lesions such as warts, molluscum, milia, and keratoses; it is also effective for treating basal and squamous cell carcinomas. The curet, a cutting instrument with a circular, loop-shaped cutting edge and a handle, is available in varying sizes. Large curets will remove masses of tissue more quickly, while smaller ones are needed to probe for small extensions of lesions into subjacent dermis; the curet 4 mm in diameter appears to be the most generally useful. A #15 scalpel blade used on edge with a scraping and not cutting motion can sometimes be used in place of a curet. The more friable the tissue, the easier it is to curet. Curettage is difficult to perform on normal skin or on lesions covered with a full thickness of intact skin. The curet is neither sharp enough nor does it have sufficient strength for this purpose, and the resulting tissue available for pathologic examination is usually fragmented and distorted.

II. **PROCEDURE**

A. Clean the area with alcohol.

B. Anesthesia is not always necessary. The process of anesthetizing can be more painful than the surgical procedure in removal of lesions such as seborrheic keratoses, molluscum, and milia. If

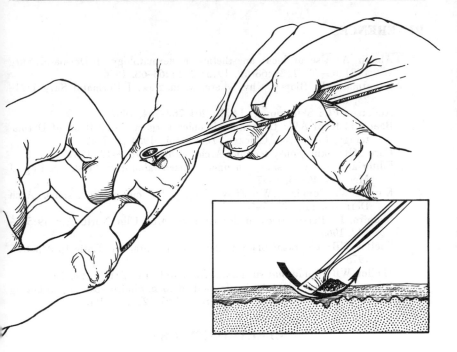

Figure 3. Curettage technique.

anesthesia is used, wait until any swelling has diminished or sub-sided, as it is difficult to scrape spongy tissue.

C. Apply the cutting edge of the curet to the lesions, and remove the tissue with a firm, quick, downward scoop (Fig. 3). The first tissue removed will come off relatively intact and should be submitted for pathologic examination if indicated. Scrape the base and margins of the lesion well. Normal dermis is re-silient and feels rough and scratchy when scraped, while most lesions are of softer composition.

D. Hemostasis is secured by pressure, hemostatic agents (ferric subsulfate, Monsel's solution), caustics (trichloroacetic acid), or electrodesiccation. Use of pressure alone yields the best cos-metic result (as with seborrheic keratoses). If electrodesiccation is used, a small spark is all that is needed for hemostasis and destruction of any remaining lesion; if there is a question of tumor, a more intense spark is used, scraping of a 3–5 mm mar-gin around the lesion is necessary, and curettage should be repeated at least twice to assure complete removal of all tissue.

REFERENCES

Abadir A: Use of local anesthetics in dermatology. J Dermatol Surg 1(2):65–70; 1(3):68–72, 1975; 2(1):63–68, 1976

Ackerman AB: Biopsy, why, where, when, how. J Dermatol Surg 1:21–23, 1975

Anderson PC: Skin biopsy. JAMA 201:762–764, 1967

Baer RL, Kopf AW: Dermatologic office surgery, Year Book of Dermatology, 1963–1964. Chicago, Year Book, 1964 pp 7–47

Caro MR: Skin biopsy technic. Arch Dermatol 76:9–12, 1957

Editorial: Biopsy of skin—an underutilized laboratory "test." N Engl J Med 277:49–50, 1967

Kopf AW, Popkin AW: Shave biopsy for cutaneous lesions. Arch Dermatol 110:637, 1974

Shapiro, L: Perspectives in dermatology. Med Clin North Am 49:531–547, 1965

Shelley WB: The razor blade in dermatologic practice. Cutis 16:843–845, 1975

Shelley WB: Epidermal surgery. J Dermatol Surg 2:125–128, 1976

Whyte HJ, Perry HD: A simple method to minimize scarring following large punch biopsies. Arch Dermatol 81:520–522, 1960

ELECTROSURGERY

I. **DISCUSSION** The small electrosurgical units most often found in physicians' offices and in hospital clinics are versatile and useful tools. They deliver a high-frequency alternating current to tissue, producing an electrical field about the tip of the treatment electrode. The high resistance of tissue to this electric current causes both mechanical disruption of cells and heat. The electrode tip delivers the current but does not itself become hot.

Electrodesiccation produces superficial destruction by dehydrating cells. This is a monoterminal high-voltage (2000 or more volts), low-amperage (100–1000 ma) operation in which the patient is not incorporated into the circuit. The needle is either held in contact with the tissue or kept a short distance away, and the current is transmitted through a spark. The lesion is destroyed by bursts of electric current.

Electrocoagulation produces more severe destruction, primarily by heat and secondarily by disruptive mechanical forces. This is a biterminal, relatively low-voltage (under 200 volts), low-frequency, high-amperage (2500–4000 ma) operation in which the patient is grounded by being placed on a large "indifferent" electrode. The treatment needle, placed in or on the tissue, delivers an intensely hot current and literally "boils" and coagulates the lesion. Electrocoagulation produces wider and deeper damage, better hemostasis, and more scarring; it is used primarily for large lesions that require extensive destruction, some neoplasms such as basal cell carcinomas, or very vascular tumors such as pyogenic granulomas.

The principal uses of electrosurgery are for (a) the destruction of benign superficial lesions such as warts, keratoses, molluscum, and skin tags; (b) hemostasis and the ablation of vascular growths; and (c) the destruction of some malignant tumors of the skin. Patients with indwelling cardiac pacemakers (especially the demand type) should not be treated with these instruments, *because high-frequency current can deactivate a pacemaker.*

II. PROCEDURE

A. Clean the skin with alcohol and let dry. Alcohol, as well as ethyl chloride sprays and some anesthetic gases, is flammable. Strict asepsis is unnecessary as the procedure is itself antiseptic.

B. Infiltrate with lidocaine with epinephrine. Treatment of some lesions, such as skin tags, is so rapid that anesthesia may not be required.

C. When tissue is needed for histologic examination, first curet the lesion, removing all the accessible pathologic tissue. The difference in texture between abnormal and normal tissue becomes difficult to "feel" after a lesion has been altered by electrosurgery. Continue the curettage until the base and borders of the lesion are firm and clean and all pockets of abnormal material have been scraped away. If there is a diagnostic question, shave excision is a superior method for obtaining intact tissue specimens for histologic study. It may be followed by curettage and electrosurgery, or by electrosurgery alone.

D. Apply the electrodesiccating current onto or into the tissue and deliver recurrent bursts of electricity (Fig. 4). It is never necessary to deliver a large spark, since this chars tissue, leads to greater tissue destruction, and offers no added therapeutic advantage. The area being treated should be as dry as possible.

    1. Use as little current as will do the job when treating spider and other angiomas and seborrheic keratoses or when ensuring hemostasis of the base of a lesion.

    2. Warts, actinic keratoses, molluscum contagiosum, and skin tags should be treated with slightly more current. The best

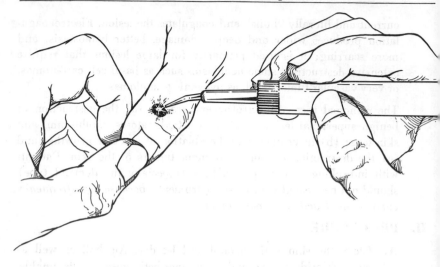

Figure 4. Electrosurgical technique.

technique for treating warts is to insert the needle electrode into the lesion and deliver current until the lesion "bubbles." The gelatinous charred tissue is removed with a curet, and a spark of less intensity is used to desiccate the base lightly. Deeper destruction will not increase the cure rate and will result in a more prolonged healing time and excessive scarring.

3. More intense current, repeated curettage, and a wider margin are needed when removing cutaneous neoplasms.

E. The wound produced by electrosurgery is best left open. Neither antibiotics nor dressings need to be applied. Reepithelialization takes place from the base and sides of the lesion and is complete in 1–6 weeks, depending on the size of the lesion and the amount and depth of tissue destruction.

REFERENCES

Burdick KI: Electrosurgical Apparatus and Their Application in Dermatology. Springfield, Ill, Thomas 1966, 60 pp

Jackson R: Basic principles of electrosurgery: a review. Can J Surg 13:354–361, 1970

Krull EA, Pickard SD, Hall JC: Effects of electrosurgery on cardiac pacemakers. J Dermatol Surg 1(3):43–45, 1975

CRYOSURGERY

I. **DISCUSSION** The application of graded degrees of cold to the skin may be used to treat many benign and neoplastic conditions. Cryogenic agents are easy to apply, usually require no anesthesia, and cause epidermal-dermal separation above the basement membrane, thus leaving no scarring after reepithelialization. The lower the boiling point of the agent, the more efficient are its freezing capabilities. The boiling point of ethyl chloride is $+13.1°C$; of Freon® 114, $+3.6°C$; of Frigiderm® (dichloro-tetra-fluoro ethane), $+3.6°C$; of solid CO_2, $-78.5°C$; of liquid nitrous oxide, $-89.5°C$; and of liquid nitrogen, $-195.6°C$. Liquid nitrogen, which is readily available from medical or industrial sources, is inexpensive and noncombustible and has become a standard therapeutic agent.

Skin is relatively resistant to freezing due to its rich vascular supply and because frozen tissue itself acts as a good insulator. Although skin freezes at 0 to $-2°C$, it is necessary to cool tissue to $-18°$ to $-30°C$ for destruction to occur. Application of liquid nitrogen to the skin with a cotton-tipped applicator stick four times within 60 sec will lower the temperature 2 mm below the cutaneous surface to $-18°C$. Direct spray of liquid nitrogen for an equal time period will cool the tissue to $-90°C$ and, after 120 sec, to $-125°C$ at 2 mm and $-70°C$ at 5 mm below the skin's surface. Such temperatures are needed only for cryosurgery of skin cancer. The degree of injury is roughly proportional to the intensity of freezing. Repeated freeze-thaw is more damaging than a single freeze. Rapid cooling and slow thawing produce the most damage.

The exact mechanism of injury is unclear, but the following changes, all of which take place in frozen tissue, may be operative at any time: (a) mechanical damage to cells by intracellular and extracellular ice formation; (b) osmotic changes related to dehydration of cells and increased concentration of electrolytes as a result of water withdrawal during ice crystal formation; (c) thermal shock, a term used to denote a precipitous fall in the temperature of living cells to subnormal temperatures above $0°C$; (d) denaturation of lipid-protein complexes within the cell membrane; (e) vascular stasis with resulting necrosis of tissue.

Freezing with liquid nitrogen is accompanied by a stinging, burning pain, which peaks during thawing about 2 min after treatment is over. It is usually unnecessary to use local anesthesia. Pressure, which increases both the rate and depth of freezing, should be applied only to lesions over thick, hyperkeratotic sites such as the feet. Freezing of lesions on the hands, feet, lips, ears, and eyelids is more painful than elsewhere. Within minutes of thawing, a triple response with redness, wheals, and surrounding flare will develop. A blister at the dermoepidermal junction forms 3–6 hr later, flattens in 2–3 days, and sloughs off in 2–4 weeks. Reepithelialization is underway within 72 hr of superficial freezing, and superinfection is rare. Melanocytes are more susceptible to cold injury than keratinocytes; mild hypopigmentation is sometimes seen in areas previously frozen with liquid nitrogen.

II. PROCEDURE

A. Nitrogen is best kept in specially made vacuum flasks and may be poured into a plastic insulated cup for immediate use. Liquid nitrogen will rarely cause normal Thermos® bottles to explode. An air vent must always be present in all storage apparatus.

B. Dip a loosely wrapped cotton-tipped applicator into the nitrogen and promptly place it onto the cutaneous lesion (Fig. 5). Larger fluffy swabs such as those used for sigmoidoscopy or gynecologic examination will hold greater amounts of nitrogen. When these are used, the cotton tip should be shaped into a point slightly smaller than the lesion under treatment.

Do not routinely apply pressure. Thick lesions should first be surgically pared and may be treated with moderate pressure. Small lesions are most successfully treated by interrupting contact between the applicator and skin frequently, preventing the zone of freezing from extending to a greater depth and width than necessary. Large lesions can be treated by rolling the applicator over the surface.

C. A 5–30-sec application is adequate for small, superficial lesions, such as lentigines, especially when located on thin skin. Most other benign growths, such as warts, keratoses, and molluscum contagiosum, require a 30–90-sec application, which may be repeated once. Within seconds, the lesion begins to turn white. Nitrogen is repeatedly applied until the white freezing front extends 1–3 mm onto the margins of normal skin (see Fig. 5). The zone of frozen tissue reaches a depth of 1.5–2 mm within 1 min of the initiation of nitrogen application and does not advance significantly farther.

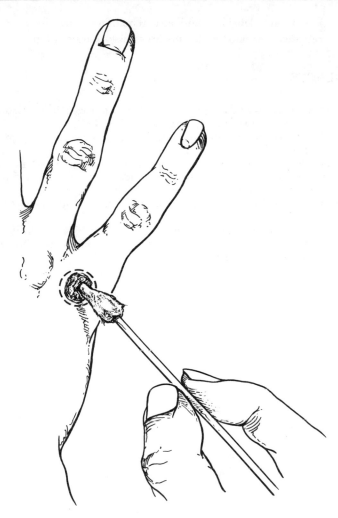

Figure 5. Cryosurgical technique. Liquid nitrogen is delivered to the lesion on a loosely wrapped cotton-tipped applicator stick (or larger cotton swab). The nitrogen should be repeatedly applied until the freezing front extends 1–3 mm around the lesion (dotted line).

D. The posttreatment lesion requires no dressings. Avoid occlusive ointments or bandages. The blister that forms may be hemorrhagic or large. If it is uncomfortable or awkward; it may be decompressed with a sterile blade or pin, leaving the roof intact. Patients with warts should be seen in 2 weeks, at which time the lesions are debrided and any remaining wart tissue is either refrozen or treated with caustics or electrodesiccation.

REFERENCES

Duperrat B, Bouquet JF: The use of liquid nitrogen in dermatological cryotherapy. Australas J Dermatol 12:5–9, 1971

Finelli PF: Ulnar neuropathy after liquid nitrogen cryotherapy. Arch Dermatol 111:1340–1342, 1975

Pearson RW: Response of human epidermis to graded thermal stress. A morphologic comparison of burns, cold-induced blisters, and pemphigus vulgaris. Arch Environ Health 11:498–507, 1965

Robertson WD: Cryotherapy in dermatology. Ohio State Med J 64:1260–1263, 1968

Torre D (ed): Cryosurgery (special issue). Cutis 16:421–518, 1975

Zakarian SA: Cryosurgery of Skin Tumors of the Skin and Oral Cavity. Springfield, Ill., Thomas, 1973, 293 pp

35
Diagnostic and Therapeutic Techniques

CYTOLOGIC SMEARS

I. **DISCUSSION** Cytologic techniques in dermatology are useful in the diagnosis of bullous diseases and solid and vesicular viral eruptions. Examination of the smear is not a substitute for a biopsy, but it does enable multiple lesions to be tested on repeated occasions and allows immediate confirmation of some disease processes.

II. **TECHNIQUE**

    A. Select an early lesion that shows no signs of trauma or infection.

    B. Separate or remove the blister top with a scalpel or sharp scissors. Absorb excess fluid with a gauze pad.

    C. Gently remove blister contents and scrape the floor of the vesicle with a #10 or #15 scalpel blade or curet. Do not provoke bleeding.

    D. Make a thin smear on a clean glass slide. (With solid lesions such as molluscum, squeeze the material between 2 slides.)

E. Air dry. If the following are available, fix tissue by dipping 4–5 times in 95% ethanol or methanol or immerse the slide in these solutions for 1–2 min.

F. Stain with Wright's, Giemsa (1 drop/1 cc water for 30 min, or undiluted Giemsa stock for 5 min), or hematoxylin and eosin.

G. **Microscopic appearance** Examine first with a low-power objective to gain an impression of cell size and depth of stain relationships; then examine with 45× or oil for the morphologic details.

1. Herpes simplex, zoster, and varicella lesions contain large, bizarre, viral mononucleate and multinucleate giant cells and the degenerative nuclear changes of "ballooning degeneration." The giant cells contain 8–10 nuclei, varying in size and shape. Occasionally an intranuclear inclusion body may be identified.

2. Molluscum contagiosum bodies appear as multiple, large, oval to round, smooth-bordered masses up to 25μ in diameter.

3. In most bullous eruptions the smear will show only inflammatory cells. In pemphigus and benign familial pemphigus, numerous rounded acantholytic epidermal cells with large nuclei and condensed cytoplasm are found.

REFERENCES

Blank H, Burgoon CF: Abnormal cytology of epithelial cells in pemphigus vulgaris: a diagnostic aid. J Invest Dermatol 18:213–223, 1952

Blank H, Burgoon CF, Baldridge GD, McCarthy PL, Urbach F: Cytologic smears in diagnosis of herpes simplex, herpes zoster and varicella. JAMA 146:1410–1412, 1951

FUNGAL SCRAPING AND CULTURE

I. **DISCUSSION** Immediate confirmation of the presence of a fungal infection may be easily accomplished by microscopic identification of organisms and is more reliable than culture. All scaling lesions from the scalp, angles of the mouth, axillae, groin, inframammary area, and feet, as well as blisters on the hands and feet, should be considered for such studies.

II. TECHNIQUE

A. Scraping examination

1. *Skin*

a. Clean the skin well with alcohol or acetone and let dry.

b. Scrape with a scalpel or edge of a microscope slide at the active edge of a lesion and collect tissue on a glass slide. With blistering eruptions the fungus is in the roof of the vesicle, which can be (a) gently dissected off with sharp scissors or scalpel, or (b) reflected back and the underside scraped with a #15 scalpel blade.

c. Small, thin fragments of tissue may be examined directly. Large pieces should be minced with a scalpel blade. Thick pieces should be discarded.

d. Gather scrapings together in the center of the slide.

e. Cover with Swartz-Medrik stain (SMS) or 10–20% potassium hydroxide (KOH) and a coverslip and heat gently, but not to boiling, for 15–30 sec.

f. SMS preparations can be examined immediately. Let KOH slides cool for 10 min (during which time the tissue is hydrolyzed and rendered clear), then press the coverslip gently to flatten the tissue and push out air bubbles.

g. Examine under a scanning lens or high-dry magnification. (It is very important to avoid getting KOH on the microscope objective, as it will etch the lens.) The diaphragm should be closed down and the condenser lowered as far as it will go. The ease of identification of hyphae varies inversely with the intensity of light passing through the slide.

h. With SMS, hyphae and spores appear blue against the red background of cells. Because the hyphae stain selectively and are more easily seen with SMS, slides may be more quickly scanned at a lower power. This stain (available through Muro Pharmacal Laboratories, Inc., 121 Liberty St., Quincy, Mass. 02169) consists of two separate solutions:

(1) The fungal stain consists of a dye, a surfactant to clear the tissues quickly, and an amount of KOH (2%) less than that which will etch glass and destroy microscope lenses.

(2) The red counterstain (rose bengal) makes it easier to identify cells.

In KOH preparations, hyphae and spores will stand out as refractile tubes and oval bodies against the background of cells and debris. It is not possible to make a species identification from any tissue scrapings.

2. *Hair and nails*

a. Examine the scalp with a Wood's lamp. If individual lesions fluoresce, pull out 10–15 hairs for examination. Otherwise, examine scales and 10–15 random hairs from the involved site. Altered, dystrophic, hypertrophic, or pigmented nails should be snipped off and minced on a slide. Subungual debris is less suitable for examination.

b. Heat on a slide or in a test tube with 10–40% KOH and let cool for 15–30 min. Tissue may then be stained with SMS or examined directly.

B. **Culture** In addition to direct examination of scales, scrapings from a suspicious lesion should be cultured at room temperature on Sabouraud's glucose agar, Sabouraud's agar with chloramphenicol and actidione (Mycobiotic®, Mycosel®), or Dermatophyte Test Medium (DTM). DTM inhibits bacteria and saprophytic molds and contains phenol red, which turns the agar from yellow to bright red when its pH becomes alkaline from dermatophyte growth. Contaminant growth does not alter the pH of the medium. Using DTM medium, if no color change takes place within 2 weeks, the culture may be discarded. If the color does change, it may be presumed that a pathogenic dermatophyte or yeast is present. Microscopic examination of the culture (culture mount) should then identify the exact species.

REFERENCES

Rebell G, Taplin D: Dermatophytes: Their Identification and Recognition (Revised Edit). Coral Gables, University of Miami Press, 1970

Swartz JH, Lamkins BE: A rapid simple stain for fungi in skin scales, nail scrapings and hairs. Arch Dermatol 89:89–94, 1964

Swartz JH, Medrik TF: Rapid contrast stain as a diagnostic aid for fungous infections. Arch Dermatol 99:494–497, 1969

Taplin D, Zaias N, Rebell D, Blank H: Isolation and recognition of dermatophytes on a new medium (DTM). Arch Dermatol 99:203–209, 1969

WOOD'S LIGHT EXAMINATION

I. DISCUSSION Wood's glass, primarily barium silicate containing 9% nickel oxide, is opaque to all light except for a band extending from 340–450 nanometers (nm). With a Wood's light such as the Blak-Ray (Ultraviolet Products Inc., San Gabriel, Ca.), when light from its high-pressure mercury arc is passed through this filter, it is principally the 365-nm radiation that is transmitted. Fluorescent bulbs (black lights) that emit a similar though slightly broader spectrum are also available. The Wood's light was first found to have medical importance in detecting fungal infections, but it is useful for many other diagnostic tasks as well. As ointments, exudates, tetracycline in sweat, makeup, deodorants, and soap may fluoresce a blue or purple color, the skin should be well cleansed before examination. The Wood's lamp may be used in the following situations.

A. Detection and control of scalp ringworm Hairs infected with *Microsporum audouini* or *M. canis* fluoresce a bright blue-green. Fluorescent hairs may be selected for microscopic examination and culture. Pteridine compounds have been postulated as the cause of this fluorescence. As normal hair regrows, a band of nonfluorescent hair will emerge. Large school populations may be screened with the Wood's lamp for tinea capitis caused by organisms acquired from man or animals. Infections acquired from soil fungi will not fluoresce, however.

B. Detection of other fungal infections Tinea versicolor may fluoresce a golden yellow color. Although this is often imperceptible, Wood's light examination nevertheless allows the accompanying pigmentary changes to be seen more vividly.

C. Detection of bacterial infections

1. Erythrasma, an intertriginous infection caused by *Corynebacterium minutissimum*, fluoresces a brilliant coral-red or pink-orange. The fluorescent substance is a water-soluble porphyrin and therefore may not be present if the area has been washed recently.

2. *Pseudomonas aeruginosa* infections give off a yellowish green color due to pyocyanin. Fluorescence due to fluorescin is detectable before obvious purulence appears and is useful in screening burn patients for infections.

D. **Delineation of pigmentary disorders** Longwave UVL is transmitted into the dermis where it gives a white to blue-white fluorescent color. Melanin present in the epidermis (but not dermis) acts to absorb longwave UVL and thus prevents this "white" color. The Wood's light therefore accentuates contrast between pigmented and nonpigmented skin, but, of more importance, it separates hypopigmented from totally amelanotic areas (the latter have true white to blue-white fluorescence). It is used for examining patients with vitiligo, albinism, leprosy, and other disorders of hypopigmentation and is also useful as a screening procedure in nurseries to look for the small, leaf-shaped, white macules indicative of tuberous sclerosis.

E. **Detection of porphyrins** Acidified urine, feces, and, rarely, blister fluid from patients with porphyria cutanea tarda will fluoresce a brilliant pink-orange.

F. **Drug detection** The teeth of people who took tetracycline in childhood while deciduous teeth were forming will fluoresce yellow, as will the nails and bones of adults taking that antibiotic.

G. **Miscellaneous** Fluorescent ingredients or markers in cosmetics, medications, or industrial compounds may be detected with the Wood's lamp.

REFERENCES

Caplan RM: Medical uses of the Wood's lamp. JAMA 202:1035–1038, 1967

Gilchrest BA, Fitzpatrick TB, Anderson E, Parrish JA: Localization of melanin pigmentation in the skin with Wood's lamp. Br J Dermatol 96:245–248, 1977

Task Force Report: Report on ultraviolet light sources. Arch Dermatol 109:833–839, 1974

Ward CG, Clarkson JG, Taplin D, Polk HC Jr: Wood's light fluorescence and *Pseudomonas* burn wound infection. JAMA 202:1039–1040, 1967

PATCH TESTING

I. **DISCUSSION**   Patch testing is used to document and validate a diagnosis of allergic contact sensitization and identify the causative agent. It may also be of value as a screening procedure in some patients with chronic or unexplained eczematous eruptions (e.g., hand and foot dermatoses). It is a unique means of in vivo reproduction of disease in diminutive proportions, since sensitization affects the whole body and may therefore be elicited at any cutaneous site. The patch test is easier and safer than a "use test" because test items can be applied in low concentrations on small areas of skin for short periods of time.

II. **TECHNIQUE**

   A. Delay patch testing until any acute inflammation has subsided. Reexposure to the antigen may cause the eruption to flare up. Neither low-dose systemic steroids nor antihistamines will influence the results.

   B. Test only with potential allergens. There are no methods available for easily assaying primary irritants.

   C. Be certain that the substances being tested will not irritate the skin. Cosmetics may be applied full strength, but items of unknown irritant potential should be diluted to 1–2% in petrolatum, mineral oil, or, less preferably, water. A standard patch test tray containing four chemical screening mixtures and 21 other items is available from Hollister-Stier Laboratories (Chem-Test® Set). Suitable dilution and vehicle data are available in the references cited at the end of this discussion and in the textbooks mentioned previously (see Preface and p. 62).

   D. Apply test substances to a disk of filter paper bound to plastic-coated aluminum (Al-Test®) and attach to the skin with adhesive tape. The Al-Test®, available through Hollister-Stier, is the standard utilized by the North American and International Contact Dermatitis groups. Alternatively, one can use a 1-inch square piece of soft cotton (Webril®) and cover with occlusive tape (Scanpore®) or cellophane and tape. A smaller patch, which may be slightly less effective, may be applied with a 1/4-inch piece of gauze, linen, cotton, or filter paper and covered with Elastopatch® and tape (or Dermacel® for those who cannot tolerate tape). Liquids and ointments may be applied directly to the cotton or gauze. Volatile liquids should be applied directly to the skin and allowed to dry before being covered. Solids must be powdered prior to application. Moisten powders and fabrics with water before application. The site of application should be normal hairless skin on the back or inner arms.

E. Leave the patches in place for 48 hr. If pain, pruritus, or irritation under a patch is noted, the patient should remove it at once. Readings should not be made until the patches have been off at least 20–30 min, as positive reactions may not show immediately. Delayed reactions are not uncommon and a final reading should be made at 4 days (96 hr).

F. The results are interpreted and noted as follows:

$? + =$ Doubtful reaction

$+ =$ Weak (nonvesicular) reaction—erythema and/or papules

$+ + =$ Strong (edematous or vesicular) reaction—erythema papules and/or small vesicles

$+ + + =$ Extreme reaction—all of the foregoing plus large vesicles, bullae, and, at times, ulceration

$IR =$ Irritant reaction

A positive patch test proves only that the patient has a contact sensitivity, but not necessarily that the eliciting substance is the cause of the clinical eruption.

G. False-negative tests may be caused by:

1. Low concentration or insufficient amount of antigen.

2. Improper testing, including inadequate occlusion, inappropriate vehicle, wrong site, incorrect reading times, or deteriorating substances.

3. Depressed reactivity due to administration of high amounts of systemic steroids or recent and aggressive topical steroid application.

4. Failure to reproduce the true conditions of exposure to antigen and lack of heat, friction, trauma.

H. False-positive tests may be related to:

1. Primary irritant reactions.

2. Tape reactions and pressure effects.

3. Reactions to occlusion: maceration, miliaria, folliculitis.

4. Contamination from another site.

5. Presence of impurities in the test material.

I. Positive reactions may sometimes take several weeks to subside. A topical corticosteroid will decrease local symptoms at test sites with active or prolonged inflammation and also shorten the healing time.

REFERENCES

Adams RM: Occupational Contact Dermatitis. Philadelphia, Lippincott, 1969, 262 pp

Agrup G, Dahlquist I, Fregert S, Rorsman H: Value of history and testing in suspected allergic contact dermatitis. Arch Dermatol 101: 212–215, 1970

Baer RL, Ramsey DL, Biondi E: The most common contact allergens 1968–1970. Arch Dermatol 108:74–78, 1973

Epstein E: Simplified patch test screening with mixtures. Arch Dermatol 95:269–274, 1967

Fisher AA: Contact Dermatitis. (2nd Edit) Philadelphia, Lea & Febiger, 1973, 448 pp

Kligman AM: The identification of contact allergens by human assays. I. A critique of standard methods. II. Factors influencing the indication and measurement of allergic contact dermatitis. III. The maximization test: a procedure for screening and rating contact sensitizers. J Invest Dermatol 47:369–374, 375–392, 393–409, 1966

Maibach HI: Patch testing—an objective tool. Cutis 13:613–619, 1974

Rudner EJ, Clendenning WE, Epstein E, Fisher AA, Jillson OF, Jordan WP, Kanof N, Larsen W, Maibach H, Mitchell JC, O'Quinn SE, Schorr WF, Sulzberger MB: Epidemiology of contact dermatitis in North America: 1972. Arch Dermatol 108:537–540, 1973

Shelley WB: The patch test. JAMA 200:874–878, 1967

ULTRAVIOLET LIGHT THERAPY

I. **DISCUSSION** (units of wavelengths: 1 cm = 10^8 angstrom [Å] = 10^7 nanometer [nm]) Ultraviolet radiation (UVL), that part of the electromagnetic spectrum that begins next to the violet end of the color spectrum (400 nm) and extends to the beginning of the x-ray region (200 nm), is often used in the therapy of psoriasis, acne, pityriasis rosea, and chronic eczematous eruptions; it may also be used in conjunction with psoralen administration for photochemotherapy of psoriasis and vitiligo. UVL causes temporary suppression of epidermal basal cell division, followed by a later increase in cell turnover. The UVL spectrum is subdivided into three bands: UVC (200–280 nm), UVB (280–320 nm), and UVA (320–400 nm). Each region has different photobiologic characteristics and will be discussed here separately.

II. SOURCES AND TECHNIQUES

A. **Sunlight** is often the optimal source of UVL. It is the least expensive and most effective under most circumstances. Sun emits radiation with a continuous emission spectrum. The ozone layer in the upper atmosphere acts as a filter and absorbs virtually all UVL shorter than 290 nm. The erythema dose for a fair-skinned person is 20 min at latitude 41° (Boston) at midday in June. The disadvantages of sunlight radiation are its variable absorption by clouds and the difficulty in controlling or monitoring its intensity.

B. **UVC radiation** from artificial sources is present in operating room germicidal lamps and in cold quartz lamps. These lamps, low-pressure, low-temperature mercury arcs, emit a band of radiation predominantly at 253.7 nm through a quartz envelope filter. The erythema dose is 30 sec at 25 cm. Its advantages are that (a) little or no pigmentation follows the erythema, and (b) severe burns cannot occur, since large increases in exposure time lead to only minimal increases in redness. Cold quartz radiation is sometimes used to produce erythema and desquamation in acne patients, particularly in pigmented individuals who wish to avoid more intense melanin pigmentation. UVC radiation can cause a painful conjunctivitis after only seconds of exposure. No one should ever look directly into these lamps or spend much time around the lamp without adequate protection (protective clothing, glasses, or sunscreens [see pp. 196, 328]).

C. **UVB radiation** is probably most responsible for most of the beneficial effects of sunlight and conventional artificial UVL therapy. There are several sources of UVB for clinical use:

1. *UVB sources*

    a. *Fluorescent sunlamp bulbs* (FS40, Westinghouse), low-pressure, low-temperature mercury arc sources, emit a continuous spectrum with a peak at 313 nm. The radiation is filtered through calcium, zinc, and thallium phosphate phosphor in the glass envelope. The erythema dose is 90–120 sec at 25 cm. These lamps are easily obtainable, relatively inexpensive (about $27 for a 4-foot bulb) and good sources of sunburn radiation

(290–320 nm). They are usually used as a bank of four bulbs for home use, or constructed into a light box lined by reflecting metal and many 4-foot and/or 2-foot lamps for office or clinic.

b. *Sunlamp bulbs* or units are low-pressure mercury lamps that emit UVL in the sunburn spectrum. They are inexpensive ($15–$30) and readily available (GE, Sylvania, or Westinghouse R-S [rapid start] bulbs; Hanovia or Sperti lamps).

c. *Hot quartz lamps,* high-pressure, high-temperature mercury arc sources, emit a discontinuous UVL spectrum with bands at 254, 265, 297, 303, 313, and 365 nm but with particular effectiveness in the erythema-producing midrange. The erythema dose is 30–60 sec at 46 cm. Overexposure can lead to severe burns. These large lamps (Hanovia) are expensive ($75–$600) and are used primarily for in-hospital and office or clinic patient care.

2. *General instructions for the patient using UVB lamps*

a. Protect the eyes with special sun goggles or moist cotton to prevent sunburn to the eyes.

b. Use a dependable timer or have someone in the room during therapy. If UVL is to be self-administered, do not used it when tired. The primary danger of sunlamp therapy is overexposure. In most instances this occurs when patients turn on the unit before going to bed and then fall asleep under the pleasant warmth of the lamp.

c. Allow the lamp to warm up for 5 min.

d. Administer UVL every day or every other day.

e. If excessive and painful erythema develops, discontinue UVL treatment until the redness completely subsides and then resume therapy at one-half the last exposure time. The object of therapy is to produce a minimal but noticeable erythema that subsides within 24 hr. Mild dryness and desquamation will follow within 1–2 days.

3. *Specific instructions for the patient*

a. *Sunlamp (R-S) therapy for facial acne*

(1) Place lamp 12 inches from the face.

(2) Treatment consists of three separate exposures of the face: left side, front, right side.

(3) Start therapy at 30-sec exposure to each aspect of the face. Increase each treatment by 30 sec a day until an erythema dose is reached, after which it is often possible to administer the same minimal erythema dose for some time. However, tanning and accommodation to UVL usually make it necessary to raise the amount of UVL exposure eventually by 30-sec increments in order to continue achieving an erythema response. Patients with darker skin may begin with a 1-min exposure and increase by 1-min increments until the erythema dose is reached, then revert to the other schedule. After reaching a 10-min exposure, continue without further increase in exposure time.

b. *Sunlamp (R-S) therapy to the body*

(1) Position the bulb 30 inches from the supine, unclothed body.

(2) Deliver UVL to four areas: upper trunk and face, lower trunk and legs, upper back, buttocks and lower legs. It is often useful to drape that half of the body not receiving light with a sheet to control dosage more accurately.

(3) Begin with an exposure time of 1 min to each area and increase by 30 sec daily until a minimal erythema dose is reached. Depending on the erythema response, the UVL exposure is either kept stable or increased by 30-sec increments until a 5-min exposure to each area is reached, then increased by 1 min each time until a 15–20 min exposure is reached.

c. *Hot quartz lamp therapy* is never self-administered. The attendant and patient must use goggles at all times.

(1) The lamp should be 30 inches away from the area being irradiated.

(2) Start with 30 sec for each exposure and increase by 30 sec daily. Hold treatment at the dose that produces a moderate erythema 24 hr later.

(3) Isolated areas may be irradiated by shielding all the surrounding area with sheeting or towels and exposing as described, but at one-half the distance. This will greatly increase the intensity of light, as the intensity is inversely proportional to the square of the distance; i.e., at one half the distance there will be four times as much light energy delivered (from a point source).

D. **UVA radiation** from sunlight or fluorescent tubes will not, by itself, cause erythema or pigmentation. However, in the presence of a circulating photosensitizer such as psoralen compounds, this longwave UVL spectrum becomes an excellent therapeutic tool. This combination of light and drug has been termed photochemotherapy, or PUVA (psoralen plus ultraviolet A) therapy (see also p. 164). In the doses used, neither the drug alone nor the light alone has any biologic activity. Absorption of electromagnetic energy in the UVA waveband in the presence of psoralens results in transient inhibition of DNA synthesis. This is presumably the mode of action of PUVA therapy for psoriasis. At this time, PUVA treatment is primarily useful in severe psoriasis and is also effective for some patients with vitiligo and mycosis fungoides. Preliminary results indicate a possible future role in treating atopic dermatitis and other inflammatory dermatoses.

1. *UVA sources*

a. *Fluorescent blacklight lamp* (FS40BL), low-pressure, low-temperature mercury arcs, emit a spectrum of 320–450 nm (peak 360 nm) filtered through the barium disilicate phosphor in its glass envelope. The peak is at 360 nm. Use of these bulbs is limited because of the low intensity of UVA emission.

b. *High-intensity UVA fluorescent bulbs* have recently been developed by GTE Sylvania and it is these bulbs that are best used in PUVA light boxes.

c. *PUVA treatment boxes* are used in hospital clinics and in some dermatologists' offices. Two hours after ingestion of 0.5–0.8 mg/kg of 8-methoxypsoralen, patients are exposed to incremental doses of UVA, starting at 1–5 joule/cm^2 (approx 2–10 min) depending on degree of melanization and on sunburn history. The treatment protocols are complicated, not yet finally standardized, and will not be discussed here.

d. *Sunlight-produced UVA* can be used with psoralens for the treatment of vitiligo and psoriasis (see p. 124 for method). This technique is dangerous because it is nearly impossible to gauge UVL exposure accurately and thus severe burns can result.

2. Biologic reaction to PUVA

a. *PUVA redness* may be absent or minimal at 12–24 hr after exposure (when UVB erythema is most intense) and may peak at 48–72 hr or later. Severe *PUVA burns* can continue to intensify for up to one week after exposure and can be treated with prednisone (see p. 197).

b. *PUVA pigmentation,* which appears clinically and histologically identical to normal UVB-induced melanogenesis (tanning) maximizes about 5–7 days after exposure, may become very intense after repeated PUVA treatments, and lasts longer than a normal suntan—weeks to many months.

c. Repeated high-dose UVA or PUVA exposure of laboratory animals causes cataracts and skin cancer just as does UVB or sun exposure. There is as yet no evidence that humans develop skin cancer after phototherapy. However, patients must be carefully observed for evidence of accelerated actinic damage, and sunglasses should be worn on PUVA treatment days to decrease UVA exposure to the lens of the eye (see p. 123).

REFERENCES

Monash S: Composition of sunlight and a number of ultraviolet lamps. Arch Dermatol 91:495–496, 1965

Parrish JA, Fitzpatrick TB, Tanenbaum L, Pathak MA: Photochemotherapy of psoriasis with oral methoxsalen and long wave ultraviolet light. N Engl J Med 291:1207–1212, 1974

Task Force Report: Report on ultraviolet light sources. Arch Dermatol 109:833–839, 1974

III
Treatment Principles and Formulary

36
Treatment Principles

DERMATOLOGIC PRESCRIPTIONS AND DRUG COSTS

The writing of dermatologic prescriptions has changed radically over the past decades. In the past, most topical preparations were compounded according to the specific instructions of the physician. Currently, there are numerous, single-component medications and fixed-composition compounds available both as prescription and over-the-counter (OTC) nonprescription drugs. As opposed to most fixed-dose medications for systemic use, where the drug ratios are often not optimum, or unnecessary medications are included, the topical agents containing several ingredients are frequently efficacious. However, there is an enormous variance in price between many items of approximately equal benefit to the patient—and it is essential to know not only the ingredients of the topicals prescribed but also the cost to the patient; at times, the cost does and should make the difference between whether a questionably effective topical or systemic medication is prescribed or discarded. Small package sizes (5–15 gm) are relatively much more costly than larger amounts (60 gm, 120 gm, 480 gm).

All drugs carry two names: the official (*generic*) and the brand (*trade,* or *proprietary*) name. The brand name is made almost universally more attractive, as it is both pronounceable and frequently carries a suggestion of the drug's alleged effects. For the first 17 years of patent monopoly on a new drug, only one company's product is available by either name unless other pharmaceutical firms have also been licensed to market the drug. Thereafter, the drug may be manufactured by several pharmaceutical houses, but the original trade name is protected forever by trademark laws and cannot be borrowed. Furthermore, pharmacies in many states are prohibited by law from substituting the generic drug when trade names are prescribed, even though the medications are identical but the costs radically different. By referring to drugs by their generic names, physicians are sometimes able to make the treatment of dermatologic disorders far less expensive. For example, the cost to the druggist for 1000 4-mg Chlor-Trimeton® is $24.00, 1000 Chlor-Trimeton® 12-mg Repetabs® $63.00 and 1000 50-mg Pyribenzamine® $31.00, while the cost of their generic equivalents is $1.25, $5.75, and $4.50, respectively.

The cost of drugs to the pharmacist is easily available and is published yearly in the *Drug Topics Red Book* and *American Druggist Blue Book.* The actual cost to the patient varies, depending on the pricing policy of the pharmacy involved. Many pharmacies simply add a fee of $2.00–2.50 to the cost of the medication, while others mark up each item by 33% or 50% based on cost (66–100% based on selling price) in order to cover overhead costs and earn a profit. If the pharmacy cost of a drug is $6.00, the patient cost would be around $8.50 if a fee is charged, or $10.00 if computed by cost plus one-third cost. There is usually a minimum fee of $1.50–2.00 for any prescription filled. This obviously makes it important not to write prescriptions for OTC products, which may then become more costly to the patient, and never to write repeated prescriptions for small amounts of medication. It is quite costly to compound topical medications simply because it takes the pharmacist considerable time, which is usually charged at $10.00/hr. Thus if a few inexpensive antipruritic agents, such as menthol and/or phenol (cost: 10–20¢) are added to 6–8 oz of a lotion such as Keri®, or Lubriderm® (cost to pharmacy: $1.50–1.75) or to 480 gm of Eucerin® cream (cost to pharmacy: $1.20), the total cost to the patient will be $10–15. Last, all drugs should always be clearly labeled as to ingredients and instructions for use. If necessary, the prescription should contain explicit instructions to the pharmacist to label all medications.

REFERENCE

Cost of prescription drugs: Med Lett Drugs Ther 17:5–6, 1975

TYPES OF TOPICAL MEDICATIONS
(see also *Dermatologic Topical Preparations*
and Vehicles, Chap. 37, p. 314) ⌐ 3/8

It is important to note that there are two variables in topical therapy. Both the medication and the vehicle chosen must be appropriate for the condition being treated. In general, acute inflammation is treated with aqueous drying preparations, and chronic inflammation is treated with greasier, more lubricating compounds, as noted in the following.

The spectrum of inflammation with the corresponding range of appropriate dermatologic vehicles

Acute inflammation: erythema, edema, vesiculation, oozing, crusting, infection, pruritus

Wet dressings (water)
↓
Powders, lotions, aerosols, sprays
↓
Creams (oil-in water emulsions), gels
↓

Chronic inflammation: erythema, scaling, lichenification, dryness, pruritus

Ointments (water-in-oil emulsions, inert bases)

I. **OPEN WET DRESSINGS** These types of dressings cool and dry through evaporation. They thus cause vasoconstriction, decreasing the vasodilatation and augmented local blood flow present in inflammation. In addition, wet dressings cleanse the skin of exudates, crusts, and debris and help maintain drainage of infected areas. They are indicated in the therapy of acute inflammatory conditions, erosions, and ulcers. Although various medicaments and antibacterial substances may be added for specific causes, water is by far the most important ingredient of wet dressings. Wet dressings covered by an impermeable cover (**closed wet dressings**) retain heat, prevent evaporation, and cause maceration (see Formulary, p. 330, for the technique of application).

II. **POWDERS** Powders promote drying by increasing the effective skin surface area. They are used primarily in intertriginous areas to reduce moisture, maceration, and friction. Powders may be inert or may contain active medications (see p. 318).

III. **LIQUIDS** **Lotions** consist of suspensions of a powder in water (see p. 314). **Tinctures** are alcoholic or hydroalcoholic solutions. As lotions and tinctures evaporate, they cool and dry; lotions leave a uniform film of powder on the skin. **Sprays** and **aerosols** act in a similar manner. Active agents are often incorporated into the aqueous phase.

IV. **CREAMS** **Creams** are semisolid emulsions of oil in water (O/W). As the proportion of grease increases and the proportion of water decreases, the preparation becomes more viscous and at some undefined ratio will no longer be considered a cream, entering the classification of ointments. A **gel** is a transparent and colorless semisolid emulsion that liquifies on contact with the skin, drying as a thin, greaseless, nonocclusive, nonstaining film.

V. **OINTMENTS** These consist of water droplets suspended in the continuous phase of oil (W/O) or of inert bases such as petrolatum. Ointments are of three types: those soluble in water, those that will emulsify with water, and those completely insoluble in water (see p. 315).

VI. **PASTES** Pastes, which are little used today, are mixtures of a powder and an ointment.

VII. **LUBRICANTS, BASES, AND PROTECTIVE COVERINGS** The following preparations are most often used as lubricants, bases in which to incorporate drugs, and protective coverings for the skin:

   A. The **oil-in-water creams,** which are water-washable ("vanishing cream") and cosmetically pleasing, account for the majority of topical items prescribed.

   B. **Water-in-oil emulsions,** which are better lubricants than oil-in-water creams, retain heat and may encourage percutaneous absorption by impeding water loss, thus increasing hydration. Because W/O preparations are occlusive, they are best not used in oozing or infected areas. To provide smooth mixtures, dispersing and emulsifying agents, surfactants, and detergents are usually added to these emulsions.

   C. **Lotions, sprays, and O/W emulsions** are most easily applied to hirsute areas and scalp.

REFERENCES

Hadgraft JW: Recent progress in the formulation of vehicles for topical applications. Br J Dermatol 87:386–389, 1972

Hellier FF: Creams, ointments and lotions. Practitioner 202:23–26, 1969

AMOUNT TO DISPENSE
(See Chart 1, p. 377)

It will become apparent on long-term patient follow-up that, when inadequate amounts of medication are dispensed, the patient will tend to apply too little, will use the drugs less frequently than prescribed (often not frequently enough to provide adequate therapy), will soon run out of medication, and then may not refill the prescription. If a medication is known to be effective and is to be used on a long-term basis, dispensing large quantities will be more economical and will insure continuous supply, resulting in better treatment.

One gm of cream will cover an area of skin approximately 10 cm × 10 cm, or about 100 sq cm. This assumes a layer 100μ in thickness. The same amount of ointment will cover an area 5–10 percent larger. Chart 1 (p. 377) gives conservative figures for the amounts needed for a single application of an ointment or cream and for application 3id for a 2-week period. If a lotion is to be used, the amounts should be doubled.

REFERENCES

British National Formulary. British Medical Association. London, Pharmaceutical Society of Great Britain, 1968, p 13

Schlagel C, Sanborn EC: The weights of topical preparations required for total and partial body inunction. J Invest Dermatol 42:253–256, 1964

37
Formulary

This section includes the topical and systemic medications most useful for treating cutaneous disease. Drugs are listed alphabetically in each instance. This is not a complete listing of all the pharmaceutical preparations available for dermatologic use, and many useful products may have been omitted. No sustained-release capsules and few aerosols or antibiotic-steroid combinations are cited here. For uniformity and ease of conversion, all package sizes are listed in metric terms (see endpaper chart 2). Costs shown are average retail cost per item to the patient, based upon the usual pharmacy markup of cost + two-thirds of cost (computed as cost/ 0.66), or manufacturer's recommended cost. Prices to the pharmacist are those listed as Average Wholesale Price (AWP) in the *Drug Topics Red Book* or *American Druggist Blue Book*. Although pharmacists can buy some drugs directly from the manufacturer at a slightly lower price ("direct price"), some manufacturers do not distribute any drugs directly and others have minimum requirements for direct orders that may exclude small orders or those from small-volume pharmacies. Thus, of the total pharmacy charge, in most instances 60% is drug cost and 40% pharmacy cost. The prices given here should be viewed only as a general guide to comparative costs and are, of course, constantly subject to change. Medications that require a prescription are so noted (R_x).

ACNE PREPARATIONS

I. DISCUSSION See Acne, p. 3.

II. PRESCRIPTION DRUGS (R_x)

A. Retinoic acid (vitamin A acid; tretinoin; Retin-A®)

1. *Structure*

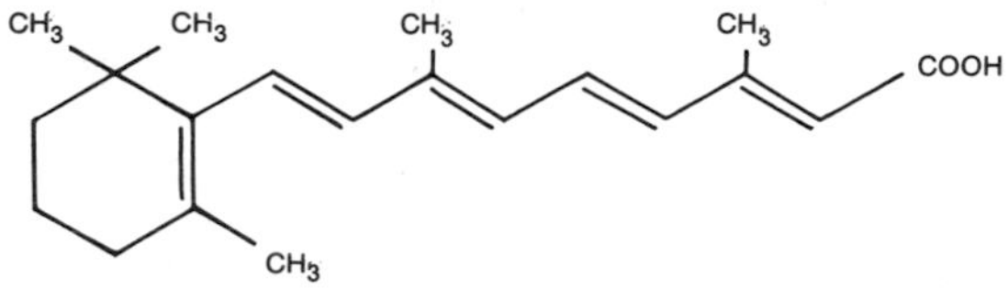

TRETINOIN

2. *Contains:* 0.05% tretinoin (vitamin A acid) in the solution and swabs, 0.1% or 0.05% in the cream, and 0.025% in the gel. The 0.05% cream or the gel are usually the least irritating. Tretinoin does not function as a vitamin in this therapy.

3. *Use:* See p. 9.

4. *Packaging and cost:*
   0.05% liquid: 28-ml bottle/$5.15
   0.05% swabs: box of 30/$6.00
   0.05% cream: 20-gm tube/$5.75
   0.1% cream: 20-gm tube/$6.00

B. Benzoyl peroxide preparations

1. *Structure*

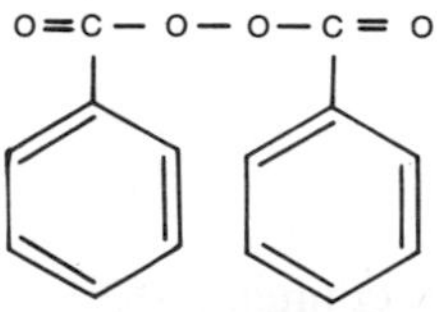

BENZOYL PEROXIDE

2. *Contain:* 5% or 10% benzoyl peroxide, oil base lotion (Benoxyl®, Persadox®; no R_x for either), alcohol gel base (Benzagel®, Pan Oxyl®), acetone gel base (Persa-Gel®), aqueous gel base (Desquam-X®)

3. *Use:* See p. 8.

4. *Packaging and cost:*
Benoxyl® 10: 30 ml/$3.30
              60 ml/$5.10
Desquam-X® 5 & 10: 45 gm/$3.00

III. OVER-THE-COUNTER (OTC) DRUGS

A. Structure of common ingredients

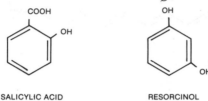

SALICYLIC ACID   RESORCINOL

B. Abrasive soaps

1. *Brasivol®*

    a. Contains: aluminum oxide particles.

    b. Use: See p. 8.

    c. Packaging and cost:
        Fine grain: 81-gm tube/$2.50
        Medium grain: 90-gm tube/$2.50
        Rough grain: 105-gm tube/$2.50

2. *Komex®*

    a. Contains: sodium tetraborate particles.

    b. Use: Apply 1–3id.

    c. Packaging and cost:
        75 gm/$2.55

3. *Pernox®*

    a. Contains: polyethylene granules, 2% sulfur, 1.5% salicylic acid.

   b. Use: See p. 8.

   c. Packaging and cost:
   60 gm/$2.35
   120 mg/$4.00

C. Cleansers

1. *Fostex® cake, cream*

   a. Contains: 2% sulfur, 2% salicylic acid.

   b. Use: See p. 9.

   c. Packaging and cost:
   112-gm cake/$1.40
   135-gm cream/$2.95

2. *Seba Nil®*

   a. Contains: 49.7% alcohol, acetone, polysorbate in saturated towelette.

   b. Use: prn for oily skin.

   c. Packaging and cost:
   Box of 24/$1.75
   Liquid: 240 ml/$2.50

D. Other drying and antiseptic topicals
Although I believe benzoyl peroxide or retinoic acid preparations are the drugs of choice, a few other acne medications are listed here for comparison of ingredients and price.

1. *Acne-Aid® cream and lotion*

   a. Contains: 2.5% sulfur, 1.25% resorcinol (cream); 10% sulfur, 10% alcohol in clear or tinted base (lotion).

   b. Use: Apply 1–2id.

   c. Packaging and cost:
   Cream: 51 gm/$2.25
   Lotion: 30 ml/$1.75
   60 ml/$2.90

2. *Acnomel® cream*

   a. Contains: 8% sulfur, 2% resorcinol, 11% alcohol in tinted vehicle.

    b. Use: Apply 1–3id.

    c. Packaging and cost:
        30 gm/$2.00

3. *Fostril® lotion*

    a. Contains: 6% polyoxyethylene lauryl ether, 2% sulfur in tinted base.

    b. Use: Apply 1–3id.

    c. Packaging and cost:
        30 ml/$2.40
        with 1% hydrocortisone (R_x) : 20 gm/$2.10

4. *Komed® lotion*

    a. Contains:

Mild	*Regular*	
2%	8%	sodium thiosulfate
1%	2%	salicylic acid
1%	2%	resorcinol
25%	25%	alcohol

    b. Use: Apply 1–3id.

    c. Packaging and cost:
        60 ml/$2.70
        with 1% hydrocortisone (R_x) : 60 gm/$4.20

5. *Liquimat® lotion*

    a. Contains: 5% sulfur, 22% alcohol in tinted lotion in 9 shades.

    b. Use: Apply 1–3id.

    c. Packaging and cost:
        45 ml/$2.00

6. *Transact® gel*

    a. Contains: 6% polyoxyethylene lauryl ether, 2% sulfur, 40% alcohol.

    b. Use: Apply 1–3id.

    c. Packaging and cost:
        30 gm/$2.55

E. Hot drying compresses

    1. *Vlem-Dome® liquid concentrate*

        a. Contains: 60.5% calcium polysulfide, 4.5% calcium thiosulfate, 4.5% sulfur (Vleminckx solution).

        b. Use: Dissolve package with 1 pint hot water and apply for 15 min nightly.

        c. Packaging and cost:
           Box of six 4-ml packets/$3.75

ANESTHETICS FOR TOPICAL ADMINISTRATION

I. DISCUSSION Topical anesthetics are useful therapeutic agents only in rare instances. This is because (a) they are ineffective if applied to epidermis that has an intact barrier layer (stratum corneum); (b) even on inflamed (e.g., sunburned) skin, only agents containing benzocaine have been shown to possibly be useful, and (c) the more effective drugs (e.g., benzocaine) are possible allergic sensitizers. A large trial on volunteers with intact or sunburned skin has shown that the wide range of local anesthetics commercially available were all useless in relieving burn discomfort or preventing experimental pain except for $\geq 10\%$ benzocaine. Mucosal surfaces lack a stratum corneum and thus topical anesthetics can be both effective and useful in some oral or anogenital disorders. Topical anesthetic use may be considered for (a) primary or recurrent herpes simplex infection of mouth or genital areas, (b) pain induced by podophyllin or alternative therapy for genital warts, and (c) aphthous stomatitis.

A. Prescription drugs

    1. *Dyclonine HCl* is a synthetic organic ketone agent related in structure to antihistamines. Onset of action is within 2–10 min and anesthesia lasts for 30–60 min.

        a. Structure

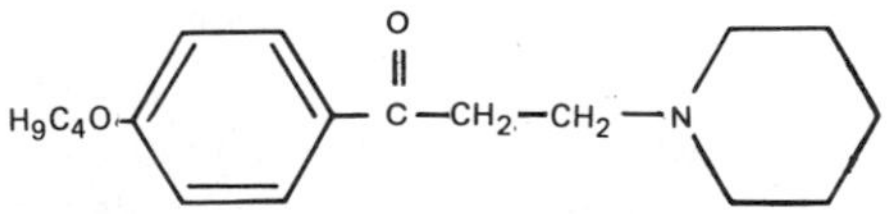

DYCLONINE

   b. Packaging (R_x) and cost:
   Dyclone®, 0.5% solution, 30 ml/$2.50
   Dyclone®, 1.0% solution, 30 ml/$3.30

2. ***Dibucaine HCl*** is an amide-type quinoline derivative and
is one of the most potent and longest acting of the commonly used local anesthetics.

   a. Structure

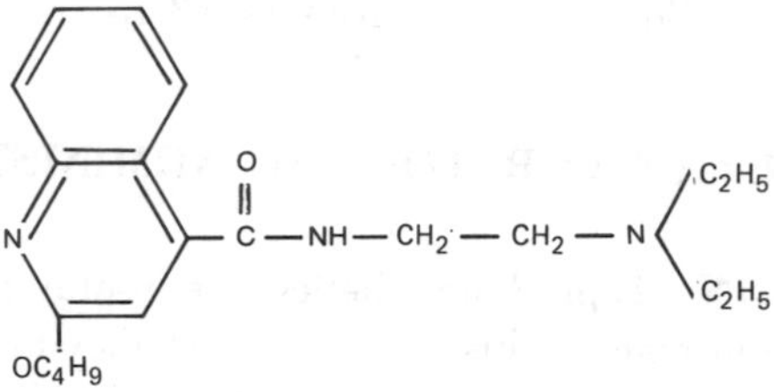

DIBUCAINE

   b. Packaging (R_x) and cost:
   0.5% solution, 30 ml/$2.50
   1.0% solution, 30 ml/$3.30

3. ***Diphenhydramine HCl (Benadryl®)*** is an effective topical agent. See pp. 22, 268 for further discussion.

4. ***Lidocaine*** is an amino acyl amide-type local anesthetic.

   a. Structure

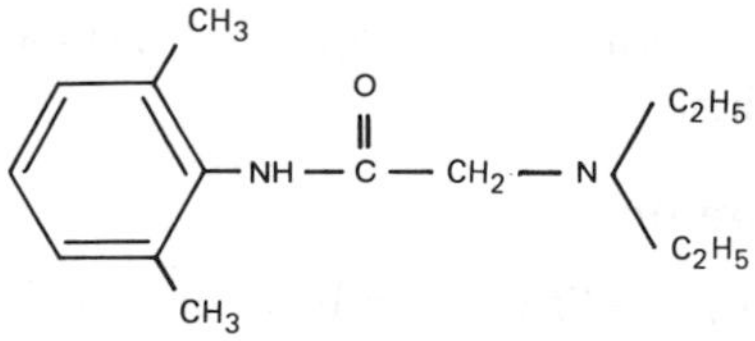

LIDOCAINE

   b. Packaging (R_x) and cost:
   Xylocaine®, 2% jelly, 30 ml/$3.50
   Xylocaine®, 2.5% ointment, 35 gm/$2.00
   Xylocaine®, 5.0% ointment, 35 gm/$3.40
   Generic 5.0% ointment, 35 gm/$1.35
   Xylocaine®, 5.0% ointment, flavored, 3.5 gm/$5.90
   Xylocaine®, 2% viscous, 100 ml/$4.25

B. Nonprescription drugs

1. **Benzocaine (*ethyl aminobenzoate*)** is poorly soluble in water and used only for topical anesthesia. Its anesthetic action is of short duration.

   a. Structure

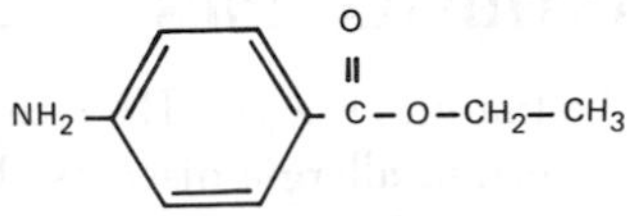

   BENZOCAINE

   b. Packaging and cost:
   Generic 5% cream, 30 gm/$0.55
   Americaine®, 20% ointment, 30 gm/$1.75
   Americaine®, 20% aerosol, 90 gm/$2.90

2. **Dimethisoquin** is an active ether-type surface anesthetic of value for treatment of cutaneous lesions. *It is less sensitizing* than drugs based on an antihistamine structure, and along with a similar compound, pramoxine (Tronothane®), *is especially useful in patients sensitive to ester- or amide-type agents.* Onset of anesthesia is rapid and its duration is 2–4 hr.

   a. Structure

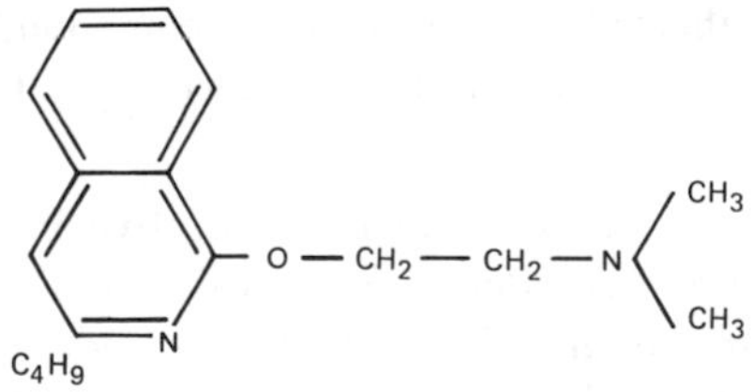

   DIMETHISOQUIN

   b. Packaging and cost:
   Quotane®, 0.5% ointment, 30 gm/$1.80
   Quotane®, 0.5% lotion with 0.1% menthol, 10% zinc oxide, 60 ml/$2.00

REFERENCES

Dalili H, Adriani J: The efficacy of local anesthetics in blocking the sensations of itch, burning, and pain in normal and "sunburned" skin. Clin Pharmacol Ther 12:913–919, 1971

Lamid S, Wang RH: The range of local anesthetics. Drug Ther (Aug): 103–113, 1975

ANTIHISTAMINES

I. **DISCUSSION** Antihistamines that are H1-receptor antagonists are useful in the control of certain allergic diseases. They completely antagonize most of the pharmacologic actions of histamine by occupying histamine receptor sites, but only if histamine has not yet reached its target receptor (competitive inhibition). Antihistamines are able to do this because they bear a close structural resemblance to histamine:

$$\text{N} \diagdown \text{CH}_2 - \text{CH}_2 - \text{N} \diagup^{\text{H}}_{\text{H}} \qquad\qquad \text{X} - \text{CH}_2 - \text{CH}_2 - \text{N} \diagup^{\text{X}}_{\text{X}}$$

HISTAMINE   MOST ANTIHISTAMINES

They do not elicit any direct effect at the receptor sites, do not react chemically with histamine, and do not prevent its release. In addition, they may diminish capillary permeability to substances other than histamine and may also have a mild local anesthetic effect. Classic antihistamines (H1 blockers) do not alter gastric acid secretion; newer H2 antagonist drugs that are able to block specific cell wall receptors not affected by the older H1 compounds affect acid secretion and have been shown to be effective in treatment of gastric ulcers.

The classic antihistamines are most effective in the management of acute urticaria and seasonal allergic rhinitis. They are also of benefit in the therapy of chronic urticaria, angioedema, and other allergic cutaneous reactions, including drug reactions. They are, however, of only limited value when given systemically for the relief of itching. Antihistamines have been shown to be no more effective than aspirin or a placebo for relief of nonhistamine-related itching (i.e., eczematous eruptions, as opposed to urticaria), but apparently there is an enormous placebo effect operating; in dealing with patients bothered by pruritus, the magnitude of this beneficial phenomenon should never be overlooked.

The several chemical classes of antihistamines show only minor variations in their properties. However, individuals frequently react differently to these preparations, and one or several antihistamines of different types may have to be tried, occasionally in combination, before the best therapeutic-sedative ratio is reached. Hydroxyzine appears to be the most effective drug in suppressing histamine-induced pruritus; in one experimental system, cyproheptadine and placebo administration necessitated a fivefold increase in the intradermal histamine dose required to produce pruritus compared to a tenfold increase following diphenhydramine and a 750-fold increase following hydroxyzine HCl.

Antihistamines are rapidly absorbed after oral or parenteral administration. Following an oral dose, symptomatic relief is noted within 15–30 min and usually lasts 3–6 hr. These drugs are metabolized mainly in the liver and excretion is nearly complete in 24 hr. Antihistamines are also used topically in antipruritic lotions, but whatever small benefit might result is greatly overshadowed by the risk of inducing an allergic contact dermatitis, and this route should be avoided. The most common untoward systemic effect is sedation, and ambulatory patients must be warned of this, especially if driving is contemplated. Gastrointestinal side-effects can also be seen. At times, atropine-like side-effects predominate, with the symptoms including excitation. Other anticholinergic effects may be dry mouth, blurred vision, and urinary retention. Patients should be cautioned about taking alcoholic beverages or barbiturates during antihistamine therapy since the depressant action of these drugs is additive.

To be used most effectively, antihistamines should be gradually increased until either clinical remission occurs or side-effects (most often sedation) become significant. It is frequently unwise to start at too high a dose, and the optimal course is often to begin at 1 tablet q4h and to increase the number of tablets administered as long as the dosage remains ineffective. It is rarely necessary to exceed 4 tablets q4h but the interval between doses may be decreased if necessary. For general use, chlorpheniramine maleate and/or hydroxyzine hydrochloride or hydroxyzine pamoate have proved consistently effective.

II. SPECIFIC AGENTS (ALL R_x)

    A. Ethanolamine derivatives, potent antihistamines, are the drugs of choice in anaphylactic reactions. However, there is a high incidence of sedation among patients who take them, and they have an additive effect with hypnotics and sedatives. With doses of 100 mg or more, hypertension, tachycardia, T-wave changes, or shortened diastole may further complicate the clinical picture.

1. *Diphenhydramine hydrochloride (Benadryl®)*

   a. Structure

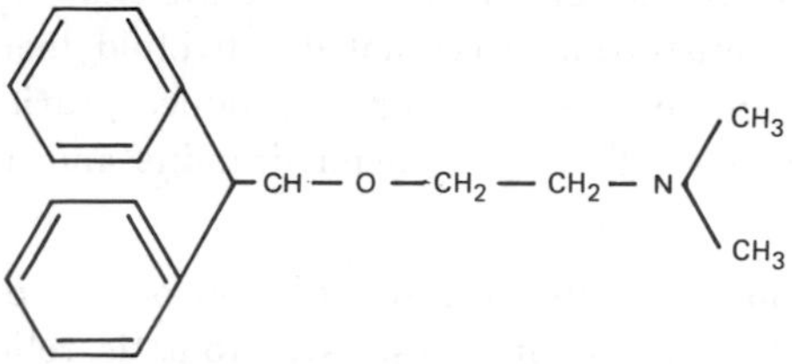

   DIPHENHYDRAMINE

   b. Dosage: 50 mg (or 1 tsp) PO q4h.

   c. Preparation and cost:
       50-mg capsules: as diphenhydramine, 1000/$9.00
                       as Benadryl®, 1000/$40.00
       Elixir (10mg/4ml): as diphenhydramine, 480 ml/$2.25
                       as Benadryl®, 500 ml/$4.90

B. **Ethylenediamine derivatives** cause less drowsiness but more gastrointestinal side-effects.

   1. *Tripelennamine hydrochloride (Pyribenzamine®)*

      a. Structure

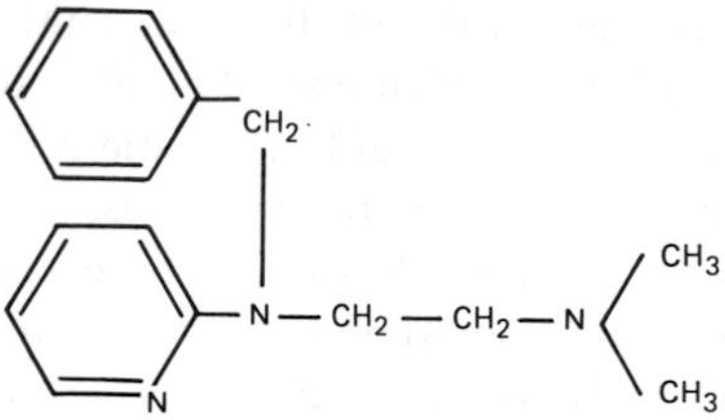

      TRIPELENNAMINE

      b. Dosage: 50 mg PO q4h.

      c. Preparation and cost:
          50-mg tablets: as tripelennamine, 1000/$6.75
                         as Pyribenzamine®, 1000/$45.00

2. *Hydroxyzine hydrochloride (Atarax®) or hydroxyzine pamoate (Vistaril®)* is an antihistamine commonly also used for its mild calming effects as a tranquilizer.

   a. Structure

   b. Use: It is the drug of choice for therapy of dermatographism and cholinergic urticaria. It is also effective alone or in combination with other antihistamines in the therapy of acute and chronic urticaria and pruritus.

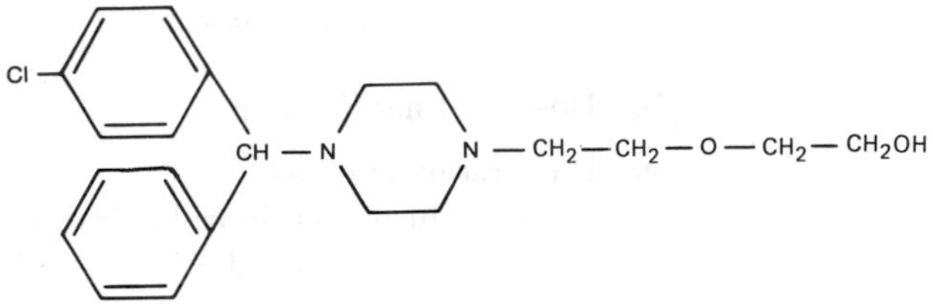

HYDROXYZINE

   c. Dosage: 25 mg PO q4h.

   d. Packaging and cost:
      10-mg tablets: as Atarax®, 100/$11.60
      25-mg tablets: as Atarax®, 100/$16.80
                     syrup, 500 ml/$10.75

C. **Alkylamine derivatives** include some of the most active antihistamines effective in low dosage. As there is no variation in the effectiveness of members of this antihistamine class, particular emphasis should be placed on the lower cost and easy availability of chlorpheniramine.

   1. *Brompheniramine maleate (Dimetane®)* (The only difference between this and chlorpheniramine is the substitution of a bromine for a chlorine atom in the first.)

      a. Dosage: 4 mg PO q4h; 1 tsp (2 mg) q4h.

      b. Preparation and cost:
         4-mg tablets: as brompheniramine, 100/$0.90
                       as Dimetane®, 100/$4.00
         Elixir (4 mg/5 ml): as brompheniramine, 500 ml/
                             $2.10
                             as Dimetane®, 500 ml/$4.50

2. *Chlorpheniramine maleate (Chlor-Trimeton®)*

a. Structure

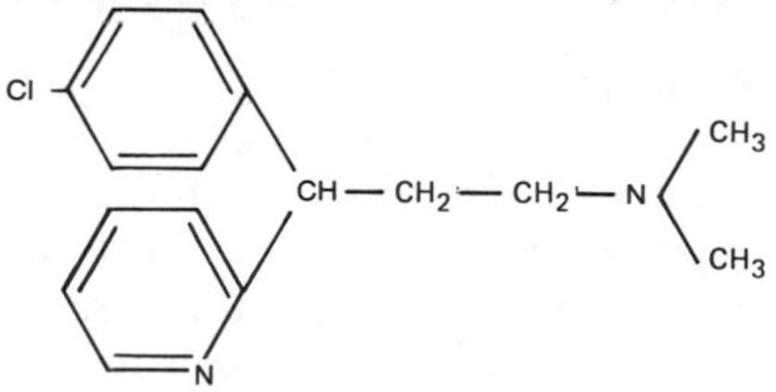

CHLORPHENIRAMINE

b. Dosage: 4 mg PO q4h.

c. Preparation and cost:
4-mg tablets: as chlorpheniramine, 1000/$1.90
as Chlor-Trimeton®, 1000/$36.00

3. *Dexchlorpheniramine maleate (Polaramine®)* is the dextrorotatory isomer of chlorpheniramine.

a. Dosage: 2 mg PO q4h.

b. Packaging and cost:
2-mg tablets: as Polaramine®, 100/$4.75

D. Phenothiazine derivatives are used primarily as central nervous system depressants, but some are useful as antihistaminics.

1. *Promethazine hydrochloride (Phenergan®)*

a. Structure

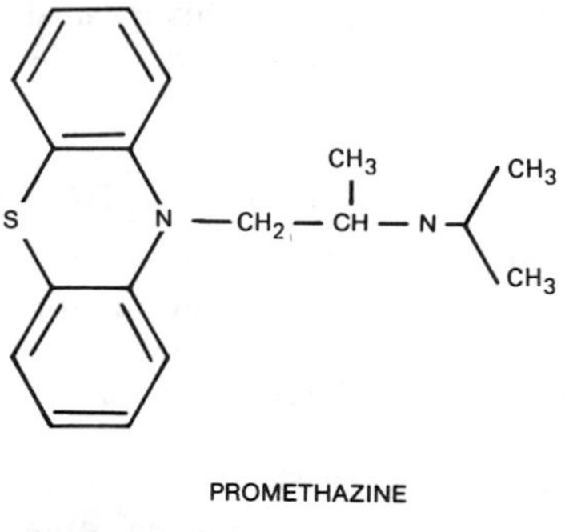

PROMETHAZINE

b. Dosage: 12.5 mg PO 4id; 25 mg PO hs.

c. Packaging and cost:
25-mg tablets: as promethazine, 1000/$14.25
as Phenergan®, 1000/$116.00

2. *Trimeprazine tartrate* (*Temaril*®)

   a. Structure

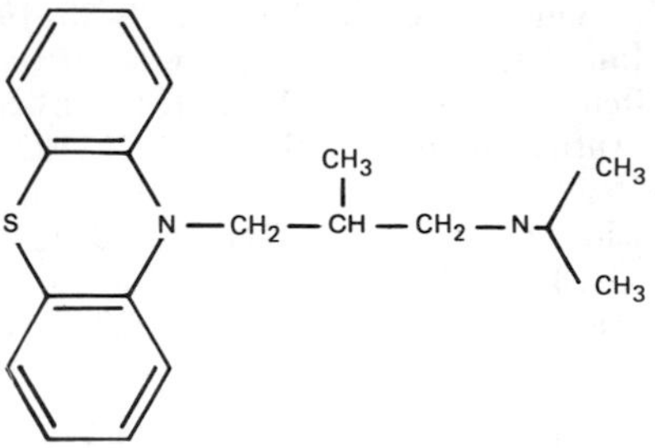

TRIMEPRAZINE

   b. Dosage: 2.5 mg PO q4h.

   c. Packaging and cost:
      2.5-mg tablets: as Temaril®, 100/$10.00

E. Propylamine derivatives

   1. *Cyproheptadine hydrochloride* (*Periactin*®) is an antihistamine in which antiserotonin activity has been demonstrated both in vivo and in vitro. As yet, however, there is no evidence that this action contributes to clinical therapeutic effects.

      a. Structure

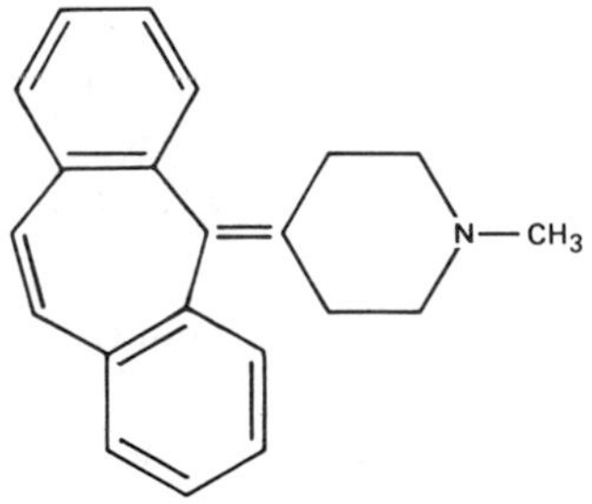

CYPROHEPTADINE

      b. Dosage: 4 mg PO q4h.

      c. Packaging and cost:
         4-mg tablets: As Periactin®, 100/$10.80

REFERENCES

Beaven MA: Histamine. N Engl J Med 294:30–35, 1976

Hagermark Ö: Influence of antihistamines, sedatives and aspirin on experimental itch. Acta Derm Venereol (Stockh) 53:363–368, 1973

Hermance WE: Antihistamines. Cutis 17:1177–1182, 1976

Rhoades RB, Leifer KN, Cohan R, Wittig HJ: Suppression of histamine-induced pruritus by three antihistaminic drugs. J Allergy Clin Immunol 55:180–185, 1975

Today's Drugs—Antihistamines. Br Med J 1:217–219, 1970

ANTI-INFECTIVE AGENTS

I. **ANTIBACTERIAL AGENTS, TOPICAL** The concept of using topical antibiotics to prevent or treat cutaneous bacterial infection seems rational, and yet it is only recently that the effectiveness of this therapy has been critically evaluated.

Numerous antibacterial agents are available for topical use. In general, those of most benefit are either combinations of the "nonabsorbable" antibiotics (bacitracin, gramicidin, neomycin) or the iodophors (e.g., povidine iodine). Use of topical antibiotics, singly or as mixtures, or broad-spectrum germicides is justified for many reasons: (1) They can treat a wide range of potential pathogens in mixed infections—frequently more than one pathogen is present and quick identification of organisms is difficult. (2) They are used in small amounts and thus permit use of drugs that are relatively toxic when given systemically. Percutaneous absorption of antibiotics from normal skin or from psoriatic or eczematous areas cannot be detected in blood or urine—the possibility of producing nephrotoxicity or ototoxicity is extremely unlikely. Neomycin is the only potential allergen, and 6 percent of individuals with chronic dermatoses are shown to be allergic by patch testing. The incidence of sensitization of normal subjects in the general population is not known. (3) The concentration of the drugs is high, though the total amounts are small; this represents large multiples of the minimum effective concentration for potential pathogens. (4) Topically administered drugs are in more direct contact with organisms so that the problems of absorption, distribution, and availability to the infected site are not involved. (5) The combined effects of bactericidal agents such as bacitracin, neomycin, and polymyxin B are predominantly synergistic, thus increasing the rate of bactericidal action and killing large numbers of bacteria more rapidly, and probably increasing the spectrum of their action. *Staphylococcus aureus* is highly susceptible to the bactericidal action of neomycin and static action of tetracyclines, while *Streptococcus pyogenes* is particularly susceptible to bacitracin and neomycin. Neomycin is approximately 50 times more active against staphylococci than bacitracin (by weight), but bacitracin is 20 times more active against streptococci. Of gram-negative invaders, all but *Proteus* species are sensitive to polymyxin B and all but *Pseudomonas* are sensitive to neomycin—thus, to cover this spectrum, combinations of two or three antibiotics may be necessary. (6) Another combined effect is to delay and depress the development of resistance or emergence of resistant mutants. This is true particularly with regard to neomycin and to gentamicin. Although outbreaks of neomycin-resistant infections have been noted in closed communities, the incidence of resistance to this antibiotic has not materially changed during the last 20 years.

With regard to treatment of infected dermatoses, agents that modify the underlying inflammatory condition (e.g., corticosteroids) seem to be as effective as topical antibiotics or antibiotic-corticosteroid combinations. Local treatment does not diminish the reservoir of pathogens in the lesion or on the rest of the body, however; systemic antibiotics would be best for that task. Similarly, impetigo should be treated with systemic antibiotics as discussed on p. 28. There is as yet no evidence to show whether topical antibiotics applied to the first wound in the skin would prevent it from becoming impetiginous, but once established, pyodermas are best treated with systemic agents.

Review of the data indicates that topical antibiotic preparations may effectively control the bacteria usually found in superficial wounds. They can reduce colony counts of bacteria and hence are effective for axillary deodorization or controlling nasal carriage of staphylococci. These antibiotics may also be useful in preventing infections in clean wounds, and when used *early*, might diminish the amount of infection, hasten healing, and reduce systemic effects of infection in infected wounds such as incisions, lacerations, or burns.

These preparations should be applied frequently (3–6id) after the skin is cleansed of adherent crusts and debris and should not be applied under occlusive dressings.

A. **Bacitracin** This polypeptide antibiotic, which is produced from *Bacillus subtilis*, interferes with cell wall growth and is bactericidal against many gram-positive organisms such as streptococci, staphylococci, and pneumococci, but is inactive against most gram-negative organisms. All anaerobic cocci, *Neisseria* and the tetanus and diphtheria bacilli are also sensitive to bacitracin. Resistance is rare, but some staphylococcal strains are inherently resistant. Hypersensitivity reactions are uncommon. Bacitracin is stable in petrolatum (but not water-miscible preparations) and is available as an ointment or as a component of antibiotic mixtures.

1. Structure

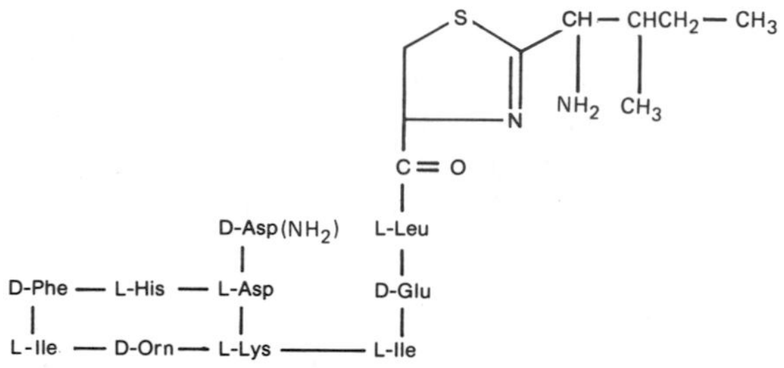

BACITRACIN

2. Use: Clean wound and apply 4–6id.

3. Packaging and cost:
500 units/gm: 15-gm tube/$0.70–$1.00

B. **Chlorhexidine** This topical antiseptic product acts rapidly but like hexachlorophene persists on the stain to give a cumulative, continuing antibacterial effect. Like iodophors and alcohol it is active against gram-positive and gram-negative bacteria, although less so against *Serratia* and *Pseudomonas*.

Packaging and cost
(as Hibiclens®: 4% chlorhexidine gluconate with 4% isopropyl alcohol) 120 ml/$3.00

C. **Gentamicin (Garamycin®)** This antibiotic is a combination of three related aminoglycoside agents obtained from cultures of *Micromonospora purpurea* and acts by interfering with the bacterial synthesis of protein. Its antibiotic spectrum is similar to that of neomycin and cross-resistance does occur. Gentamicin is active against gram-negative organisms including *Escherichia coli* and a high percentage of strains of species of *Pseudomonas* and other gram-negative bacteria. *Proteus* organisms show a variable degree of sensitivity. Some gram-positive organisms, including *S. aureus* and group A beta-hemolytic streptococci, are also affected. In general, higher concentrations are needed to inhibit streptococci than are needed to inhibit staphylococci and many gram-negative bacteria. The most important use of gentamicin is in the treatment of systemic gram-negative infections, particularly those due to *Pseudomonas* organisms. Widespread topical use is unwarranted, since equally effective drugs are available, and widespread utilization will increase the background of gentamicin-resistant organisms.

1. *Structure*

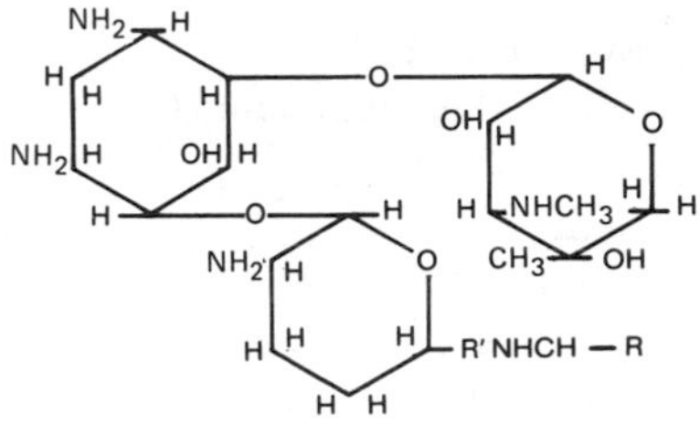

GENTAMICIN SULFATE

GENTAMICIN	R	R'
C_1	CH_3	CH_3
C_2	CH_3	H
C_{1A}	H	H

2. *Use:* Clean lesion and apply 4–6id.

3. *Packaging and cost* (R_x):

15-gm cream or ointment: as Garamycin®/$2.70

D. **Iodophors** These consist of a water-soluble organic complex of iodine with a carrier that slowly liberates iodine on contact with reducing substances in body tissues. These broad-range germicidal antiseptics are effective against bacteria, fungi, viruses, protozoa, and yeasts. They are water-soluble, nonirritating, and nonstinging; they are often used for preoperative skin cleansing and surgical scrubbing and as treatment for skin infections and burns. These effective agents are available in many vehicles, and in many circumstances they are the antimicrobial agent of choice. The solubilizing carrier substances include polyvinyl-pyrrolidone (povidone-iodine, as in Betadine® products, or available as generics) and poloxamer-iodine complex.

1. *Structure*

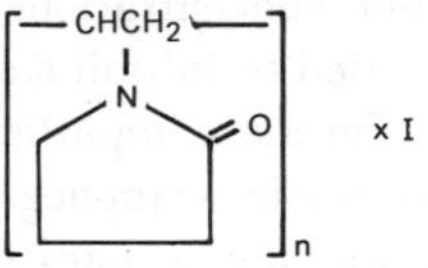

POVIDONE-IODINE

2. *Packaging and cost* (as Betadine® microbicidal antiseptics):

Solution: 15 ml/$1.05
Aerosol spray: 90 ml/$4.05
Surgical scrub: 960 ml with pump/$10.15
Douche: 240 ml/$3.90
Ointment: 30 gm/$2.80
Shampoo: 120 ml/$2.70
Skin cleanser: 120 ml/$2.70
Vaginal gel (R_x): 90 gm/$4.50
as generic: Surgical scrub: 500 ml/$2.60
Solution: 500 ml/$3.15

E. **Neomycin sulfate** This is obtained from species of the actinomycete *Streptomyces*, is an aminoglycoside antibiotic (as are streptomycin, gentamicin, and kanamycin) effective against most gram-negative organisms. Group A streptococci are relatively resistant. This antibiotic, as do all aminoglycosides, acts by inhibiting protein synthesis. Neomycin is responsible for a greater incidence of allergic contact sensitivity than any other topical antibiotic. This diagnosis often remains hidden, since morphologically the eruption is of a mild eczematous nature, and it frequently appears as if the original cutaneous disease were unaffected by treatment.

1. *Structure*

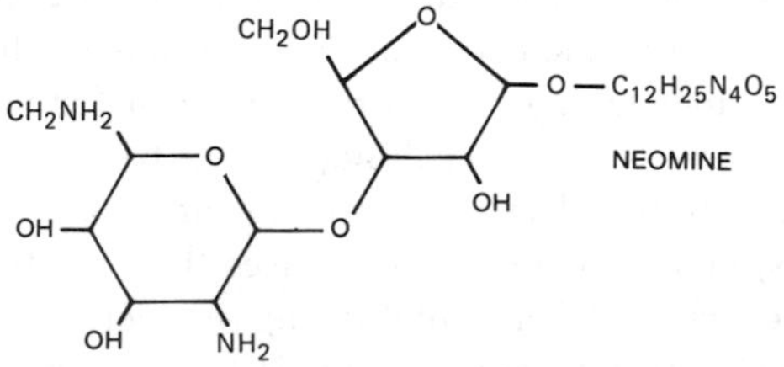

NEOMINE

NEOMYCIN B

2. *Use:* Apply 4–6id.

3. *Packaging and cost:*
   15-gm ointment/$0.75

F. **Polymyxin B** Polymyxin B is one of a group of cyclic polypeptides, elaborated by *Bacillus polymyxa.* The drug is a surface-active agent and is thought to alter the lipoprotein membrane of bacteria so that it no longer functions as an effective barrier, and thereby allows the cell contents to escape. Polymyxin B is effective against *Pseudomonas* and other gram-negative bacteria except the *Proteus* and *Serratia* species and has little effect on gram-positive organisms.

G. **Tyrothricin** Tyrothricin, containing **gramicidin** and **tyrocidine,** is a mixture of polypeptide antibiotics bactericidal for common gram-positive organisms but generally inactive against gram-negative organisms. Gramicidin uncouples oxidative phosphorylation, while tyrocidine decreases bacterial cell respiration, with concomitant leakage of amino acids into the surrounding medium. Tyrothricin has the advantage of a wide gram-positive spectrum, no sensitizing properties or tissue toxicity, and rarity of acquired resistance. It is frequently found as a component of antibacterial mixtures for topical use.

H. **Combination topical preparations**

1. *Neo-Polycin® ointment*

   a. Contains: per gm, 8000 units polymyxin B sulfate, 400 units zinc bacitracin, 3 mg neomycin sulfate (as base).

   b. Dosage: Apply 4–6id.

   c. Packaging and cost:
      as generic, 15-gm tube/$0.90
      as Neo-Polycin®, 15-gm tube/$2.35

2. *Neosporin® Aerosol*

   a. Contains: per 90 gm, 100,000 units polymyxin B sulfate, 8000 units zinc bacitracin, 70 mg neomycin sulfate (as base).

   b. Dosage: Apply 4–6id.

   c. Packaging (R_x) and cost:
      90-gm can/$3.50

3. *Neosporin® ointment*

    a.   Contains: per gm, 5000 units polymyxin B sulfate, 400 units zinc bacitracin, 3.5 mg neomycin sulfate (as base).

    b.   Dosage: Apply 4–6id.

    c.   Packaging and cost:
        as generic, 15-gm tube/$0.90
        as Neosporin®, 15-gm tube/$1.85

4. *Neosporin® powder*

    a.   Contains: per gm, 5000 units polymyxin B sulfate, 400 units zinc bacitracin, 3.5 mg neomycin sulfate (as base).

    b.   Dosage: Apply 4–6id. Neosporin® powder is particularly useful in the therapy of erosions and ulcers.

    c.   Packaging (R_x) and cost:
        10-gm shaker-top container/$2.30

5. *Neosporin G® cream*

    a.   Contains: per gm, 10,000 units polymyxin B sulfate, 3.5 gm neomycin sulfate (as base), and 0.25 mg gramicidin.

    b.   Dosage: Apply 4–6id.

    c.   Packaging (R_x) and cost:
        15-gm tube/$1.65

6. *Polysporin® ointment*

    a.   Contains: per gm, 10,000 units polymyxin B sulfate with 500 units zinc bacitracin.

    b.   Packaging and cost:
        15 gm/$1.75

7. *Spectrocin® ointment*

    a.   Contains: per gm, 0.25 mg gramicidin, 2.5 mg neosporin sulfate (as base).

    b.   Packaging and cost:
        15 gm/$1.65

REFERENCES

Anderson V (ed): Over-the-counter topical antibiotic products: Data on safety and efficacy. Int J Dermatol 15:2 [Suppl], 118 pp, 1976

Leyden JJ, Kligman AM: The case for topical antibiotics. Prog Dermatol 10:13–16, 1976

Leyden JJ, Kligman AM: Criticism of "the case against topical antibiotics." Prog Dermatol 11:7–8, 1977

Rasmussen JE: The case against topical antibiotics. Prog Dermatol 11:1–4, 1977

Rasmussen JE: Criticism of "the case for topical antibiotics." Prog Dermatol 11:5–7, 1977

II. ANTIFUNGAL AGENTS

A. Discussion   See Fungal Infections, p. 86.

B. Prescription drugs

    1. *Acrisorcin (Akrinol®)* cream is effective in vitro against a variety of bacteria, fungi, and protozoa. Clinically, it is used solely for the topical therapy of tinea versicolor.

        a. Dosage: See p. 101.

        b. Packaging (R_x) and cost:
            50-gm tube/$3.90

    2. *Amphotericin B (Fungizone®)* is one of the polyene group of antifungal antibiotics used topically in the treatment of superficial *Candida albicans* infection and is the therapy of choice for most systemic fungal infections. It is ineffective against dermatophytes. The drug is yellow-orange, odorless, and may stain skin.

        a. Structure

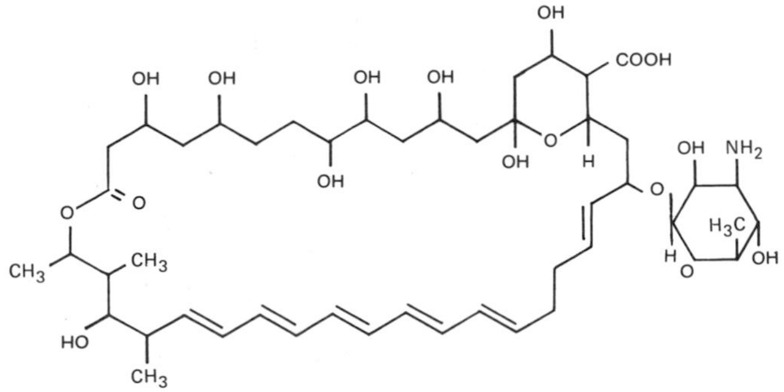

AMPHOTERICIN B

b. Dosage: Apply 4–6id.

c. Packaging (R_x) and cost:
as Fungizone®: 3% cream and ointment, 20 gm/
$5.20
3% lotion, 30 ml/$7.05

3. *Candicidin (Candeptin®, Vanobid®)* is a polyene anti-fungal antibiotic similar chemically and in spectrum to amphotericin B. It is used topically only in the treatment of monilial vulvovaginitis.

   a. Packaging (R_x) and cost:
   Ointment: 75 gm × 2/$8.90
   Vaginal tablets: package of 28/$6.50

4. *Chlordantoin (Sporostacin®)*, an odorless and non-staining synthetic mercaptan derivative, is used in the topical treatment of monilial vulvovaginitis.

   a. Packaging (R_x) and cost:
   Cream: 95 gm/$5.75

5. *Clotrimazole (Lotrimin®)* is a synthetic imidazole agent used for treatment of superficial fungal infections and *C. albicans* infections. It inhibits the growth of most dermatophyte species, is as active as nystatin against *C. albicans,* inhibits growth of some gram-positive bacteria, and in high concentrations is active against *Trichomonas* species. Its mechanism of action is not yet clear but probably involves damage to the cell wall in a fashion similar to that of the polyene antibiotics.

   a. Structure

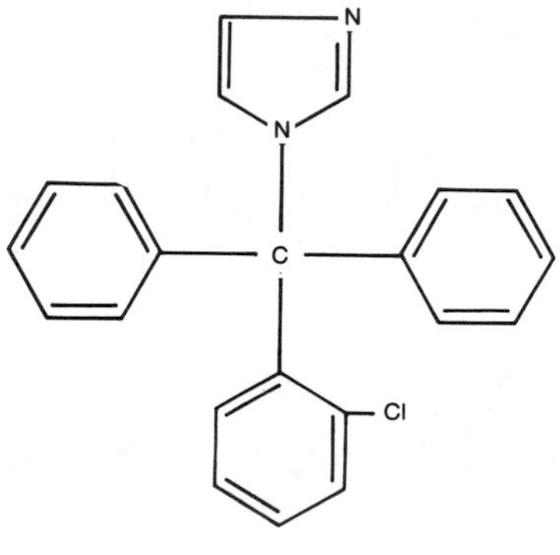

CLOTRIMAZOLE

b. Dosage: Apply 2–3id until eruption clears (see p. 00).

c. Packaging (R_x) and cost:
 Cream: 15-gm tube/$4.10
     30-gm tube/$7.10
 Solution: 10 ml/$3.60
      30 ml/$7.60
 Vaginal tablets (Gyne-Lotrimin®): pkg of 7/$8.30

6. ***Griseofulvin*** is an antifungal antibiotic effective against all dermatophyte fungi, but not against *C. albicans* or tinea versicolor. Its gastrointestinal absorption is variable but is enhanced by use of the microcrystalline preparation (see Fungal Infections, p. 97).

 a. Structure

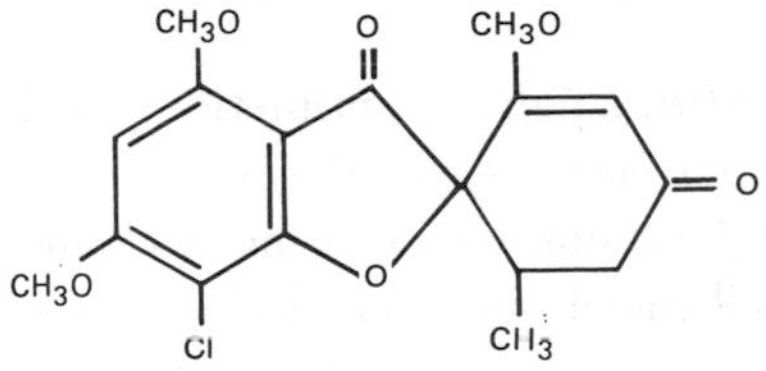

 GRISEOFULVIN

 b. Dosage: See Fungal Infections, pp. 97, 98.

 c. Packaging (R_x) and cost:

 (1) as Fulvicin-U/F®, Grifulvin V®, Grisactin®:
    100 250-mg caps/$18.15
    100 500-mg caps/$34.35

 (2) as Gris-PEG® (ultramicrosize dispersion in polyethylene glycol; 125 mg Gris-PEG = 250 microcrystalline griseofulvin):
    100 125-mg tabs/$14.10

 (3) as generic: 100 250-mg caps/$13.90

 (4) as suspension (125 mg/5 ml): 120 ml/$4.90

7. ***Haloprogin (Halotex®)*** is a synthetic chlorinated iodopropynyl trichlorophenyl ether antifungal agent used in the topical treatment of dermatophyte infections and tinea versicolor. It is also active in vitro against staphylococci, streptococci, and *C. albicans*.

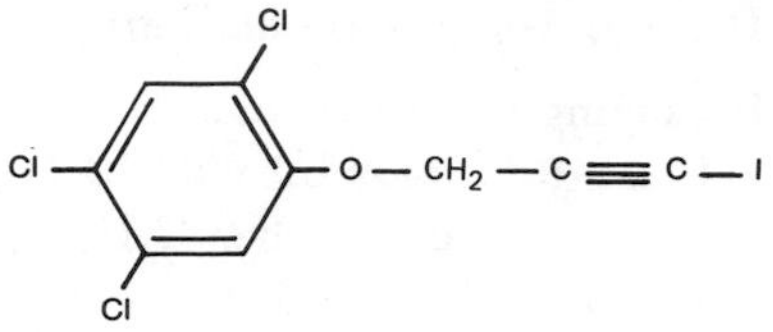

HALOPROGIN

a. Structure

b. Dosage: Apply 3id.

c. Packaging (R_x) and cost:
    1% cream: 30 gm/$6.30
    1% solution: 10 ml/$3.15
                  30 ml/$6.75

8. *Nystatin,* a polyene antibiotic derived from a species of the actinomycete *Streptomyces noursei,* binds to sterols in fungal membranes, causing a change in the permeability of cell membranes and leakage of cell components. It is nontoxic and available for oral, vaginal, and topical administration. Nystatin is poorly absorbed from the gastrointestinal tract and will thus rid the oral and gastrointestinal mucosa of *Candida* but have no effect on systemic or cutaneous lesions when given orally. Nystatin is unstable to heat, light, moisture, and air. Aqueous-alcohol suspensions are stable for 10 days under refrigeration.

a. Dosage: See Fungal Infections, p. 88.

b. Packaging (R_x) and cost:

    (1)   Nystatin (Candex®, Mycostatin®, Nilstat®)
               Ointment and cream (100,000 units/gm):
                    15 gm/$3.20
               Powder (100,000 units): 15 gm/$3.80
               Tablets (500,000 units): 100/$19.90
               Oral suspension (100,000 units/ml): 60 ml/
                    $7.30
               Vaginal tablets: 15/$3.75
               Lotion (100,000 units/ml): 30 ml/$7.60

   (2)   Nystatin, 1% iodochlorhydroxyquin (Nysta-form®)
       Ointment: 15 gm/4.00

   (3)   Nystatin, neomycin sulfate, gramicidin, 0.1% triamcinolone acetonide (Mycolog®)
       Cream and ointment:
         5 gm/$2.80
         15 gm/$5.65
         60 gm/$18.10

9. *Miconazole* (MicaTin®, Monistat®) is a synthetic imidazole antifungal compound effective against most dermatophyte species and against *C. albicans*. It destroys fungi presumably by inhibiting cell wall synthesis.

  a. Structure

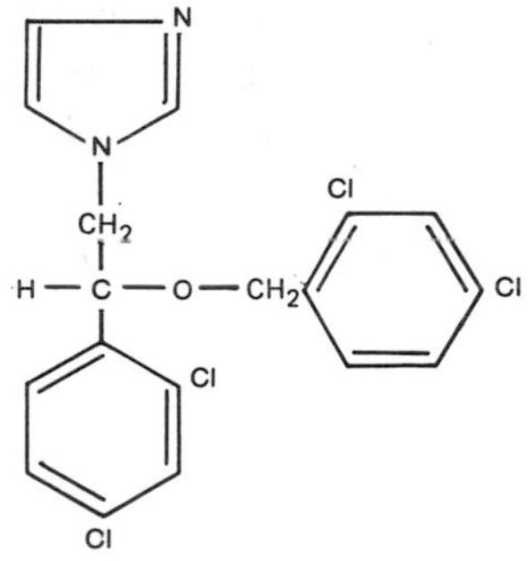

MICONAZOLE

  b. Dosage: Apply 2–3id until eruption clears (see p. 95).

  c. Packaging (R_x) and cost:
     as MicaTin®: 2% cream: 30 gm/$5.55
     as Monistat®: 2% vaginal cream: 85-gm tube with applicator/$8.10

10. *Tinver*® contains 25% sodium thiosulfate ($Na_2S_2O_3$), 1% salicylic acid, and 10% alcohol and is used in treatment of tinea versicolor.

  a. Dosage: See p. 101.

  b. Packaging (R_x) and cost:
     150-ml lotion/$4.65

11. **Thymol** is an alkyl derivative of phenol with bactericidal and fungicidal properties. It is chiefly of value as a fungicide.

a. Structure

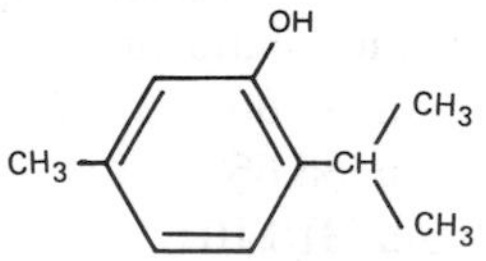

THYMOL

b. Dosage: See p. 89.

C. OTC preparations

1. **Benzoic (12%) acid and salicylic (6%) acid (Whitfield's) ointment** is a potent keratolytic agent and is used in the treatment of dermatophyte infections. It has, however, a strong potential for causing irritant reactions. It is also available in half-strength (6%/3%) concentration.

a. Structure

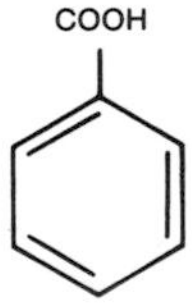

BENZOIC ACID

b. Dosage: Apply 2–4id.

c. Packaging and cost:
30 gm/$0.60

2. **Carbol-fuchsin solution (Castellani's paint)** is a dark purple liquid that appears red on the skin. It has local anesthetic, bactericidal, and fungicidal properties and is applied topically in the treatment of subacute and chronic superficial fungal infection. It is particularly effective in intertriginous inflammation.

a. Structure

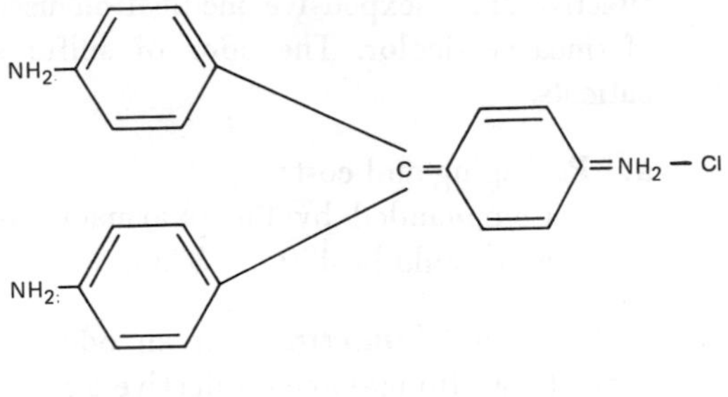

FUCHSIN (PARAROSANILINE HYDROCHLORIDE)

b. Contains:

Boric acid	1.0%
Phenol	4.5%
Resorcinol	10.0%
Fuchsin	0.3%
Acetone	5.0%

    in water

c. Dosage: Apply 1–3id with swab. Clean skin with soap and water prior to application.

d. Packaging: Must be compounded by a pharmacist.

3. *Gentian (crystal, methyl) violet (methylrosaniline chloride)*, 0.5–3%, is used in the treatment of infections due to yeasts and molds. This triphenylmethane dye has also been effective in therapy of Vincent's angina and secondarily infected dermatoses and dermatophytoses.

a. Structure

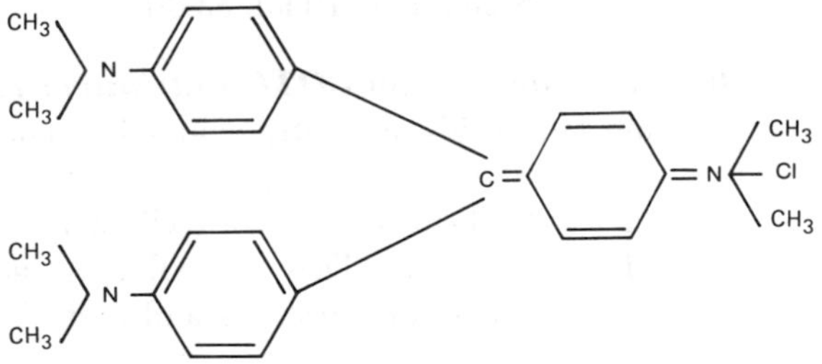

GENTIAN VIOLET (METHYLROSANILINE CHLORIDE)

b. Dosage: Apply with cotton 2id.

c. Packaging and cost:

    1% solution: 30 ml/$0.70

4. **Sodium thiosulfate ($Na_2S_2O_3 \cdot 5\,H_2O$), 25%,** is an effective and inexpensive medication used in the treatment of tinea versicolor. The odor of sulfur sometimes offends patients.

  a. Packaging and cost:
  Compounded by the pharmacist to order, a typical cost would be 480 ml/$3.00.

5. **Tolnaftate (*Tinactin®*)** is an odorless and nonstaining synthetic antifungal agent effective against all dermatophyte fungi and tinea versicolor. However, it is ineffective against *C. albicans* and bacteria.

  a. Structure

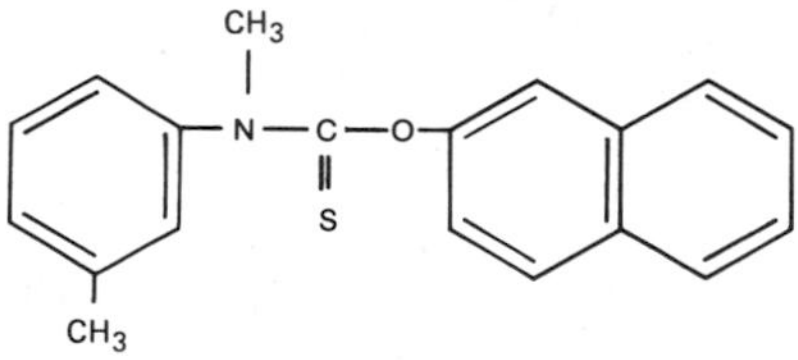

TOLNAFTATE

  b. Dosage: Apply 2–3id until the eruption has cleared (2–6 weeks) (see p. 00).

  c. Packaging and cost:
  Cream: 15 gm/$3.80
  1% powder: 45 gm/$2.00
  1% solution: 10 ml/$3.30

6. There are numerous **OTC antifungal remedies** that contain fatty acids and fatty acid salts (undecylenic acid $CH_2 = CH(CH_2)_8COOH$, proprionic acid), organic acids and their salts (benzoic acid, salicylic acid), and miscellaneous other compounds. They are all only moderately effective. Some common preparations and costs follow.

  a. *Desenex®*
  Ointment (5% undecylenic acid, 20% zinc undecylenate)
  Powder (2% undecylenic acid, 20% zinc undecylenate)

Packaging and cost:
Ointment: 54 gm/$2.50
Powder: 90 gm/$2.30

b. *Sopronol®*
Solution (12.3% sodium proprionate,
10% sodium caprylate)
Ointment (12.3% sodium proprionate,
10% sodium caprylate, 5% zinc caprylate)
Powder (5% sodium proprionate,
5% sodium caprylate, 10% zinc caprylate)

Packaging and cost:
Solution: 60 ml/$1.00
Ointment: 30 gm/$1.20
Powder: 150 gm/$2.10

c. *Verdefam®*
Solution (2% sodium proprionate, 2% sodium caprylate, 3% proprionic acid, 5% undecylenic acid,
5% salicylic acid, 0.5% copper undecylenate)
Cream (1% sodium proprionate, 1% sodium caprylate, 3% proprionic acid, 2% undecylenic acid,
3% salicylic acid, 0.5% copper undecylenate)

Packaging and cost:
Solution: 60 ml/$1.95
Cream: 30 gm/$1.95

REFERENCES

Holt RJ: Topical pharmacology of imidazole antifungals. J Cutan Pathol 3:45–59, 1976
Smith GB: New topical agents for dermatophytosis. Cutis 17:54–58, 1976

III. ANTIVIRAL AGENTS

A. Adenine arabinoside (vidarabine) (VIRA-A®) is a purine
nucleoside which interferes with the early steps of viral DNA
synthesis of herpes simplex, zoster-varicella, and vaccinia viruses.

1. *Dosage:* Apply 3id into conjunctual sac for herpes simplex
keratitis.

2. *Packaging and cost:*
3.5 gm/$9.30

B. **Idoxuridine (2'-Deoxy-5-iodouridine) (Dendrid®, Herplex®, Stoxil®)** This is an antiviral agent that interferes with viral DNA synthesis. It is of proven value in the treatment of dendritic keratitis and may sometimes be helpful for herpes infections of the skin and mucous membranes.

1. *Structure*

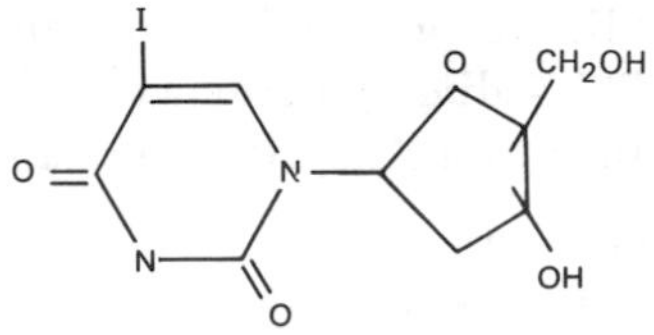

IDOXURIDINE

2. *Dosage:* See Herpes Simplex, p. 109.

3. *Packaging (R_x) and cost:*
   0.5% ointment (Stoxil®) : 4 gm/$5.30
   0.1% solution (Stoxil®) : 15 gm/$5.30

IV. **SCABICIDES AND PEDICULICIDES** (For discussion, see Infestations, p. 127.)

A. **Benzyl benzoate, 20–25%,** is effective in scabies and in the treatment of pediculosis when accompanied by scabies. It is, however, not recommended for the treatment of uncomplicated pediculosis.

1. *Structure*

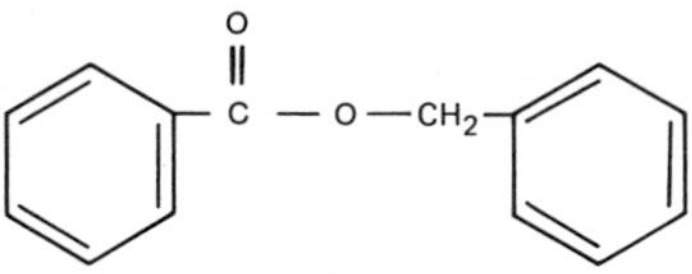

BENZYL BENZOATE

2. *Packaging and cost* (as 50% emulsion) :
   500 ml/$3.70

B. **Chlorophenothane, USP (DDT)** (10% powder, 10% solution [R_x]) eradicates body lice and bedbugs and is an excellent insecticide for flies, mosquitoes, ants, cockroaches, and spiders.

1. *Structure*

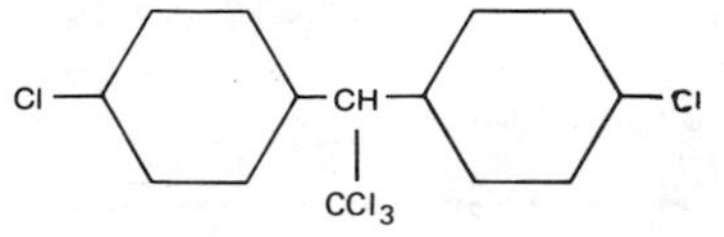

DDT

C. **Crotamiton (N-ethyl-o-crotonotoluide) (Eurax®)** is used for the prevention and treatment of scabies and is also an effective antipruritic agent.

1. *Structure*

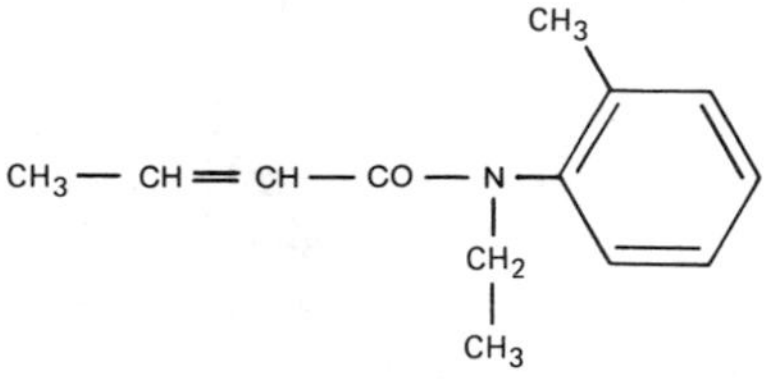

CROTAMITON (N-ethyl-o-CROTONOTOLUIDE)

2. *Packaging (R_x) and cost:*
10% cream: 60 gm/$1.75

D. **Gamma benzene hexachloride (Gamene®, Kwell®)** This is a highly toxic scabicide and pediculicide.

1. *Structure*

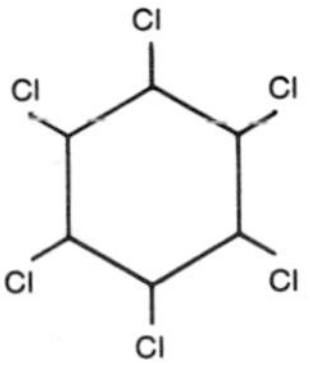

GAMMA BENZENE HEXACHLORIDE

2. *Packaging (R_x) and cost* (as Kwell®):
Cream: 60 ml/$3.20
Lotion: 60 ml/$3.00; 500 ml/$10.30
Shampoo: 60 ml/$3.10

E. **Malathion®** (0.5% lotion, 1% powder) is effective in the prevention and treatment of pediculosis.

1. *Structure*

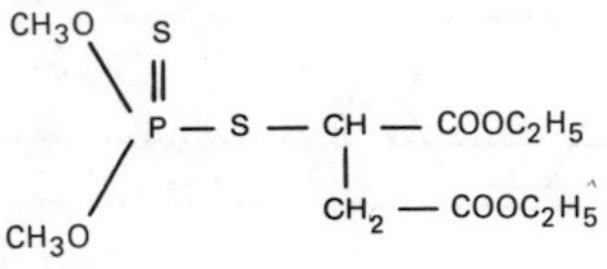

CH$_3$O   S
$\backslash$ $\parallel$
    P — S — CH — COOC$_2$H$_5$
/ |
CH$_3$O   CH$_2$ — COOC$_2$H$_5$

MALATHION

F. Pyrethrin compounds are used for the treatment of pediculosis.

1. *Packaging (R_x) and cost:*
Gel (A-200 Pyrinate®) : 30 gm/$2.30
Liquid (A-200 Pyrinate®, RID®) : 60 ml/$2.40
Liquid (RID®) : 120 ml/$4.50

V. MISCELLANEOUS

A. Iodochlorhydroxyquin (Vioform®), containing 40% iodine, was originally developed as a substitute for iodoform as an antiseptic dusting powder. While its most effective use is in the treatment of amebiasis, it also has antibacterial and mild antifungal effects and may be used alone or with steroids in the treatment of eczematous and impetiginized processes and some dermatophyte, yeast, and *Trichomonas* infections. However, more specific agents are available. The medication may stain the skin, hair, and clothing yellow and may induce contact allergy.

1. *Structure*

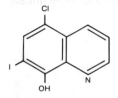

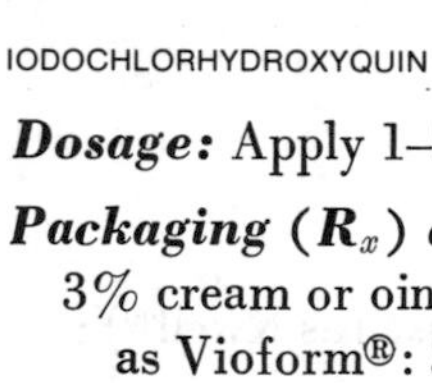

IODOCHLORHYDROXYQUIN

2. *Dosage:* Apply 1–3id.

3. *Packaging (R_x) and cost:*
3% cream or ointment:
   as Vioform®: 30 gm/$2.00
   as iodochlorhydroxyquin: 30 gm/$1.10
3% cream with 1% hydrocortisone:
   as Vioform® hydrocortisone: 20 gm/$5.70
   as iodochlorhydroxyquin hydrocortisone: 20 gm/$1.50
Powder, as Vioform®: 15 gm/$3.60

B. Mafenide (α-amino-p-toluenesulfonamide, **Sulfamylon®**) is a synthetic antibacterial agent related chemically, but not pharmacologically, to the sulfonamides. The drug appears to interfere with bacterial cellular metabolism and is not antagonized by para-aminobenzoic acid, pus, or serum. It is bacteriostatic against many gram-positive and gram-negative organisms, including staphylococci, streptococci, and *Pseudomonas* species. After percutaneous absorption the drug is metabolized; it acts as a weak carbonic anhydrase inhibitor and may therefore cause systemic acidosis.

Mafenide is used primarily in the treatment of burn wounds. It may be painful on application, and active allergic contact sensitivity may develop.

1. *Structure*

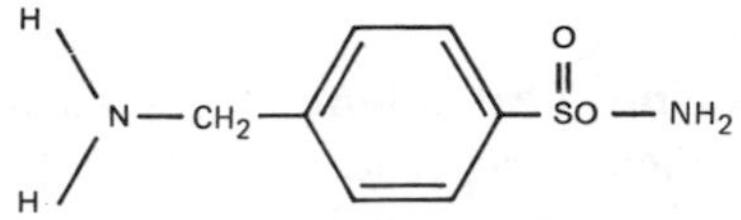

MAFENIDE

2. *Dosage:* Apply 2id with hand in a sterile glove.

3. *Packaging* (R_x) *and cost:*
Cream (as acetate):
60 gm/$2.40
120 gm/$4.30

C. Mercurial compounds have bacteriostatic effects, most likely mediated through inhibiting sulfhydryl enzymes, but fall far short of being ideal antibacterial compounds. Mercurial compounds may be absorbed and can sensitize; more effective and less hazardous antiseptic agents are available.

1. *Insoluble mercury compounds* are used as antibacterial and antiparasitic agents. *Yellow mercury oxide ointment* has been used for pediculosis involving the eyelashes; *ammoniated mercury*, containing 78% mercury, has been utilized in pyoderma and scaling processes.

2. The ***organic mercurial antiseptics*** are more bacteriostatic and less irritating and toxic than inorganic salts. Merbromin (Mercurochrome®), containing 25% mercury, is not particularly strongly active and further suffers from having its activity decreased in the presence of organic material. Thimerosal (Merthiolate®), containing 49% mercury, has the same drawbacks but is more effective.

D. Nitrofurazone (Furacin®), a synthetic nitrofuran derivative with a broad antibacterial spectrum, can be used for prophylaxis and treatment of infections of the skin. It is rarely used by dermatologists, however, as it carries a high risk of acquired contact sensitivity.

1. *Structure*

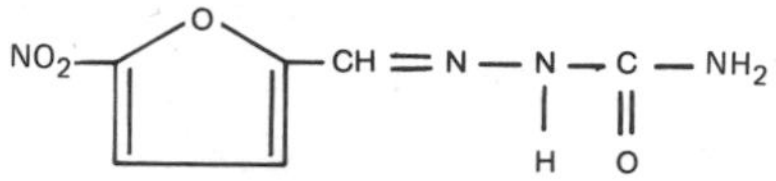

NO₂—furan ring—CH = N — N — C — NH₂, with H below the second N and O below the C

NITROFURAZONE

E. Silver sulfadiazine (Silvadene®) represents an effort to combine the beneficial properties of silver nitrate and sulfonamides such as mafenide primarily in the prevention and treatment of wound sepsis in patients with second- and third-degree burns. It is bactericidal against many gram-positive and gram-negative bacteria as well as *C. albicans* and is reasonably effective against *Pseudomonas aeruginosa* and *S. aureus*. Bacteria susceptible to sulfadiazine but resistant to silver nitrate, as well as those sensitive to silver nitrate but resistant to sulfadiazine, have shown good response to silver sulfadiazine. It does not stain, is unlikely to produce electrolyte imbalance, and does not cause systemic acidosis. Some patients note a stinging sensation on application, and because this compound can be absorbed, systemic sulfonamide-type reactions may occur.

1. *Structure*

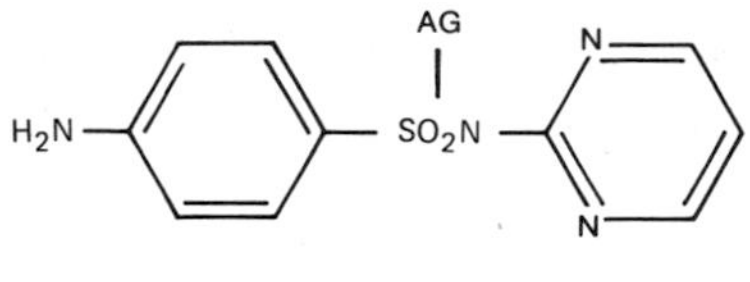

H₂N—benzene ring—SO₂N—AG—pyrimidine ring (with N atoms)

SILVER SULFADIAZINE

2. *Dosage:* Apply 1–2id.

3. *Packaging (R_x) and cost:*
400 gm/$20.50

ANTI-INFLAMMATORY AGENTS

I. **TOPICAL CORTICOSTEROIDS**   Corticosteroids are the most potent and effective local anti-inflammatory medications available and also have a striking ability to inhibit cell division. They are the therapy of choice in all inflammatory, pruritic eruptions (e.g., dermatitis and eczema) and are also effective in hyperplastic disorders (e.g., psoriasis) and infiltrative disorders (e.g., sarcoid, granuloma annulare). Since 1952, when these preparations first became commercially available, hundreds have been marketed. Their continuous wide usage has been assured by their numerous desirable qualities: broad applicability in treating a wide variety of common eruptions, rapidity of action in small amounts, ease of use, absence of pain or odor, lack of sensitization, unlimited stability, compatibility with almost all commonly used topical medications, and rarity of untoward clinical systemic effects from percutaneous absorption.

The effectiveness of a topical corticosteroid is related to the potency of the drug and its percutaneous penetration. Approximately 1% of a hydrocortisone solution will penetrate normal skin on the forearm. There is a marked regional variation in corticosteroid penetration; compared to the forearm data, hydrocortisone is absorbed 0.14 times as well through the plantar foot arch, 0.83 times through the palm, 1.7 times through the back, 3.5 times through the scalp, 6.0 times through the forehead, 13 times through the cheeks at the jaw angle, and 42 times through scrotal skin. If the skin is completely hydrated, absorption will be increased four- or fivefold. Inflamed skin, such as is found with atopic dermatitis, allows increased percutaneous penetration; with conditions such as exfoliative psoriasis there seems to be little barrier to absorption at all. Small changes in molecular structure result in enormous alterations in clinical effectiveness. Cortisone has no anti-inflammatory action, while fluorinated corticosteroids may be highly effective. The potency of topical corticosteroids is most often assessed in vivo by their ability to produce vasoconstriction on human skin, and results of this bioassay correlate well with clinical trials. Other potency assays include suppression of experimentally induced allergic contact dermatitis (e.g., to Rhus antigen) or irritant dermatitis (produced by kerosene or croton oil), or reduction in size of histamine-induced wheals. Antimitotic activity may be assessed by in vitro fibroblast inhibition and/or in vivo epidermal mitotic assay. The adverse effects of the fluorinated steroids include the production of cutaneous telangiectasia, striae, epidermal and dermal atrophy, a rosacea-like facial eruption, and senile-type purpura.

In 1960 it was discovered that placing corticosteroids under occlusion with thin, pliable plastic wraps dramatically increased their efficacy (up to 100-fold); occlusion causes hydration of the stratum corneum, increases the surface area of skin almost 40 percent, and appears to induce a reservoir of corticosteroid in the horny layer that persists for several days after application. Percutaneous absorption of steroids under wrap, particularly through altered skin, always occurs. It should be assumed that all patients under substantial occlusive therapy have temporary suppression of the pituitary-adrenal axis. Normal function returns within days to weeks after dressings are discontinued, depending on the duration, extent, and intensity of prior therapy. Undesirable effects from occlusive therapy include infection, miliaria, folliculitis, a disagreeable odor, interference with heat exchange, increased ease of sunburn, and atrophy and striae.

Injection of small amounts of corticosteroids (betamethasone sodium phosphate and betamethasone acetate suspension, triamcinolone acetonide, triamcinolone diacetate, triamcinolone hexacetonide, and methylprednisolone) into cutaneous lesions has the advantage of achieving high local concentration with prolonged depot effects and no systemic side-effects. Intralesional use is of particular value in the treatment of acne cysts, psoriatic plaques, circumscribed neurodermatitis, keloids, and, occasionally, chronic plaques of nummular eczema, insect bite reactions, alopecia areata, and nail disorders. Local adverse reactions include atrophy (especially when the concentration is too high or the steroid is injected too high in the dermis), hypopigmentation of deeply pigmented skin, growth of occasional tufts of hair in susceptible individuals, infection, and ulceration. Usually, a 1:4 dilution of the steroid (i.e., to 2.5 mg/ml triamcinolone acetonide) will provide enough steroid to reduce inflammation while avoiding these problems.

II. DOSAGE CONSIDERATIONS

 A. Dose-response relationship It is usually possible to observe a clear dose-response relationship in the use of topical corticosteroids. Compounds vary markedly in their potency and efficacy, and most products are available in standard concentrations and diluted 1:2 or 1:4 concentrations; some may also be obtained in high-potency concentrations. Efficacy may also be strikingly altered by method of use (e.g., prior hydration, occlusion).

Ointment vehicles generally give better biologic activity to the incorporated steroids than do cream or lotion vehicles. In most instances, initial therapy should be with one of the more potent compounds, and maintenance therapy with either a less concentrated fluorinated compound or with 1% hydrocortisone. At least 33–50 percent of patients can be managed with medium- to low-strength topical corticosteroids and this should always be tried. When possible, apply medications to moist skin after bathing or soaking the area in water. Rub in medications thoroughly several times daily (1–3id).

B. **Tachyphylaxis** Repeated application of potent topical steroids may result in a diminished effect of that preparation. This may occur within 1 week of initial use, but the ability to fully respond returns within a week of stopping drug application.

C. **Relative potency** It is possible to list the potency of topical corticosteroid preparations based on bioassay tests and literature reviews. The table on page 296 is modified with Stoughton (1975). There are no significant differences within each group.

D. **Occlusive therapy** Some conditions, such as psoriasis, lichen simplex chronicus, and hand eczema, respond poorly, if at all, to creams alone. The use of **occlusive (airtight) dressings** will increase the efficacy of these preparations. Patients should be instructed to:

1. *Wash the area well.*

2. *While the skin is still moist,* rub medication into lesions.

3. *Cover the area with a plastic wrap* (Saran Wrap®, Stretch n'Save®), plastic gloves for hands, plastic bags for feet, bathing cap for scalp, vinyl exercise suit for large areas of the legs or torso. Tubular plastic dressings (see Fig. 6) are also useful.

4. *Seal edges with tape* or cover plastic with an ace bandage, a long stocking, panty hose, or any dressing that will insure close adherence to skin. Blenderm® tape (3M Co.) will stick particularly well to skin. Paper tape may be less irritating.

Topical Corticosteroid Potency (modified from Stoughton, 1975)

Most potent 1	Fluocinonide cream, ointment, gel 0.05% (Lidex® cream and ointment, Topsyn® gel) Halcinonide cream 0.1% (Halog®)
2	Betamethasone benzoate gel 0.025% (Benisone®, Flurobate®) Betamethasone diproprionate cream 0.05% (Diprosone®) Betamethasone lotion, ointment 0.1% (Valisone®) Triamcinolone acetonide cream 0.5% (Aristocort®)
3	Fluocinolone acetonide cream (HP) 0.2%, ointment 0.025% (Synalar®) Flurandrenolide ointment 0.025% (Cordran®) Triamcinolone acetonide ointment 0.1% (Aristocort®; Kenalog®)
4	Betamethasone 17-valerate cream 0.1% (Valisone®) Fluocinolone acetonide cream 0.025% (Synalar®) Flurandrenolide cream 0.05% (Cordran®) Triamcinolone acetonide cream 0.1%, lotion 0.025% (Kenalog®)
5	Flumethasone pivalate cream 0.03% (Locorten®) Desonide cream 0.05% (Tridesilon®)
Least potent 6	Preparations containing dexamethasone, flumethalone, hydrocortisone, methylprednisolone, or prednisolone

5. *Use for 4–12 hr.* Overnight application is usually sufficient to induce clinical remission, but such a technique may also be used during the day. Occlusion for even a few hours, however, may be very beneficial.

As noted previously, significant percutaneous absorption of steroids will occur with occlusive therapy, and patients undergoing stressful procedures (i.e., operations) should be supplemented with IV corticosteroids.

III. **PACKAGING (ALL R$_x$) AND COST** As topical corticosteroids are stable preparations, buying in bulk is feasible and will frequently result in significant cost savings to the patient. Some pharmacies and institutions will buy 5-lb containers and repackage, with resultant enormous decreases in unit cost.

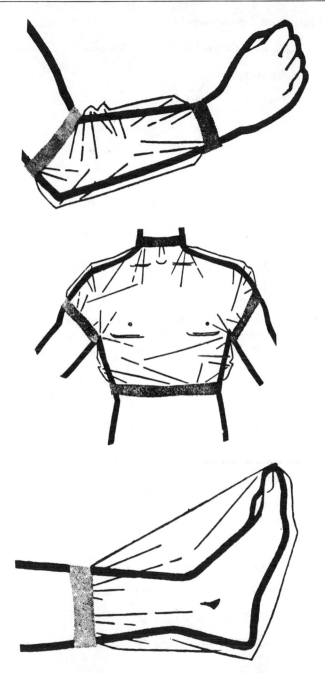

Figure 6. Plastic dressings applied to (A) arm, (B) body, (C) foot.

A. Fluorinated compounds

1. *Betamethasone benzoate* (*Benisone*®, *Flurobate*®)

a. Structure

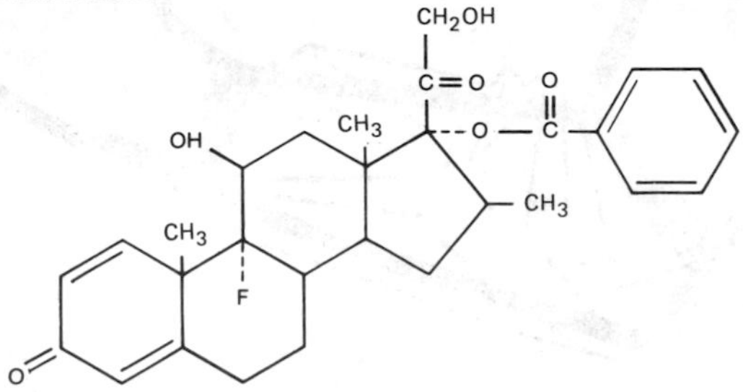

BETAMETHASONE BENZOATE

b. 0.025% gel: 15 gm/$4.00, 60 gm/$11.00

c. 0.025% cream: 15 gm/$3.70, 60 gm/$10.30

2. *Betamethasone valerate* (*Valisone*®)

a. Structure

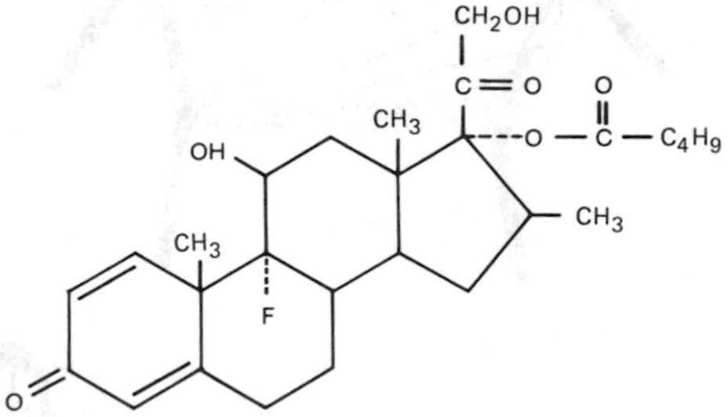

BETAMETHASONE VALERATE

b. 0.01% cream: 15 gm/$2.25, 60 gm/$5.20

c. 0.1% cream or ointment: 15 gm/$4.00, 45 gm/$7.65

d. 0.1% lotion: 20 ml/$4.60, 60 ml/$9.05

e. 0.15% aerosol: 85 gm/$4.00

3. *Fluocinolone acetonide* (*Fluonid*®, *Synalar*®)

a. Structure

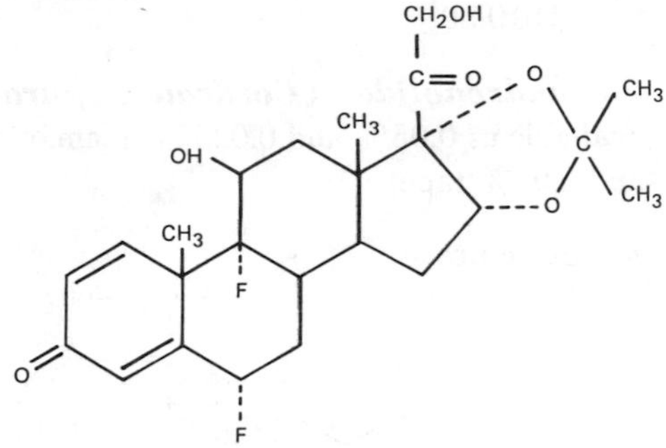

FLUOCINOLONE ACETONIDE

b. 0.025% cream, ointment, and emollient cream (Synemol®): 15 gm/$3.40, 60 gm/$9.45, 120 gm/$17.00

c. 0.01% cream: 15 gm/$2.40, 60 gm/$4.80, 120 gm/$8.60

d. 0.2% (HP) cream: 5 gm/$5.65, 12 gm/$11.40

e. 0.01% solution: 20 ml/$2.60, 60 ml/$6.30

(Institutions may purchase five 425-gm jars of full-strength [0.025%] or ten 425-gm jars of 0.01% cream or ointment for $75.00.)

4. *Fluocinonide (Fluocinolone acetonide acetate; Lidex® cream and ointment, Topsyn® gel)*

a. Structure

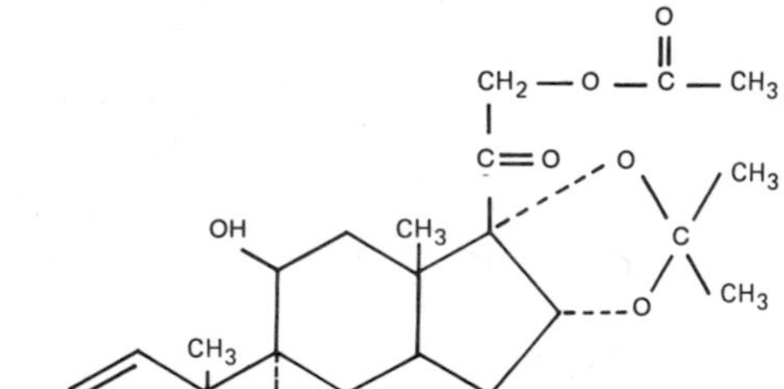

FLUOCINONIDE
FLUOCINOLONE ACETONIDE ACETATE

    b. 0.05% cream, ointment or gel: 15 gm/$4.00, 60 gm/ $10.50

5. *Flurandrenolide (Cordran®, flurandrenolone)* is available as 0.05% and 0.025% cream, ointment, and lotion, and 0.05% tape.

    a. Structure

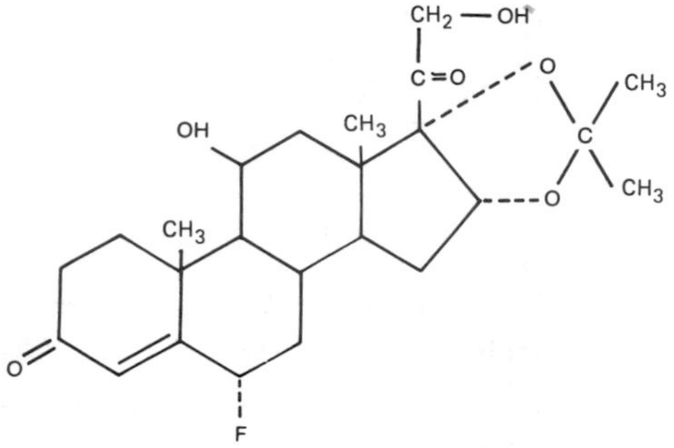

FLURANDRENOLIDE

    b. Cordran® tape 4 mcgm/sq cm:
        small roll, 60 cm × 7.5 cm/$4.00
        large roll, 200 cm × 7.5 cm/$8.65

6. *Halcinonide (Halog®)*

    a. Structure

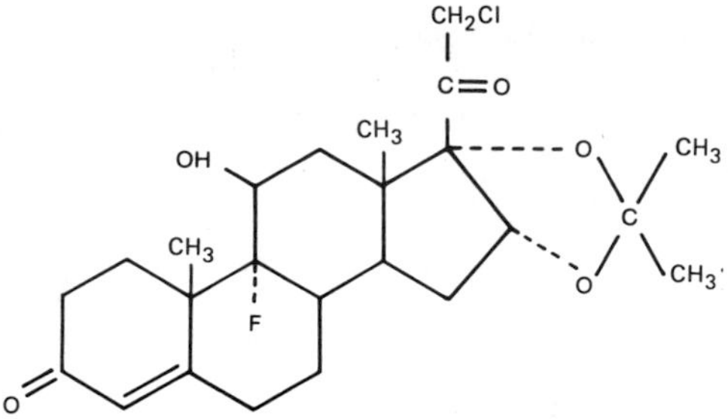

HALCINONIDE

    b. 0.1% cream: 15 gm/$4.80, 60 gm/$11.30

7. *Triamcinolone acetonide (Kenalog®, Tramacin®) or triamcinolone diacetate (Aristocort®)*

a. Structure

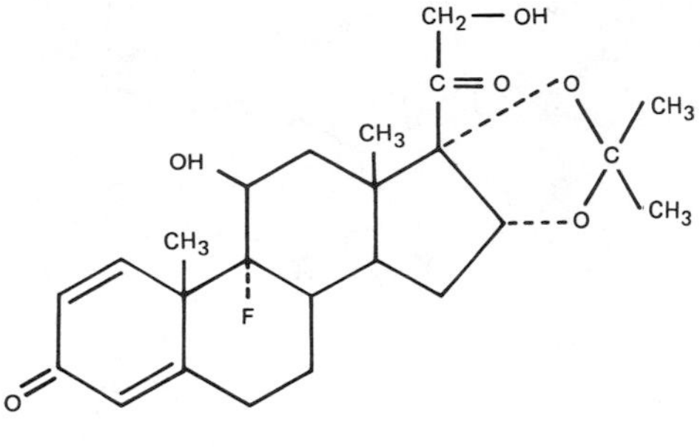

TRIAMCINOLONE ACETONIDE

b. 0.025% cream or ointment: 15 gm/$2.25
60 gm (as Kenalog®)/$5.15
75 gm (as Aristocort®)/$5.45
240 gm (½ lb)/$16.75

c. 0.1% cream or ointment: 15 gm/$3.50
60 gm (as Kenalog®)/$8.20
75 gm (as Aristocort®)/$8.90

d. 0.5% cream or ointment (as Aristocort®): 15 gm/$7.65

e. 0.1% in Orabase (as Kenalog®): 5 gm/$3.60

f. Spray, 0.1%: 50 gm/$3.40, 150 gm/$6.30

g. Lotion, 0.1%: 60 ml/$9.90
0.025%: 60 ml/$7.35

h. Aqueous suspension for injection:
10 mg/ml, 5 ml/$4.70
40 mg/ml, 1 ml/$3.80
40 mg/ml, 5 ml/$26.00

(2400 gm [5.25 lb] of 0.1% triamcinolone may be purchased directly by institutions or pharmacies for $94.00, or 2400 gm of 0.025% for $26.00.)

B. Nonfluorinated compounds

1. *Desonide (Tridesilon®)*

a. Structure

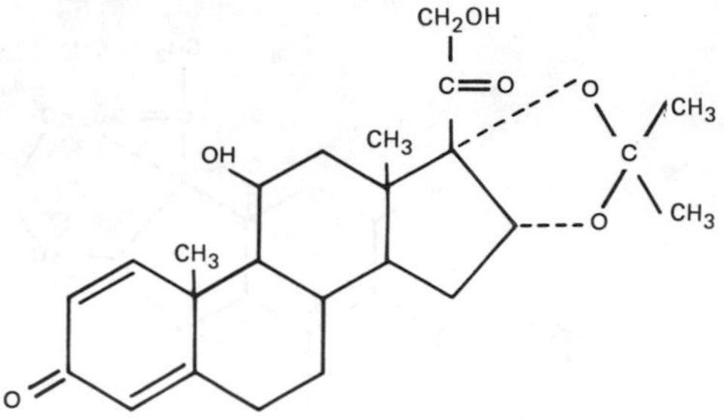

DESONIDE

b. 0.05% cream and ointment: 15 gm/$3.30, 60 gm/$9.30

2. *Hydrocortisone* may be purchased as a generic drug.

a. Structure

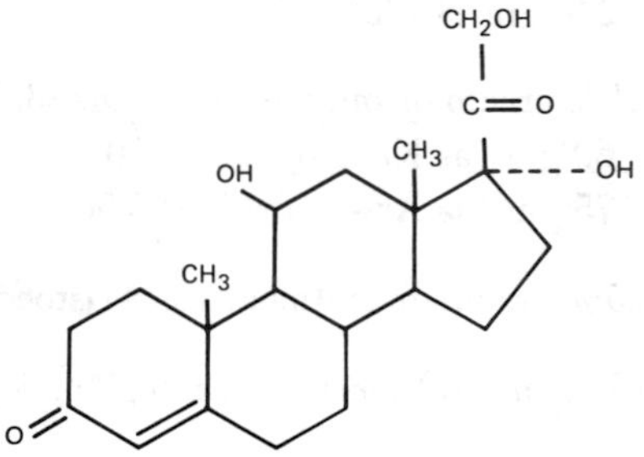

HYDROCORTISONE

b. 1% cream or ointment:
  15 gm (as Hytone®) /$2.65
  30 gm (as Hytone®) /$3.60
  30 gm (as generic) /$1.50–2.50
  120 gm (as Nutracort®) /$9.70
1% lotion
  30 ml (as Hytone®) /$3.60
  120 ml (as Nutracort®) /$9.70
1% gel
  120 gm (as Nutracort®) /$6.10
2.50% cream
  15 gm (as Hytone®) /$2.95
  30 gm (as Hytone®) /$5.75

C. **Steroid combinations** There are hundreds of topical corticosteroid preparations available in different vehicles and in combination with antibiotics (most frequently, neomycin), other antiseptics (iodochlorhydroxyquin), and other agents (tars, keratolytic agents). Some combinations are useful, but there is more flexibility and control over therapy, often at a lower cost to the patient, if separate identifiable agents are used.

REFERENCES

Chernosky ME, Schmidt JD: Atrophy, telangiectasia, and purpura after topical fluorinated corticosteroid therapy. Cutis 13:383–386, 1974

du Vivier A: Tachyphylaxis to topically applied steroids. Arch Dermatol 112:1245–1248, 1976

Eaglstein WH, Farzad A, Capland L: Topical corticosteroid therapy: efficacy of frequent application. Arch Dermatol 110:955, 1974

Jarratt MT, Spark RF, Arndt KA: The effects of intradermal steroids on the pituitary-adrenal axis and the skin. J Invest Dermatol 62:463–466, 1974

Maibach HI, Stoughton RB: Topical corticosteroids. In Steroid Therapy. Edited by DL Azarnoff. Philadelphia, Saunders, 1975, pp 174–190

Marples RR, Rebora A, Kligman AM: Topical steroid-antibiotic combinations. Assay of use in experimentally induced human infections. Arch Dermatol 108:237–240, 1973

Munro DD, Wilson L (eds): Steroids and the Skin. Proceedings of a Conference held in Edinburgh in October 1975. Br J Dermatol 94 (suppl 12), 138 pp, 1976

Scoggins RB, Kliman R: Percutaneous absorption of corticosteroids: systemic effects. N Engl J Med 273:831–840, 1965

Stoughton RB: Perspectives in topical glucocorticosteroid therapy. Prog Dermatol 9:7–10, 1975

ANTIPERSPIRANTS AND MEDICATIONS USED IN THE TREATMENT OF HYPERHIDROSIS

I. FOR HYPERHIDROSIS OF PALMS AND SOLES

A. **Aldehydes** Aldehydes induce anhidrosis probably by producing a blockage within the stratum corneum. Either formalin (5–10%) or nonalkalinized glutaraldehyde applied with a cotton swab is effective. Unbuffered generic glutaraldehyde is available as a 50% solution through drug supply houses; 2% glutaraldehyde is most easily used as Cidex® (Arbrook Co.).

1. *Glutaraldehyde* solution is applied three times a week for 2 weeks, and then once weekly or as needed. A 10% solu-

tion is used for the feet. This will cause a temporary brown discoloration to appear, but this will diminish as frequency of application decreases. A 2% solution, which will not stain, may be used on the palms; however, this concentration produces only slight diminution in sweating.

2. *Methenamine* is a structure that, when applied to the skin, hydrolyzes to ammonia and formaldehyde. A 5% methenamine stick or 10% solution is effective in mild to moderate hyperhidrosis.

    Structure

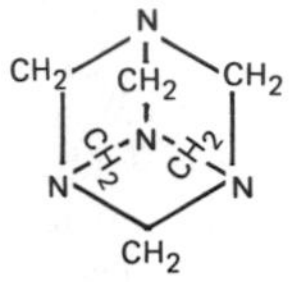

    METHENAMINE

B. Aluminum compounds may be used as noted below.

C. Iontophoresis with anticholinergic drugs such as glycopyrrolate will induce hypohidrosis of palms or soles for 4–6-week periods. The drugs are safe, and sensitization does not occur.

    1. *Structure*

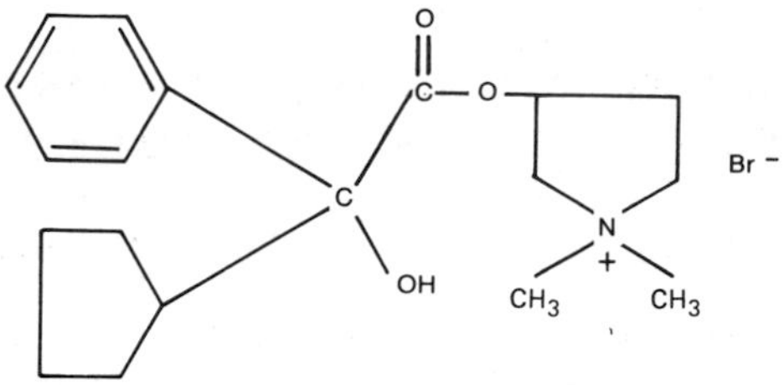

    GLYCOPYRROLATE

D. Systemic anticholinergic drugs are usually not tolerated in the required doses but may be tried (glycopyrrolate [Robinul® PH 2 ml] 3–5id initially, then decrease). Sedatives or tranquilizing drugs are sometimes helpful.

II. FOR AXILLARY HYPERHIDROSIS

A. **Glutaraldehyde** is generally not effective in the axillae.

B. **Aluminum compounds**

1. Apply 20% solution of aluminum chloride in 80% absolute anhydrous ethyl alcohol (Drysol®; 37.5 ml/$3.75) to *absolutely dry* axillae at bedtime and cover with plastic wrap. Do not wash the area closer than 2 hr before applying. Use a shirt (not tape) to keep wrap in place 6–8 hr (overnight) and wash medication off in the AM. Use for two consecutive nights or more the first week until the desired anhidrosis is achieved, then 1–3 times weekly thereafter. For treatment of palms and soles, initial treatment may have to be for 3–5 nights and follow-up treatment more often (q4–5d). For regular use, plastc wrap can be sewn into the foot of a sock or used inside a glove.

C. **Scopolamine hydrobromide** 0.025% applied topically can be an effective antiperspirant. Higher concentrations produce side-effects such as diplopia.

D. **Systemic anticholinergic and sedative (tranquilizing) drugs** may be of value.

E. **Excision** of the sweat gland–containing axillary vault is a simple surgical procedure and is the management of choice in some patients with severe hyperhidrosis.

REFERENCES

Abell E, Morgan K: The treatment of idiopathic hyperhidrosis by glycopyrronium bromide and tap water iontophoresis. Br J Dermatol 91:87–91, 1974

Cullen SI: Topical methenamine therapy for hyperhidrosis. Arch Dermatol 111:1158–1160, 1975

Eiseman G: Surgical treatment of axillary hyperhidrosis as an out-patient procedure. Cutis 16:69–72, 1975

Gordon BI: "No sweat." Cutis 15:401–404, 1975

Gordon HH: Hyperhidrosis: treatment with gluteraldehyde. Cutis 9:375–378, 1972

Kinmont PPC: Deodorants. Practitioner 202:88–94, 1969

Munro DD, Verbov JL, O'Gorman DJ, du Vivier A: Axillary hyperhidrosis. Its quantification and surgical treatment. Br J Dermatol 90:325–329, 1974

Papa CM, Kligman AM: Mechanisms of eccrine anhidrosis. II. The anti-perspirant effects of aluminum salts. J Invest Dermatol 49:139–145, 1967

Sato K, Dobson RL: Mechanism of the antiperspirant effect of topical glutaraldehyde. Arch Dermatol 100:564–569, 1969

ANTIPRURITIC AGENTS

I. **DISCUSSION** Pruritus is a symptom, not a disease, but the intense discomfort it can produce should not be underestimated. Complete investigation into the systemic or cutaneous cause of the itching is of primary importance, but whatever the cause, the complaint requires prompt and effective therapy. Topical corticosteroids and emollients are often useful. This section will discuss some of the more traditional dermatologic antipruritic agents and formulations. Pruritus is a complicated sensation involving neurophysiologic and psychologic considerations not yet fully understood; this naturally increases the difficulty of treatment. See also Antihistamines, p. 266.

A. **Camphor** is a ketone that, when applied in 1–3% concentration, has mild antipruritic effects through its anesthetic properties.

   Structure

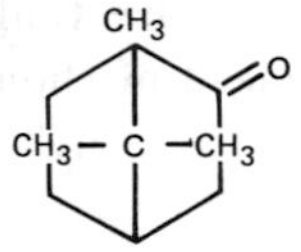

   CAMPHOR

B. **Menthol,** a cyclic alcohol (derived from peppermint, other mint oils, or prepared synthetically), relieves itching by substituting a cool sensation. It is used in 0.25–2% concentration.

   Structure

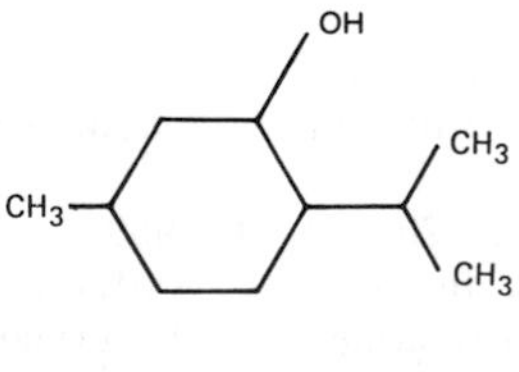

   MENTHOL

C. **Phenol** in dilute solution (0.5–2%) decreases itch by anesthetizing the cutaneous nerve endings.

Structure

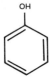

PHENOL

D. **Salicylic acid** (1–2%) and **tars** (coal tar solution, 3–10%) are also occasionally useful, although their mode of action is not known.

Structure

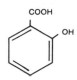

SALICYLIC ACID

E. Local **anesthetics** are often used to allay pruritus by blocking nerve impulses at sensory nerve endings. See also section on Anesthetics, p. 263.

F. **Dermatologic antipruritic formulations**

   1. *Lotions, liniments, emulsions*

      *a. Calamine lotion, USP (drying):

calamine (zinc oxide with 0.5% ferric oxide for coloring)	8 gm
zinc oxide	8 gm
glycerin	2 ml
bentonite magma (suspending agent)	25 ml
calcium hydroxide solution, to make	100 ml

      *b. Phenolated calamine, USP:

        1% phenol added to the above

---

* N.B. Menthol, phenol, or camphor may be added to any of the calamine lotions.

*c. Alcoholic calamine lotion (more drying) :

calamine	10 gm
zinc oxide	10 gm
bentonite	2 gm
talc	10 gm
glycerin	10 gm
alcohol	40 ml
water, to make	100 ml

*d. Calamine liniment (less drying) :

calamine	15 gm
peanut oil	50 ml
calcium hydroxide, to make	100 ml

e. Menthol lotion with phenol (Schamberg's) :

menthol	0.5 gm
phenol	1 gm
zinc oxide	20 gm
calcium hydroxide solution	40 ml
peanut oil, to make	100 ml

f.

menthol	0.25 gm
phenol	1 gm
in Eucerin®, to make	100 gm

g.

menthol	0.5–1.0 gm
phenol	0.5–1.0 gm
benzyl alcohol	5–10 gm
olive oil	5 ml
propylene glycol	5 ml
camphor water, to make	100 ml

h.

menthol		0.25 gm
*phenol		0.50 gm
*coal tar solution		5.0 gm
zinc oxide		15.0 gm
talc		15.0 gm
glycerin		10.0 ml
isopropanol 25% (less drying)–70% (more drying)	q.s.	100 ml

2. *Gels, ointments, and oils*

    a.   camphor
            menthol
            benzyl alcohol, 9%
            isopropyl alcohol, 30%
            in mildly drying, greaseless gel base

            Packaging and cost:
            60-gm tube (as Topic®)/$2.00

b.		
	phenol	1 gm
	menthol	0.25 gm
	salicylic acid	1 gm
	coal tar	2 gm
	hydrophilic ointment, to make	100 gm

c.		
	phenol	0.5 gm
	menthol	0.5 gm
	camphor	0.5 gm
	liquid petrolatum, to make	100 ml

d.		
	salicylic acid	3%
	phenol	1%

            Packaging and cost (as Panscol®):
               ointment, 100 gm/$6.90
               lotion, 120 ml/$5.00

3. *Impregnated pads*

a.		
	glycerin	10%
	witch hazel (contains gallic acid, tannin, and volatile oils)	50%
	water	40%

        (1)   Dosage: Apply prn as replacement for toilet tissue or as cleansing and antipruritic wipe in prevention and therapy of pruritus ani and other perineal pruritic processes.

        (2)   Packaging and cost:
                  as Tucks®: box of 40/$2.25
                            box of 100/$3.50

4. *Miscellaneous antipruritic preparations* (some contain potential allergic sensitizers such as benzocaine and diphenhydramine).

    a. Calamatum® contains benzocaine (0.5% in spray, 3% in ointment) calamine, zinc oxide, menthol (in aerosol), camphor, phenol (in ointment), isopropanol.

        (1) Packaging and cost:
            aerosol, 150 ml/$2.00
            ointment, 45 gm/$2.00

    b. Caladryl® contains 1% diphenhydramine, 1% camphor, calamine, 10% isopropyl alcohol (spray).

        (1) Packaging and cost:
            lotion, 180 ml/$1.90
            spray, 120 ml/$1.90

    c. Hazel-Balm® aerosol foam contains 80% witch hazel extract, 20% lanolin derivative, 0.1% benzethonium.

        (1) Packaging and cost:
            60 ml/$3.20

REFERENCES

Ayres S: The fine art of scratching. JAMA 189:1003–1007, 1964

Epstein E, Pinsky JB: A blind study. Arch Dermatol 89:548–549, 1964

Fischer RW: Comparison of antipruritic agents administered orally. A double blind study. JAMA 203:418–419, 1968

Herndon JH: Itching—the pathophysiology of pruritus. Int J Dermatol 14:465–484, 1975

Lyell A: The itching patient. A review of the causes of pruritus. Scott Med J 17:334–347, 1972

Shapior A: Itching. In Signs and Symptoms—Applied Pathologic Physiology and Clinical Interpretation. (Fifth edition) Edited by CM MacBryde, RS Blacklow. Philadelphia, Lippincott, 1970, p. 960

CLEANSING AGENTS

I. **DISCUSSION** Soaps are alkaline (pH 9–10) sodium or potassium salts of fatty acids. They emulsify fats with water and help remove foreign particles from the skin. Their surfactant and alkaline properties may, however, lead to primary irritation of intact or already damaged skin.

    A. **Neutral soaps** or soaplike preparations have a pH of 7.5 or less. Preparations include: Acidolate®, Aveenobar® (contains

50% oatmeal), Dove®, Lowila® Cake, Neutragena®, pHiso-Derm®, Soy-Dome®.

B. **Superfatted soaps** contain increased fat or oil to presumably prevent excessive defatting of skin. They are useful because the addition of fat makes them less effective detergents. Preparations include Basis®, Emulave®, Oilatum Soap®.

C. **Shampoos** are liquid soaps or detergents used for cleansing and/or therapeutic measures. Individual preparations are discussed elsewhere (see pp. 174, 325).

    1. *Selenium sulfide suspension* (SeS_2; Exsel®, Iosel®, Selsun®) is a mixture of selenium monosulfide and a suspension of solid selenium and amorphous sulfur. It is used in the control of seborrheic dermatitis, dandruff, and tinea versicolor.

        a. Packaging and cost:
           Selsun (R_x), 2.5% suspension, 120 ml/\$3.65
           Exsel (R_x), 2.5% suspension, 120 ml/\$3.00
           Iosel (R_x), 2.5% suspension, 240 ml/\$4.85
           Selsun Blue, 1% cream, 105 gm/\$2.50
                  1% lotion, 120 ml/\$2.30

REFERENCE

Blank IH: Action of soaps and detergents on the skin. Practitioner 202: 147–151, 1969

COSMETICS AND COVERING AGENTS

I. HYPOALLERGENIC COSMETICS

A. So-called **hypoallergenic** cosmetics abound, but only a few manufacturers will supply the physician with a list of the non-allergenic ingredients of their products. The term *hypoallergenic* means only that all product ingredients are chemically pure, but *not* that they are less likely to cause allergic reactions. Pharmaceutical companies specifically involved in the manufacture of less allergenic compounds include Almay®, Ar-Ex® Products Co., Marcelle®, and the Texas Pharmacal Company (Allercreme®).

II. COVERING AGENTS

A. Covermark® (Lydia O'Leary) is a tinted, inert, opaque makeup that is highly effective in covering pigmentary, vascular, and scarring lesions. It is, in addition, an effective sunscreen. A waterproof form is available.

Packaging and cost:
   Cream: 22.5 gm/$3.50
            85.5 gm/$8.00
   Stick form, as Spotstick®/$1.75

B. Erace® (Max Factor) is an effective covering agent available in lipstick form.

C. Covering agents and stains for vitiligo are discussed on p. 125.

REFERENCES

Hodgson G: Cosmetics. Practitioner 202:134–146, 1969

Klarmann EG: Cosmetic Chemistry for Dermatologists. Springfield, Ill., Thomas, 1962

Toxicology and Applied Pharmacology: Evaluation of Safety of Cosmetics. Edited by CS Weil, A Rostenberg. New York, Academic, Suppl 3, 1969

DEPILATORIES AND REMOVAL OF EXCESSIVE HAIR

I. HYPERTRICHOSIS

A. Mild hypertrichosis, most often familial in nature, is a cause for cosmetic concern for many women. It is mandatory that endocrine or local factors be ruled out before dismissing excessive hair as a simple cosmetic difficulty.

II. HAIR REMOVAL

A. There are several ways in which to decrease the amount or appearance of excessive hair.

1. *Bleaching* fine hair will make it less obvious. A 6% solution of hydrogen peroxide, commonly known as 20 volume peroxide, is most often used. It may be used alone, but the addition of an alkali, usually 10 drops of ammonia per 30 ml of peroxide, immediately before use will activate the hydrogen peroxide and permit more intense bleaching.

2. **Plucking** hair is painful but effective. Each pluck will start another growing cycle in the hair root.

3. **Wax epilation** is essentially just widespread plucking. A warm wax is placed on the skin, allowed to dry, and then, as it is peeled off, the hairs are pulled out.

4. **Shaving** is quick and effective and does *not* cause the hair to regrow more rapidly or more abundantly.

5. **Rubbing with a pumice stone** will remove fine hair.

6. **Depilatories** disintegrate and destroy hair on topical application by degrading disulfide bonds. The hair is left as a gelatinous mass, which is easily wiped off the skin. Two active ingredients are currently used:

   a. *Sulfides of alkali metals and alkaline earths* are the most effective, but they also develop a disagreeable hydrogen sulfide odor and are more irritating than thioglycollate products. Preparations available include Magic Shaving Powder® and Royal Crown Shaving Powder®. Both contain barium sulfide and calcium hydroxide.

   b. *Thioglycollate-containing agents* require increased contact time, but are more easily perfumed and are less irritating than other preparations. Preparations available include Better Off®, Nair®, Neet®, Nudit®, Shimmy Shins®, Sleek®, Surgi Cream®.

7. **Electrolysis** is the only permanent method of hair removal. In this procedure the hair bulb is destroyed by a high-frequency electric current, and the hair will not grow back later. When performed in a skillful fashion, this is a useful technique. Pitlike perifollicular scarring and regrowth of incompletely destroyed hairs may follow electrolysis. Self-use, home electrolysis units (PermaTweez, $19.50; General Medical Co., 1935 Armcost Ave., Los Angeles, Calif., 90025) are instruments that most patients may easily learn to use to yield effective results.

REFERENCE

Sternberg TH: Clinical study of self-use electrolysis. Derm Digest 20–27 (July) 1976

DERMATOLOGIC TOPICAL PREPARATIONS AND VEHICLES
(See also p. 255)

Lotions, creams, ointments, and powders can be used alone or may act as vehicles for pharmacologically active substances. Ideally, they are nontoxic, stable, and do not sensitize with repeated use.

I. LOTIONS, CREAMS, OINTMENTS, AND POWDERS

A. Lotions are suspensions of a powder in water that require shaking before application. Many are now held in more or less permanent suspension by suspending or surface-active agents. They provide a protective, drying, and cooling effect and may act as a vehicle for other agents. The addition of alcohol increases the cooling effect. If an astringent, such as aluminum, is present, it will precipitate protein and dry and seal exudating surfaces.

1. *Calamine lotion* (See Antipruritic Agents, p. 306.)

2. *Alcohol, zinc oxide, and talc lotion* (more drying):

zinc oxide	15 gm
talc	15 gm
glycerin	10 gm
alcohol	30 ml
water, to make	100 ml

3. *Burow's emulsion,* modified (less drying):

zinc oxide	10 gm
talc	10 gm
olive oil	45 ml
anhydrous lanolin	10 gm
aluminum acetate solution	2.5 ml
water, to make	100 ml

B. Oil-in-water and water-washable creams are easily washable and will take up water but are not in themselves soluble.

1. *Hydrophilic ointment, USP* contains polyoxyl 40 stearate as an emulsifying and wetting agent, stearyl alcohol as a stabilizer, and parabens (parahydroxybenzoic acid) as preservatives. If hydrophilic ointment is used under occlusion, an irritant contact dermatitis may result. Sodium lauryl sulfate is the provocative agent.

   a. Contains:

methylparaben	0.025 gm
propylparaben	0.015 gm
sodium lauryl sulfate	1.0 gm
stearyl alcohol	25 gm
white petrolatum	25 gm
propylene glycol	12 gm
polyoxyl 40 stearate	5 gm
water, to make	100 ml

   b. Packaging and cost:
480 gm/$1.75

2. Commercially available oil-in-water emulsion bases include Cetaphil®, Dermabase®, Keri®, Lubriderm®, Multibase®, Neobase®, Syntex®, Unibase®, Vanibase®, WIBI®.

C. Ointments These bland bases may have an antimitotic effect on stripped epidermis, perhaps related to the effects of physical occlusion. The "stickiest" preparations are the most inhibitory.

1. *Water-soluble ointments (Polyethylene glycols) (Carbowax®)* are completely water soluble and may also act as lubricants or as water-soluble bases.

2. *Emulsifiable ointments*

   a. *Water-in-oil absorbent ointments* are difficult to wash off and are insoluble in water, but will take up water in significant amounts.

     (1) *Hydrous wool fat, USP (lanolin)*, although insoluble in water, is capable of absorbing twice its weight in water. It is a yellow-white preparation containing 28% water and is the purified, fat-like substance from the wool of sheep, *Ovis aries* Linné.

       Anhydrous lanolin, a brown-yellow absorbent ointment that contains less than 0.25% water, is more greasy and occlusive.

      (a) Packaging and cost:
30 gm/$0.75, 480 gm/$3.50

(2) *Cold cream, USP* (*rose water ointment*) is a pleasant-smelling, soft base used chiefly because of its cosmetic appearance and for its lubricating, emollient, and cooling effects (hence its name, cold cream). These preparations are good vehicles for the incorporation of many substances. The official cold cream is a water-in-oil (W/O) emulsion, but there are many variations that approach oil-in-water (O/W) emulsions. These creams are the basis of many cosmetic products such as cleansing, night, moisturizing, and eye creams.

(a) Contains:

spermaceti	12.5 gm
white wax	12.0 gm
mineral oil	56.0 gm
sodium borate	0.5 gm
water	19.0 ml
	100.0 gm

(b) Packaging and cost:
480 gm/$3.00

b. Similar bases consisting of oils and emulsifying agents but no water are termed *absorbent ointments*. They are difficult to wash off and are insoluble in water, but they will soak up water to become water-in-oil emulsions.

(1) *Hydrophilic petrolatum, USP* is characterized by its ability to take up large amounts of water. It is less greasy than petrolatum but more greasy than hydrophilic ointment.

(a) Contains:

cholesterol	3 gm
stearyl alcohol	3 gm
white wax	8 gm
white petrolatum, to make	100 gm

(b) Packaging and cost:
480 gm/$2.75

(2) Commercially available hydrophilic (W/O) bases include Eucerin® (which is equal parts Aquaphor® and water), Hydrosorb®, Nivea® oil and

cream, Polysorb®, Qualatum®, Aquaphor® and Hydrosorb®, the latter four when hydrated.

3. ***Water-repellent ointments*** consist of inert oils, are insoluble in water, are difficult to wash off, will not dry out, and change little with time.

   a. *Petrolatum, USP* is a semisolid mixture of hydrocarbons obtained from petrolatum and is the most commonly used base for ointments. *White petrolatum (decolorized petrolatum)* is more esthetically appealing and is most often used.

      (1) Packaging and cost:
      480 gm/$1.00

   b. *Liquid petrolatum, USP (mineral oil, liquid paraffin)* is a mixture of purified hydrocarbons obtained from petrolatum.

      (1) Packaging and cost:
      480 ml/$1.00

4. ***Silicone (dimethicone) ointments*** are excellent water-protective agents because they have an extremely low surface tension and penetrate crevices in the skin to form a plastic-like barrier. Further, they are nontoxic, inert, stable, and water-repellent. As such, they are useful as barrier creams in industry or wherever constant or frequent exposure to aqueous compounds is a problem. They will not, however, protect well against solvents, oils, or dusts. Silicone preparations are available as sprays, liquids, ointments, and creams.

   a. Structure

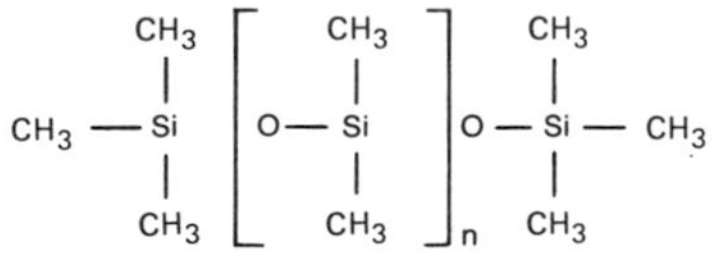

$$CH_3 - \underset{\underset{CH_3}{|}}{\overset{\overset{CH_3}{|}}{Si}} \left[O - \underset{\underset{CH_3}{|}}{\overset{\overset{CH_3}{|}}{Si}} \right]_n O - \underset{\underset{CH_3}{|}}{\overset{\overset{CH_3}{|}}{Si}} - CH_3$$

   DIMETHICONE

   b. Packaging and cost:
   30% silicone ointment (Silicote®), 30 gm/$2.50
   33.3% silicone aerosol spray (Silicote®), 90 ml/$3.00

As there are no all-purpose effective protective agents, it is essential to choose a particular cream for protection against a specific hazard, i.e., against dusts and particulate matter, aqueous compounds, or solvents.

D. **Pastes** are made by incorporating a fine powder into an ointment. The base is usually petrolatum, and the powders, which constitute 20–50 percent of the paste, are usually zinc oxide, talc, starch, bentonite, aluminum oxide, or titanium dioxide. Pastes are more absorptive, less greasy, and less effective vehicles than ointments and are less efficient at preventing water evaporation. However, they are excellent protective compounds and may be used in subacute and chronic dermatoses. Pastes should be applied evenly with a tongue blade or finger and may be removed most easily with a cloth soaked in mineral or vegetable oil.

Zinc oxide paste, USP (Lassar's):
zinc oxide	25 gm
starch	25 gm
white petrolatum, to make	100 gm

E. **Powders** increase evaporation, reduce friction, and provide antipruritic and cooling sensations. Zinc oxide or stearate, magnesium stearate, talc, cornstarch, bentonite, and titanium dioxide may either be used as dusting powders or incorporated into pastes or shake lotions. Talc is the most lubricating, but it does not absorb water; starch is less lubricating and absorbs water; zinc oxide has absorptive properties intermediate between the two. Talc can cause a granulomatous reaction in wounds, and starch may be metabolized by organisms and cause an increase in *Candida* overgrowth.

Talc, USP (talcum) is hydrous magnesium silicate that sometimes contains a small amount of aluminum silicate.

Packaging and cost:
454 gm/$2.00

REFERENCES

Bergstresser PR, Eaglstein WH: Irritation by hydrophilic ointment under occlusion. Arch Dermatol 108:218–219, 1973
Tree S, Marks R: An explanation for the "placebo" effect of bland ointment bases. Br J Dermatol 92:195–198, 1975

INSECT REPELLENTS

I. **DISCUSSION** See Bites and Stings, p. 32.

II. Effective preparations contain either *diethyltoluamide* (*deet*) or *ethyl hexanediol* (*E-H*). The amount of active ingredient is highest in the liquid products.

A. **Diethyltoluamide products**

   1. *Mosquitone® lotion* (McKesson), 50% deet
      52.5 ml/$0.70–$0.75

   2. *Off® liquid* (S. C. Johnson), 50% deet
      45 ml/$0.60–$0.85

   3. *Cutter Insect Repellent Cream®*, 30% deet
      30 ml/$1.90

B. **Ethyl hexanediol (E-H) products**

   1. *6–12® plus liquid* (Union Carbide), 75% E-H
      45 ml/$1.00

   2. *6–12® plus stick*, 65% E-H
      30 ml/$1.00

   3. *6–12® plus towelettes*, 46% E-H
      package of 10/$1.00

   4. *Walgreen's Spray®*, 20% E-H
      42 ml/$0.40

KERATOLYTIC AND DESTRUCTIVE AGENTS

I. **PREPARATIONS FOR PSORIASIS, SEBORRHEIC DERMATITIS, AND OTHER SCALING ERUPTIONS**

A. **Anthralin,** a synthetic substance prepared from anthracene, is used in the therapy of psoriasis. It is most effective when incorporated into a thick paste containing salicylic acid. Anthralin reduces epidermal mitotic activity. It may act as an irritant and will stain skin and clothing (see p. 162).

1. *Structure*

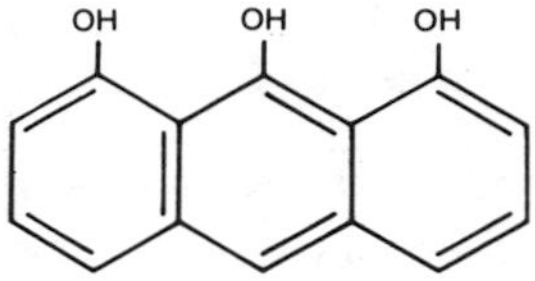

ANTHRALIN

2. ***Anthera®*** ointment contains anthralin 0.2%, salicylic acid 0.2%.

Packaging and cost:
   120-gm jar/$6.00

3. ***Anthra-Derm Ointment®*** contains anthralin (0.10%, 0.25%, 0.50%, 1%) petrolatum, and a fatty acid ester.

Packaging and cost:
   45 gm/$2.60

4. ***Lasan® Unguent*** contains 0.4% anthralin in a water-washable base.

Packaging and cost:
   120-gm jar/$7.10

B. **Cantharidin** (Spanish fly, Russian flies) causes intraepidermal vesiculation and is used in the treatment of warts and other benign cutaneous lesions (see p. 214).

1. Structure

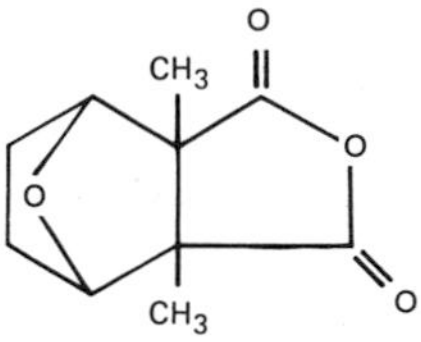

CANTHARIDIN

2. Packaging (R_x) and cost:
   Cantharone® (0.7% cantharidin, in equal amounts of flexible collodion and acetone): 7.5 ml/$5.65
   Verrusol® (1% cantharidin, 5% podophyllin, 30% salicylic acid): 7.5 ml/$4.20 (sold to physicians only)

C. **Caustics** are used alone or with electrosurgery for the superficial treatment of benign and malignant cutaneous lesions (warts, keratoses, xanthelasmas, basal cell carcinoma) and are also utilized in cosmetic therapy for aging, wrinkled facial skin.

1. *Mono-, di-, and trichloroacetic acids* (CCl_3COOH [trichloroacetic acid]) are rapid and effective local cauterizing agents. They are strongly corrosive and act by precipitation and coagulation of skin proteins. Saturated solutions are often used. The monochloroacetic derivative is more deeply destructive than the trichloroacetic preparation; 35–50% trichloroacetic acid is the most useful preparation for general use.

2. *Silver nitrate* ($AgNO_3$) in solid form or in solutions stronger than 5%, is used for its caustic action; 5–10% solutions may be applied to fissures or excessive granulation tissue. *Silver nitrate sticks* consist of a head of toughened silver nitrate ($>94.5\%$) prepared by fusing the silver salt with sodium chloride. It is dipped in water and applied as needed.

   Packaging and cost:
   100 sticks/$2.50

D. **Fluorouracil (Efudex®, Fluoroplex®, 5-FU)** is a pyrimidine antagonist that interferes with DNA synthesis by inhibiting thymidylate synthetase activity. It is used topically, primarily for the treatment of multiple actinic keratoses (see p. 146).

1. Structure

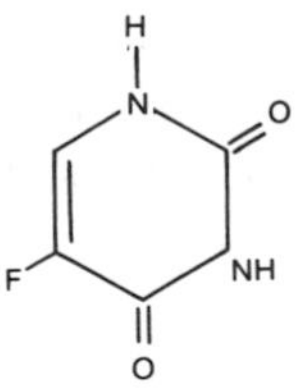

   FLUOROURACIL

2. Packaging and cost:
   Cream (Fluoroplex®), 1%: 30 gm/$5.40
   Cream (Efudex®), 5%: 25 gm/$5.70
   Solution (Fluoroplex®), 1%: 30 ml/$5.40

Solution (Efudex®), 2%: 10 ml/$3.50
Solution (Efudex®), 5%: 10 ml/$5.00

E. Podophyllum resin (podophyllin) is obtained from *Podophyllum peltatum* (called also mandrake or May apple) and is used in the treatment of condyloma acuminatum and other warts. In vitro, podophyllin inhibits RNA synthesis. Podophyllotoxin, an active component of podophyllum resin, also has specific affinity for, and prevents the normal assembly of, the microtubule protein of the mitotic spindle. Podophyllin can induce severe erosive changes in adjacent tissue, which thus must be protected from its action. It is applied as a 25% suspension in compound tincture of benzoin or in alcohol (see p. 215).

Structure

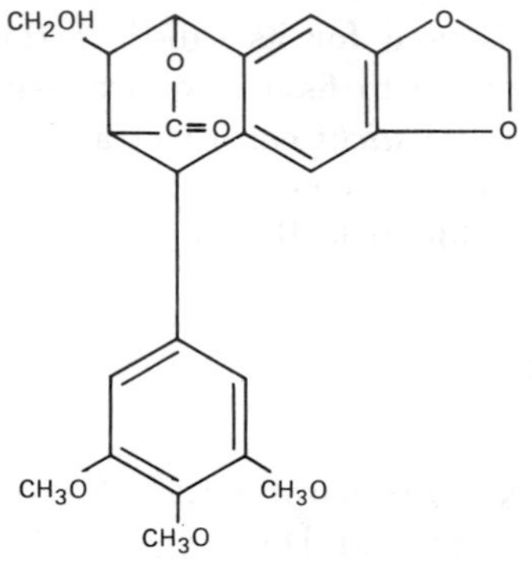

PODOPHYLLOTOXIN

F. Propylene glycol solutions (40–60%, v/v, $CH_3CH(OH)CH_2OH$, propylene glycol) applied to the skin under plastic occlusion hydrate the skin and cause desquamation of scales. Addition of 6% salicylic acid produces a very effective keratolytic preparation (Keralyt® gel). Overnight occlusion is used nightly until improvement is evident, at which time the frequency of therapy can be decreased to every third night or once weekly. This therapy is well tolerated, is nonirritating, and has been most successful in patients with X-linked ichthyosis and ichthyosis vulgaris (see p. 77). Patients with other abnormalities of keratinization with hyperkeratosis, scaling, and dryness may also benefit.

Packaging and cost:
30 gm (Keralyt® gel)/$3.40

G. **Resorcinol (resorcin),** a phenol derivative, is less keratolytic than salicylic acid. This drug is an irritant and sensitizer and is said to be both bactericidal and fungicidal. Solutions containing 1–2% have been used in preparations for seborrhea, acne, and psoriasis.

Structure

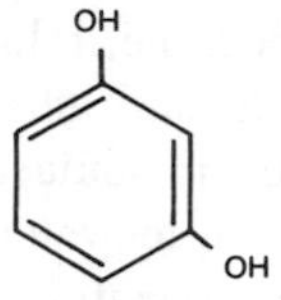

OH

OH

RESORCINOL

H. **Salicylic acid** is keratolytic and at concentrations between 3% and 6% causes shedding and softening of scaling and of the horny layer. It produces this desquamation by solubilizing the intercellular cement that bonds scales in the stratum corneum. In concentrations greater than 6% it can be destructive to tissue. Salicylic acid is used in the treatment of superficial fungal infections, acne, psoriasis, seborrheic dermatitis, and other scaling dermatoses. When combined with sulfur, some believe a synergistic keratolytic effect is produced. Common preparations include a 3% and 6% ointment with equal concentration of sulfur; 6% propylene glycol solution (Keralyt®); 5–20% with equal parts lactic acid in flexible collodion for warts; in a cream base at any concentration for keratolytic effects; as a 60% ointment for plantar warts; and in a 40% plaster on velvet cloth for the treatment of calluses and warts (40% salicylic acid plaster).

1. Structure

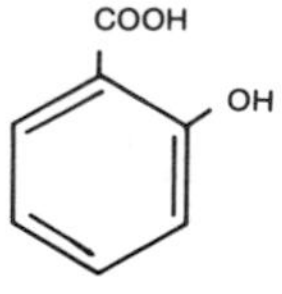

COOH

OH

SALICYLIC ACID

2. Packaging and cost:
Duofilm®, 16.7% salicylic acid, 16.7% lactic acid in flexible collodion: 15 ml/$3.65

I. **Sulfur** is incorporated into many preparations used in the treatment of acne, rosacea, ringworm, psoriasis, seborrheic dermatitis, and infestations. Sulfur inhibits the growth of microorganisms, particularly fungi and parasites; it may also be keratolytic, especially in combination with salicylic acid.

J. **Tar compounds** Coal tars, by-products of the destructive distillation of bituminous coal, contain benzene, toluene, naphthalene, anthracene, xylene, phenol, cresols, and other aromatic compounds; bases such as pyridine; and ammonia and peroxides. They are almost black, slightly soluble in water, and partially soluble in many solvents. Tars for dermatologic use are also obtained from shale, petroleum, and wood.

Tars can suppress DNA synthesis of normal or hyperplastic skin. They promote return to normal keratinization in patients with eczematous and hyperplastic diseases and are antipruritic and astringent. Tars are often used in combination with sulfur, salicylic acid, and topical steroids. Their effects are heightened if the skin is irradiated with ultraviolet light after the tar has been removed (see p. 163).

1. *Coal tar products* are available over the counter or may be compounded to USP, NF, or other formulas. Zetar® and Doak® tar compounds are available as ointments, bath oils, emulsions, shampoos, and lotions.

a. *Pragmatar®:*

coal tar distillate	4%
precipitated sulfur	3%
salicylic acid	
in o/w base	3%

Packaging and cost:
30 gm/$2.00

b. *Estar® gel:*

tar (equivalent to crude coal tar)	
in hydro-alcoholic base	5%

Packaging and cost:
90 gm/$4.50

c. *Tar ointment, USP:*

coal tar	1 gm
polysorbate 80	0.5 gm
zinc oxide paste, to make	100 gm

d. *White's tar ointment:*

coal tar	5 gm
polysorbate 80	2.5 gm
starch	45 gm
zinc oxide	5 gm
petrolatum, to make	100 gm

e. *Bath preparations* include Alma-Tar®, Ar-Ex®, Balnetar®, Lavatar®, Polytar®, Supertah®, Tar Distillate "Doak", Tarbonis®, Tarsum®, Zetar®.

f. *Shampoos* containing tar include Alma-Tar®, DHS® tar shampoo, Ionil T®, Pentrax®, Sebutone®, Tersa-Tar®, Vanseb-T®, Zetar®.

2. *Coal tar solution (liquor carbonis detergens; LCD)* is prepared by extracting coal tar with alcohol and polysorbate (Tween) 80, an emulsifying agent. Each 100 ml of the solution represents 20 gm of coal tar. When mixed with water, a fine dispersion of coal tar results. LCD may be incorporated (at 2–5%) in creams or ointments, in tincture of green soap for a shampoo (10%), or added (60 ml) to the bath for antipruritic and other effects.

3. *Ichthammol (Ichthyol®)* is obtained by the destructive distillation of certain bituminous schists (shale rock). It is less irritating than coal or wood tars, is water soluble, stains linens, and is used at 2–5% in the treatment of some subacute and chronic dermatoses.

4. *Juniper tar, USP (Cade oil)* is obtained by destructive distillation of the heartwood of *Juniperus oxycedrus*. It contains hydrocarbons, including phenolic compounds and aromatic compounds, and is used in the management of chronic eczema and psoriasis. It is available in an ointment, shampoo, bath solution, and soap.

K. **Urea-containing preparations** are said to have a softening and moisturizing effect on the stratum corneum and at times may provide good therapy for dry skin and the pruritus associated with it. They appear to have an antipruritic effect separate from their hydrating qualities. Urea compounds dissolve hydrogen bonds as well as epidermal keratin; thus their effect in dry hyperkeratotic diseases such as ichthyosis vulgaris and psoriasis is not only to make the skin more pliable but also to help remove adherent scales, to some degree.

Packaging and cost:
  Aquacare® (2% urea)
    cream: 75 gm/$2.25
    lotion: 240 ml/$3.15
  Aquacare HP® (10% urea) cream: 75 gm/$2.65
  Calmurid® (10% urea) cream: 105 gm/$3.50
  Carmol® (20% urea) cream: 90 gm/$2.85
  Carmol HC® (10% urea with 1% hydrocortisone)
    cream (R_x): 30 gm/$4.00

REFERENCES

Baden HP, Alper JC: A keratolytic gel containing salicylic acid in propylene glycol. J Invest Dermatol 61:330–333, 1973

Edinbinden JM, Parshly MS, Walzer RA, Sanders SL: The effect of cantharidin on epithelial cells in tissue culture. J Invest Dermatol 52:291–303, 1969

Freedberg IM: Effects of podophyllin upon macromolecular metabolism. J Invest Dermatol 45:539–546, 1965

Goldsmith LA, Baden HP: Propylene glycol with occlusion for treatment of ichthyosis. JAMA 220:579–580, 1972

Lorenc E, Winkelmann RK: Evaluation of dermatologic therapy. I. Sulfur and petrolatum. Arch Dermatol 83:761–767, 1961

Perez-Figaredo R, Baden H: The pharmacology of podophyllin. Prog Dermatol 10:1–4, 1976

Stoughton RB, DeQuoy P, Walter JF: Crude coal tar plus near ultraviolet light suppresses DNA synthesis in epidermis. Arch Dermatol 114:43–48, 1978

Strakosch EA: Studies on ointments. II. Ointments containing salicylic acid. Arch Dermatol 47:16–26, 1943

Strakosch EA: Studies on ointments. III. Ointments containing sulfur. Arch Dermatol 47:216–225, 1943

PIGMENTING AND DEPIGMENTING AGENTS, SUNSCREENS

I. **DISCUSSION** (See Hyperpigmentation and Hypopigmentation, p. 118.)

II. AGENTS THAT CAUSE HYPOPIGMENTATION

A. Hydroquinone products

1. *Structure*

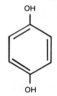

HYDROQUINONE

2. *Packaging and cost:*
Artra® cream, 2%: 30 gm/$1.00
Eldopaque® ointment with opaque base, 2%:
    15 gm/$4.50
Eldopaque Forte® ointment with opaque base, 4%:
    15 gm/$5.00
Eldoquin® lotion, 2%: 15 ml/$4.50
Eldoquin Forte®, 4%: 30 gm/$9.90

B. Monobenzone products should be used only when permanent depigmentation is desired.

1. *Structure*

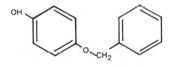

MONOBENZONE

2. *Packaging and cost:*
Benoquin® (R_x) 20% ointment: 15 gm/$4.50

III. AGENTS THAT INDUCE HYPERPIGMENTATION AND REPIGMENTATION

A. Trioxsalen (Trisoralen®, trimethylpsoralen) followed by UVA exposure is used to repigment vitiliginous areas, protect against sunburn, enhance pigmentation (see p. 123), and in photochemotherapy.

Structure

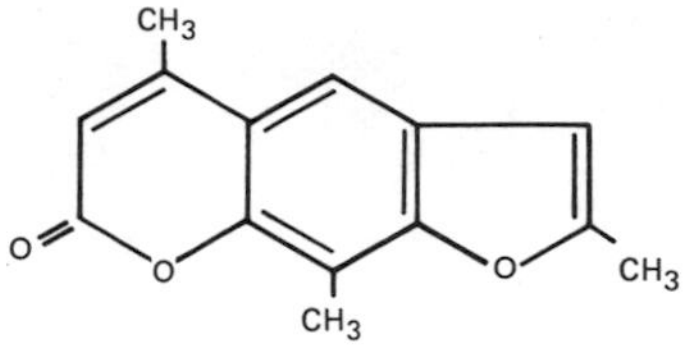

TRIOXSALEN

B. **Methoxsalen (methoxypsoralen, Oxsoralen®)** has effects similar to trioxsalen. Methoxsalen is superior to trioxsalen in producing erythema and tanning; it is not known if either is more effective in the therapy of vitiligo. Methoxsalen is also available as a 1% lotion.

1. *Structure*

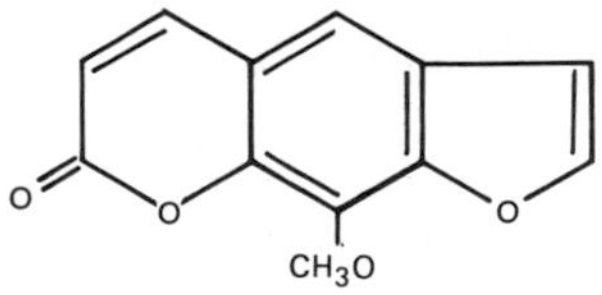

METHOXSALEN

2. *Packaging and cost:*
   Oxsoralen® 10-mg tablets: 100/$27.00
   Oxsoralen® 1% lotion: 30 ml/$10.50

IV. **SUNSCREENS** (See also p. 195.)

A. **Para-aminobenzoic acid (PABA) preparations** absorb UVL between 280–320 nm. This acid will stain white fabrics, especially cotton. The esters of PABA are slightly less effective and do not stain as much.

1. *Structure*

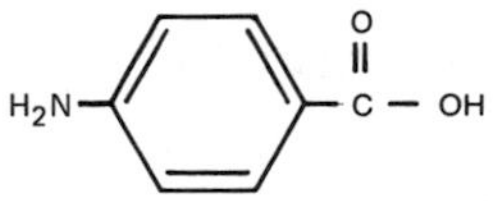

PARA-AMINOBENZOIC ACID

2. *Packaging and cost:*
   Blockout® (5% PABA esters in 70% alcohol): 120 ml/ $2.00

Pabafilm® (5% PABA esters in 70% alcohol) : 120 ml/ $3.30

Pabanol® (5% PABA in 70% alcohol) : 120 ml/$2.80

PreSun® (5% PABA in 55% alcohol) : 120 ml/$3.35 lotion, gel, 90 gm/$3.35

B. **Benzophenone compounds** absorb UVL well from 250–365 nm and somewhat from 365–400 nm. They are less effective than PABA compounds in the UVB sunburn spectrum.

1. *Structure*

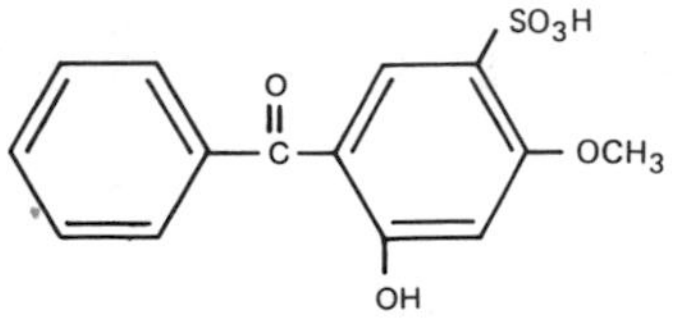

SULISOBENZONE

2. *Packaging and cost:*

Piz Buin Exclusiv Extrem Creme (4% ethyl hexyl paracinnamate, 3% 2-hydroxy-4-methoxy benzophenone, 2% phenyl benzimidazole sulfonic acid) : 45 gm/$3.00

Solbar® (3% oxybenzone and 3% dioxybenzone) : 75 gm/$3.25

Uval® (10% sulisobenzone) : 75 gm/$3.20

C. **Others**

1. *RVP (red veterinary petrolatum)* has UVL-absorbing qualities to 340 nm and is also a water-protective agent because of its greasy base. It is available as a sunshade with zinc oxide added (RVPaque®) and for lip protection with 5% PABA.

Packaging and cost:

RVP® (95% RVP) : 60 gm/$2.70

RVPaba® lipstick (20% RVP, 5% PABA) : 4.2 gm/$1.50

2. *Sunshades* physically block light and usually contain titanium dioxide or zinc oxide powders. They are not very effective unless a thick coat is applied.

Packaging and cost:

A-Fil® (5% menthyl anthranilate, 5% titanium dioxide, in two shades) : 45 gm/$1.95

Reflecta® (contains titanium dioxide) : 120 ml/$2.75

RVPaque® (20% zinc oxide, 3% RVP, 1.5% cinoxinate) : 15 gm/$2.50

RVPlus® (10% titanium-mica platelets, 30% RVP) : 60 gm/$3.30

Solar® cream (4% PABA, 5% titanium dioxide) : 30 gm/$3.35

WET DRESSINGS, BATHS, ASTRINGENTS

I. WET DRESSINGS

A. The effects of wet dressings have been previously discussed (see p. 255).

1. *Open wet dressings* are indicated in acute inflammatory states with exudation, oozing, and crusting. They are applied as follows:

a. The patient should be in a comfortable position, usually in bed, with an impermeable material under the area to be compressed to prevent wetting the mattress.

b. The dressings, which need not be sterile, should consist of 2–4-inch-wide Kerlix®, soft gauze (not 4 × 4's), or soft linen such as old sheeting or pillowcases, handkerchiefs, or shirts.

c. Moisten dressings by immersing them in the solution and then gently wringing them out. They should be sopping wet, but not dripping. Solutions should be warm or tepid. Cover with a soft towel or cloth that will allow evaporation.

d. Apply or wrap around the skin loosely. Multiple layers, at least 6–8, should be applied to prevent rapid drying and cooling.

e. Dressings should be removed, remoistened, and reapplied every 10–15 min, for between 30 min and 2 hr 3id. It is difficult to completely moisten dressings in place, and resoaking is often needed to remove accumulated and adherent exudate and crusts. If frequent changes are impracticable, an IV bottle with the wet dressing solution may be suspended over the bed and the material slowly fed into the dressing through IV tubing. Alternatively, the dressing should simply be removed every 2–3 hr and reapplied. It is usually difficult for patients to care for their own dressings.

f. After dressings are removed, a lotion, powder, liniment, or paste may be applied to the skin. Occlusion of exudative skin with ointments should be avoided.

g. Dressing material should be discarded daily, but some, such as Kerlix®, may be laundered and reused.

h. If large areas of skin are compressed at once, chilling and hypothermia may result. In general, no more than one-third of the body should be treated at any time.

2. *Closed wet dressings* will cause maceration and retain heat and are used in the treatment of conditions such as cellulitis and abscesses. The foregoing instructions should be followed, but warm dressings should be covered with plastic, oilcloth, or other impermeable material.

B. **Solutions for wet dressings** are either astringents or antiseptic agents. Astringents precipitate protein and thereby decrease oozing. The principal astringents are salts of aluminum, zinc, lead, iron, bismuth, tannins, or other polyphenolic compounds.

1. *Aluminum acetate* ($Al [OCOCH_3]_3$, *Burow's solution*), containing approximately 5% aluminum acetate, is diluted 1:10 to 1:40 for use. Probably the most widely used astringent for wet dressings, it is easy to use, does not stain, and is drying, soothing, and mildly antiseptic.

Domeboro® powder packets or tablets quickly dissolve in water to make fresh aluminum acetate available. One packet or tablet in 1 pint of water yields a 1:40 dilution (two packets a 1:20 dilution); 30-min evaporation, however, will concentrate a 1:40 solution to 1:10, at which point the aluminum salts may become too irritating and drying.

    a. Packaging and cost:
      as Domeboro®:
        12 packets/$2.25
        12 tablets/$2.25
      as Bluboro® (aluminum acetate, boric acid, FD&C blue dye)
        12 packets/$2.25

2. ***Potassium permanganate*** (KM_NO_4) is an oxidizing agent that is rapidly rendered inactive in the presence of organic material. The oxidizing action of the chemical is purportedly responsible for its germicidal activity. It is also an astringent and a fungicide. This preparation stains the skin and clothing, and undissolved crystals will cause a chemical burn. It is used less commonly now than formerly (primarily as an antifungal agent) and may be little better than water as a wet dressing. A 1:4000 to 1:16,000 dilution is used on weeping or denuded surfaces (one crushed 65-mg tablet to 250 ml → 1000 ml; one 330-mg tablet to 1500 ml → 5.0 L). For use as a medicated bath, 650 mg (about 2 tsp) should be dissolved in 200 L (a full bathtub) of water to produce about a 1:25,000 dilution. Skin stains may be removed with a weak solution of oxalic acid or sodium thiosulfate.

3. ***Normal saline (0.9% sodium chloride)*** may be approximated by adding 1 level tsp of salt to 480 ml water.

4. ***Copper and zinc sulfates and camphor (Dalibour solution, Dalidome®)*** is an effective, nonstaining, blue astringent.

5. ***Boric acid*** is not of any use as a topical agent; it is toxic when absorbed and has caused poisoning in children through percutaneous absorption.

6. ***Silver nitrate, 0.1–0.5%,*** is an excellent germicide and astringent. Its germicidal action is due to precipitation of bacterial protein by liberated silver ions. It may cause pain if applied in concentrations greater than 0.5%. A 0.25% solution may be prepared by adding 1 tsp of the stock 50% aqueous solution to 1000 ml of cool water. Silver nitrate stains skin dark brown after exposure to air and will stain black any metal container (including the teaspoon) and everything else that it touches.

7. **Compresses with 1% acetic acid** reduce the microbial count in infected wounds and are used primarily for infections involving *Pseudomonas aeruginosa.*

II. BATHS

A. **Baths and soaks** are useful in treating widespread eruptions. Evaporation is impeded, and thus there is less drying and cooling. Nevertheless, baths and soaks may be very soothing, antipruritic, and somewhat anti-inflammatory. The tub should be half full (about 100 L, or 25 gallons of water) and the duration of exposure limited to 30 min. Many of the bath oils make the tub very slippery.

1. *Soothing and antipruritic colloid additives*

   a. Oatmeal contains 50% starch with about 25% protein and 9% oil. Mix 1 cup Aveeno® oatmeal and 2 cups of cold tap water, shake, and pour into tub of lukewarm water. Oilated Aveeno® contains an additional 35% mineral oil and lanolin derivative for emollient action.

   Packaging and cost:
   Aveeno®, 480 gm/$3.00
   Oilated Aveeno®, 240 gm/$3.00

   b. *Starch baths* are best prepared by mixing 2 cups of a hydrolyzed starch, such as Linit®, with 4 cups of cold tap water to form a paste, then adding this to a tub of lukewarm water. A mixture of equal parts of sodium bicarbonate (baking soda) and starch is often used as a soothing colloidal bath powder.

2. *Bath oils* are added to tub water to help prevent drying of the skin. Most contain a mineral or a vegetable oil and also a surfactant. Theoretically, the patient adsorbs a portion of the oil around him. There are two types of bath oils: those that are dispersed throughout the bath, and those that lie on the surface of the water and coat the surface of the body as the patient leaves the tub. If nothing else, bath oils are pleasant, but patients occasionally note mild pruritus immediately after their use. All of the following are pleasing preparations; some patients will prefer one to another: Alpha-Keri®, Ar-Ex®, Domol®, Kauma®, Lubath®, Lubath-ML®, Lubriderm®, Syntex®.

REFERENCES

Hedberg M, Miller JK: Effectiveness of acetic acid, betadine, amphyll, polymyxin B, colistin and gentamicin against *Pseudomonas aeruginosa*. Appl Microbiol 18:854–855, 1969

Quinones CA, Winkelmann RK: Changes in skin temperature with wet dressing therapy. Arch Dermatol 96:708–711, 1967

Wilkinson DS: Dermatological dressings. Practitioner 202:27–36, 1969

General References

AMA Drug Evaluations. Chicago, American Medical Association, 1973, 1032 pp

American Hospital Formulary Service. Washington, American Society of Hospital Pharmacists, 1971

Burack R, Fox F: The 1976 Handbook of Prescription Drugs. New York, Pantheon, 1976, 451 pp

Drug Topics Red Book. Oradell, N.J., Topics, 1977, 175 pp

Frazier CN, Blank IH: A Formulary for External Therapy of the Skin. Springfield, Ill., Thomas, 1954

Goodman LS, Gilman A (eds): The Pharmacological Basis of Therapeutics. (5th Edit) New York, Macmillan, 1975, 1704 pp

Griffenhagen GB, Hawkins LL (eds): Handbook of Non-Prescription Drugs. Washington, D.C., American Pharmaceutical Association, 1973

Lerner MR, Lerner AB: Dermatologic Medications. (2nd Edit) Chicago, Year Book, 1960, 208 pp

Lewis AJ (ed): Modern Drug Encyclopedia and Therapeutic Index: A Compendium (13th Edit). New York, Yorke Medical Group, 1975

Maddin SW (ed): Current Dermatologic Management (2nd Edit). St. Louis, Mosby, 1975, 404 pp

The United States Pharmacopoeia. 19th Rev. Easton, Pa., Mack, 1974, 824 pp

Index

Chart 1. *Amount of Topical Medication Needed for Single or Multiple Application(s)*

Area Treated	One Application (gm)	3id Application for 2 Weeks (gm [oz])
Hands, head, face, anogenital area	2	90 [3]
One arm, anterior or posterior trunk	3	120 [4]
One leg	4	180 [6]
Entire body	30–60	1.26–2.52 kg [42–84 oz; 2½–5 lb]

Chart 2. *Metric Measures with Approximate Equivalents*

Liquid Measure
4000.0 ml = 1 gallon (4 qt)
1000.0 ml
(1 liter) = 1 quart
  (32 oz)
 500.0 ml = 1 pint (16 oz)
 250.0 ml = 8 fluid ounces
  30.0 ml = 1 fluid ounce
  15.0 ml = 1 tablespoon
   5.0 ml = 1 teaspoon
   4.0 ml = 1 dram
   0.06 ml = 1 minim, the rough
      equivalent of 1 drop

Weight
454 gm = 16 oz (pound)
30 gm = 1 oz
 4 gm = 60 grains (gr) (1 dram)
 1 gm = 15 gr
60 mg = 1 gr

Length (exact equivalents)
1 meter = 39.37 in
30.48 cm = 1 ft
 2.54 cm = 1 in
 1 cm = 0.39 in
 1 mm = 0.04 in

Note: A. 1 milliliter (ml) ≃ 1 cubic centimeter (cc); B. Most of these approximate dose equivalents have been approved by the Food and Drug Administration. They may be used as a convenience in prescribing, but must not be used for compounding specific pharmaceutical formulas.